Reflective helping in
HIV and AIDS

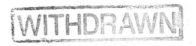

Reflective helping in HIV and AIDS

Edited by
CHARLES ANDERSON AND
PATRICIA WILKIE

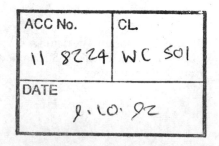
OPEN UNIVERSITY PRESS
Milton Keynes · Philadelphia

Open University Press
Celtic Court
22 Ballmoor
Buckingham
MK18 1XW

and

1900 Frost Road, Suite 101
Bristol, PA 19007, USA

First published 1992

British Library Cataloguing-in-Publication Data

Reflective helping in HIV and AIDS.
  I. Anderson, Charles II.   Wilkie, Patricia
  616.97

  ISBN 0–335–15632–0
  ISBN 0–335–15631–2 pbk

Library of Congress Cataloging-in-Publication Data

Reflective helping in HIV and AIDS/Charles Anderson and Patricia
  Wilkie, eds.
     p.   cm.
  Includes index.
  ISBN 0–335–15632–0 (hb). 0–335–15631–2 (pb)
     1. AIDS (Disease)   2. AIDS (Disease)—Patients—Counseling of.
  I. Anderson, Charles, 1952–   .   II. Wilkie, Patricia, 1938–
  RC607.A26R453   1991
  362.1'9697'92—dc20   91-14733
                                                                CIP

Typeset by Inforum Typesetting, Portsmouth
Printed in Great Britain by St Edmundsbury Press
Bury St Edmunds, Suffolk

Contents

Looking at particular needs

The needs of the helper

Sources of information and services

List of contributors

CHARLES ANDERSON is a psychologist and a lecturer in the Department of Education, University of Edinburgh. He is a consultant on training and counselling to Scottish AIDS Monitor, a trustee of Scottish AIDS Monitor and a trustee of Milestone Venture Trust. He has considerable experience in the training of voluntary helpers in the area of HIV.

ALAN FERRY is a lecturer in the Community Services Department, Cardonald College. He is a qualified social worker, and has worked as a social worker in the area of addictions. From 1985 to 1988, he was the co-ordinator of Possil Drug Project, Glasgow, and from 1988 to 1990 drug development co-ordinator, East Glasgow.

DR ALEXANDER McMILLAN, MD, FRCPE is a consultant physician and head of the Department of Genitourinary Medicine, Edinburgh Royal Infirmary. He is also a part-time senior lecturer in the Genitourinary Medicine Unit, Department of Medicine, University of Edinburgh.

DR ALISON RICHARDSON is a top grade clinical psychologist, HIV/AIDS and Drugs Service, Lothian Health Board. She is also involved in research work in the area of HIV infection and in voluntary work in the community.

DR NORAH SMITH has a private counselling practice in London and is an associate therapist, Wellspring, Edinburgh. She is also training as a Jungian analyst at the Society of Analytical Psychology, London.

PATRICIA WILKIE is a research fellow in the Division of General Practice, St George's Hospital Medical School, London. Formerly a research fellow in the Department of Psychology, University of Stirling and research fellow/ haemophilia HIV counsellor, Haemophilia Unit, Glasgow Royal Infirmary.

PROFESSOR DAVID WILKIE, FFA, FIA is a partner of R. Watson & Sons, Consulting Actuaries, Reigate, honorary visiting professor at the Actuarial Science Departments of Heriot-Watt University and the City University, member of the Institute of Actuaries AIDS Working Party, member of the Department of Health Committee under the chairmanship of Sir David Cox on the forecasting of HIV infection and AIDS in England and Wales (1988), and of the similar committee under the chairmanship of Professor Nicholas Day (1990).

Acknowledgements

We would like to acknowledge the ideas, inspiration and support that we have received from many people we know who are living with HIV, and from a large number of colleagues.

The royalties from this book will be divided equally between the Terrence Higgins Trust and The Milestone Venture Trust.

Introduction

CHARLES ANDERSON AND PATRICIA WILKIE

In 1981, only a small number of cases of what was later to be described as Acquired Immune Deficiency Syndrome (AIDS) had been officially reported in the USA. Now, in 1991, HIV infection has claimed very many lives worldwide. During the past decade, it has become clear that the effects of HIV infection are not simply limited to the life-threatening conditions identified in the official definitions of AIDS. People with HIV infection very often remain healthy and free from symptoms for many years. Dr McMillan comments, in Chapter 3, that 'The variability in the effects of HIV infection has led some clinicians in recent years to prefer to think in terms of a range, a spectrum, of HIV-related illnesses and conditions, rather than in terms of sharply defined stages of illness.' This variability in the effects of HIV infection means that helpers in this area need to be well prepared to meet the very different sets of needs of individuals living with HIV who are asymptomatic and well, individuals who are experiencing some HIV-related symptoms and individuals who are faced by very serious health problems.

People with HIV-related illnesses have to meet a number of challenges. They have to cope with the pain and the problems in everyday living which accompany any serious illness. At the same time, they need to deal with the social stigma that has been attached to HIV infection and AIDS. Many individuals living with HIV have required the courage to meet very directly expressed prejudices and discrimination. Individuals who discover that they have been infected with HIV but who are well, have to find ways of dealing with the stress and anxiety which accompanies knowing that one may possibly become unwell and even face life-threatening illness at some point in the future. It can be very taxing to live for a very long period of time with considerable uncertainty about the future. The partners, family and friends of people living with HIV can also experience great distress and practical problems as a result of uncertainty about the future and coping with the illness of a loved one. They also require emotional support, counselling and practical help.

Many individuals now find themselves playing a helping role for someone who is affected in some way or other by HIV infection. They include volunteers working for an HIV agency, such as the Terrence Higgins Trust or Scottish AIDS Monitor, and professional helpers employed by statutory agencies. Quite often, helpers in the area of HIV are themselves HIV antibody positive, or have a partner or close friend who is living with HIV. This book aims to:

- assist helpers in the area of HIV to clarify their purposes;
- present helpers with knowledge about HIV and related matters which they will require;
- look in detail at how best to respond to the needs of individuals who are living with HIV and coping with illness;
- aid helpers to gain greater awareness of the needs of particular groups of clients; and
- encourage people with a helping role to look at how their own needs can be met appropriately.

In this Introduction, it seemed more useful to identify common themes rather than to give a chapter-by-chapter précis of the book. The chapters in the section of the book entitled 'Medical, psychiatric and epidemiological aspects of HIV' present current knowledge concerning the nature of the HIV virus, its transmission, and HIV-related illnesses including psychiatric and neuropsychological problems. Information is also presented in this section on the spread of the disease and the forecasting of its future course. The chapters in the section 'Coping with HIV' look in some detail at issues involved in HIV antibody pre-test counselling, at coping with the immediate impact of an HIV antibody positive diagnosis, at the longer-term challenges of living with HIV and the difficulties of coping with illness. Although a considerable amount of information and a fairly wide range of helping actions are presented in these two sections, it needs to be emphasized that the authors do not believe that it is possible or desirable to follow a 'cook-book' approach to helping in HIV. The accent throughout the book as a whole, and particularly in the first section on 'Clarifying purposes', is on the need for helpers to think carefully about their purposes and to be vigilant about the way in which they are responding to individuals with HIV infection. The aim is to encourage reflection about general aims, particular purposes and the effect of specific helping techniques and actions.

Using power responsibly

Another important theme of the book is the need for helpers to ensure that they make responsible use of the power which comes from the fact that they are likely to be better informed about HIV and related matters than many of their clients. Chapter 6 on 'Giving information, handling information', in particular, looks at how helpers can ensure that the power which comes from knowledge about HIV is used responsibly. Helpers are asked to examine carefully how they interpret and represent 'the facts about HIV', and to consider how their own convictions about HIV-related issues may influence the way in which they give information. Chapter 6 also considers how clients can be enabled to gain sufficient information and skills to make rational choices.

Throughout the book there is a concern to emphasize the need to respect the ground rules of good practice in helping, to make sure that the power which comes from the trust that a client places in a helper is not abused. The requirements to be aware of the vulnerability of some clients, to respect confidentiality, to obtain consent, to act with 'due care' and to be aware of one's own limitations are highlighted in Chapter 1. These requirements are also considered at a number of points in the chapters within the section 'Coping with HIV'.

Power can also be misused if models of adjustment are forced on a client. The book encourages helpers to look very carefully at what they regard as 'good adjustment' to illness and to stressful experiences, and to appreciate that individuals vary greatly in how they wish to cope with illness and stress. Helping responses need to be tailored very carefully to meet the particular goals and social situation of each individual who is living with HIV. Chapter 1 emphasizes that social expectations about how one should adjust to illness and uncertainty differ widely across cultures, and helpers must take care to meet the needs of a person living with HIV in a way which is appropriate to his or her cultural context.

A related concern which appears explicitly, or more implicitly, in a number of chapters, is the need for helpers to avoid imposing hasty or simplistic interpretations of their situation on individuals who are living with HIV. It is argued that helpers need to use a framework of ideas to understand the situation of an individual living with HIV which takes full account of his or her personal history, present situation, values, motives, social context and cultural background. There is a concern throughout the book that helping should be firmly guided by an attempt to understand the situation of an individual who is HIV antibody positive from within his or her own perspective on the world. For example, a fairly lengthy section in Chapter 8 looks at the need to try to understand how a particular individual is constructing meaning out of the experience of being HIV antibody positive; and also explores a number of different possible ways in which an individual may make sense of an HIV antibody positive diagnosis.

Chapter 6 stresses the need to reduce any differentials in power that exist between a helper and a person who is living with HIV by being willing to share information fully and openly, and to pass on skills. Learning new skills is only one way in which someone living with HIV can gain a greater degree of control over the direction of his or her life and be enabled to cope with uncertainty. A number of chapters highlight the need for a worker in the area of HIV to have a wide repertoire of general helping techniques and particular helping actions to be able to respond flexibly and appropriately to a client. Responding flexibly to the needs of a client does not mean, however, trying out various helping actions in a haphazard manner. Helpers need to make a 'principled' choice of how they should respond on a particular occasion. In other words, it is important that they are able to give a clear justification for why they responded in a particular way.

Looking at the social context of helping

The section 'Looking at particular needs' tries to give some sense of how the social situation and the specific problems faced by different groups of clients may determine how they meet the challenges posed by HIV. The chapters here look at how HIV has affected women, gay men, drug users, haemophiliacs and the partners of people who are living with HIV. The chapter on haemophilia also considers the challenges faced by children coping with HIV. Throughout these chapters there is a concern to get readers to focus on how coping with HIV is influenced by social circumstances and by the social pressures or stigma experienced by particular groups of individuals. In the sections 'Clarifying purposes' and 'Coping with HIV', there is also an attempt to set helping efforts firmly within a social context, to look at how the reactions of significant people in the life of a person living with HIV can be either a source of strength or a source of distress. Chapter 1 gives an explicit warning of the dangers of thinking about the problems faced by an individual who is living with HIV in too 'individualistic' a fashion, as deriving largely from problems of 'internal' adjustment to a new difficult situation. It reminds readers of the fact that some of the distress experienced by people with HIV infection has its source in the social world, in real hurts that they receive from other people.

This focus on the social context in which helping takes place includes a consideration of the active part that a helper may play in the social world of a person who is living with HIV infection. Within the area of HIV infection it is difficult for a helper to play the part of a detached observer of the client's interactions with the world about him or her. It is pointed out in Chapters 1, 8 and 9 that a helper on occasion may need to act as an advocate or agent for a client who is living with HIV, say, to assist communication with doctors, or to fight for benefits and services to which the individual is entitled. It is stated that there is a need for helpers to be honest with their clients about the extent to which they are able to act on their behalf.

Care in the use of language

Setting helping in HIV within a social context also requires that attention is given to the way in which HIV and AIDS have been represented within the media and throughout society. A number of chapters comment on the destructive power of the images and metaphors that have been used to describe HIV and AIDS, and the stigmatizing way in which people with HIV infection have been portrayed. Helpers need to gain a clear recognition of the harmful effects of these stigmatizing and frightening images, and to be able to work with people living with HIV to strip these images of their destructive power.

An important theme of the book is the need to use clear, precise language and language which is tailored to the personal characteristics and experience of individual clients. In addition, Chapter 6 alerts helpers to the need to use terms which people living with HIV themselves prefer to use to represent their situation. Information concerning certain aspects of HIV and its effects remains somewhat uncertain. Chapter 6 describes the need to balance the desire to present information in a clear, concrete manner with a concern not to oversimplify complex or uncertain knowledge. In areas where knowledge remains uncertain, helpers also require to be honest about the limitations of current understanding.

The personal qualities of the helper

It has already been stated that the book as a whole emphasizes the need for helpers to have a wide repertoire of helping strategies and actions which they can use in a flexible manner to respond appropriately to the needs of individual clients. This does not mean, however, that the book views helping in the area of HIV as simply a technical matter of applying appropriate helping techniques to enable individuals to deal, say, with particular troublesome thoughts or to solve relationship problems. Equal emphasis is placed on the personal qualities that are required for effective helping in the area of HIV. Helping actions are likely to be perceived by people living with HIV as uncaring or patronizing if they are not accompanied by a genuine interest, warmth and acceptance of the person. An earlier section of this Introduction has indicated the importance that is placed within the book on the need for helpers to act with integrity and to use power responsibly. This aim to act in an honest, responsible manner, is more likely to be achieved if helpers in the area of HIV set aside time to reflect on their general purposes and on the nature of their day-to-day practice.

January 1991

Clarifying purposes

ONE

Aspects of helping in HIV:
A personal view

CHARLES ANDERSON

Introduction

This chapter discusses some aspects of training for a helping role in the area of HIV, and then looks at a number of issues which the author believes need to be considered if effective helping is to be achieved. Among the points which are highlighted are the need to adopt a flexible counselling approach, to check that the ground rules of good practice are being observed, to use an explanatory framework which stays close to the client's own experience, and to avoid imposing particular models of adjustment on the client.

Aspects of training in HIV

The need for fairly lengthy training courses

Even when there has been very careful selection of volunteers, or when experienced professional helpers are training to work in the area of HIV, there is still a need for a considerable amount of preparation. Helping in the area of HIV can be very demanding. Helpers often find themselves in difficult or stressful situations; and they must prepare themselves to cope well with such situations. They need to feel comfortable and be able to work effectively with clients who have widely varying lifestyles. They are also required to be prepared to meet the different sets of needs experienced by people who are HIV antibody positive but are asymptomatic and well, people who are beginning to have health problems, and people who are seriously ill.

Initial training programmes also need to be designed to cover a wide range of topics. Sessions will be required on information concerning HIV and information-handling skills; and sessions which allow participants to explore particular aspects of themselves and their reactions to others, such as their experience of loss and bereavement, issues surrounding sexuality and attitudes to drug use. Training will probably be required which focuses on developing particular counselling skills and encouraging a reflective, self-critical approach to counselling work.

Sessions are also needed on how HIV affects particular groups of clients, and what these groups may regard as appropriate counselling responses. It is necessary to look in separate sessions at how HIV is affecting women, gay men, drug users, ethnic minorities and at the needs of partners and families of people who are HIV-infected. Some organizations may also wish to look at work with HIV positive clients who are in prison. Other important content areas to include in an initial training course for helping work in HIV infection are welfare rights and patient advocacy.

Using an initial training course to build support mechanisms

A fairly extensive course, which may also be spread over a considerable period of time, has the advantage that it tests the commitment of voluntary helpers and allows them to make a realistic assessment of their own suitability for this area of work. A lengthy training course also provides the opportunity to build strong support groups for helpers (see Chapter 15). A wide definition of what support means in counselling can be provided within a training course. Support can be presented not only in affective terms, of giving individual members care and understanding when they are dealing with stressful helping situations, but also in terms of joint problem solving. A training course can highlight the problem-solving functions of a support group. A support group can discuss a difficult situation that is faced by an individual member, provide a variety of possible interpretations of this situation and carefully assess what might be the best course of action to take.

A delicate balance needs to be struck during a training course between encouraging individual trainees to have sufficient confidence in their ability to act in a self-directed manner with their clients, and ensuring that they will also be prepared to accept support and be open to alternative interpretations of their actions and decisions.

Tailoring a training course to local circumstances

The preceding paragraphs have suggested content areas that it is useful to include in any training course for counselling in HIV infection. However, the suggestions for content were not made in a very prescriptive way. Any training course will have to be designed to meet the needs of a particular locality; and the shape of a course designed to fit the context of London might need to be considerably remodelled to meet the requirements of a very different area in the UK.

Meeting the changing challenges that HIV poses

Any training course also needs to be continuously remodelled to take account of changes in the epidemiology and treatment of HIV, and in the responses of statutory agencies to HIV. For example, if the treatment of HIV improves considerably in the next few years, the emphasis in training courses for helpers may need to move more to considering how best to support individuals who have a much improved life expectancy but face problems of chronic ill-health over a long period of time.

Particular considerations in designing a training course for helpers in the area of HIV

Trainers in the area of HIV may feel that it is important to spend a lot of time on exercises in counselling skills. It certainly may be necessary to provide many opportunities for participants in a course to sharpen up their existing counselling skills or to acquire new skills. However, the manner in which skills training is carried out requires careful thought. Particularly where voluntary helpers are being trained, it is important that training in the use of particular communication or listening skills is not done in a fashion which leads some participants to devalue their existing strengths and everyday repertoire of helping skills. Trainers can aim to make participants in a course more aware of the helping skills which they already possess and to encourage them to use existing skills in a more disciplined and sensitive manner.

Practising counselling skills may also have a very limited impact on the day-to-day performance of helpers in the area of HIV, if it is divorced from the context of their use. As far as possible, the practising of helping skills should be related to some situation which a helper in the area of HIV might meet.

An introduction to counselling which focuses narrowly on the practice of a set of discrete skills, on communication skills with clients, may risk spending insufficient time in improving the quality of interpretations of clients' problems and the quality of joint work with a client in solving problems (Robinson and Halliday, 1987). It is worth spending a considerable amount of time on a training course encouraging participants to be flexible in their interpretations of a client's problems, and to form a picture of the client's situation which stays close to the client's own account of his or her experience. Discussion of role-plays and counselling exercises can be used to get the participants in a training course to reflect on the way in which they are interpreting a particular problem situation, to consider a number of different perspectives on the same situation and to attempt to see matters from the client's own point of view. A later section of the chapter looks in detail at a number of questions concerning the responsible use of the skills of interpretation and of particular interpretive frameworks in helping work in the area of HIV infection.

Many training courses for helpers in HIV work which are run in the UK and elsewhere give a very active participatory role to the trainees, and provide considerable opportunity for experiential learning in counselling. Customarily, participants are given sufficient time for general self-exploration, for work on grief and loss, and exploration of their attitudes towards particular groups of clients.

However, it is much less common to get trainees to examine their conceptions of what constitutes 'good adjustment' to a situation of uncertainty and loss. A later section of this chapter looks in some detail at ideas concerning 'good adjustment'. It is also not common to push prospective helpers to explore the extent to which they are able to accept adjustment responses which diverge considerably from their own notions of what constitutes 'good adjustment' to difficult situations. This type of exploration of values and beliefs about how to adjust to situations of loss and uncertainty, may need to be given a more central place in the training of helpers in the area of HIV (Anderson and Lockley, 1990).

The exploration of general and particular attitudes forms an important part of the work of preparation for helping in the area of HIV infection. However, the value of this work in examining attitudes and beliefs may be lessened if it is not done in a sufficiently focused manner. The exploration of attitudes is not solely for the benefit of the personal growth of the trainees. Trainees may need to be directed to consider in very concrete terms how particular attitudes and assumptions which they possess may affect their work with people who are IIIV antibody positive, and how they may need to change in certain ways if they are to provide an appropriate response to the needs of people with HIV infection.

Realistic role preview

An attempt can be made to give participants on a course a sense of the demands that may be placed on them as helpers by the use of videos of work with clients, and the role play or discussion of a wide variety of different scenarios. Where this preview takes the form of the discussion of a possible scenario, the scenario constructed needs to be open to a number of different interpretations and courses of appropriate action if it is to be a realistic representation of a helping situation. One set of situations which it is valuable to preview, are occasions where a helper may need to work in a cooperative way with volunteers or professionals from other agencies but still maintain client confidentiality and remain the agent of the client.

This previewing of helping situations is useful in increasing the confidence of trainees, and in helping trainees to define the role of a helper and to come to an understanding of the nature of the helping relationship. It also serves as a means of stimulating the exploration of trainees' everyday assumptions concerning the nature of helping and allows them to look at the possible effects of their values and beliefs in the context of helping in HIV infection.

The need for a flexible response and a wide repertoire of helping actions

Helpers in the area of HIV need to be flexible in their approach if they are to put into practice the aims of responding to the expressed needs of clients, of assisting clients to deal with emotional and practical problems, and of enabling clients to exercise greater control over their lives.

Many helpers in the area of HIV will already have gained considerable skills and experience within a particular theoretical approach to counselling. This experience, and the particular theoretical framework of understanding a client's problems which they bring to their work in HIV, will give a strong foundation to their day-to-day helping activities. However, if they are to be truly responsive to the wide range of problems and needs faced by people affected by HIV, they will probably also need to make judicious use of ideas and ways of working from other approaches to counselling. Initial training courses for helpers in HIV can be used to highlight this need for a flexible response and a wide repertoire of helping actions. To illustrate the need for a wide repertoire of helping responses, the following sections give a brief indication of how aspects of some of the leading approaches to counselling can be put to good use in the area of HIV infection.

Looking first at the *person-centred approach* to counselling, the ethos of most humanistic approaches to counselling would seem to be particularly appropriate in the area of HIV. The person-centred approach, in common with other humanistic approaches to helping, places emphasis on respect for the individual's own goals and capacity for self-direction. It also stresses the need to avoid imposing any prescriptive interpretive framework on a client. The central principles which guide practice in the person-centred approach are:

- the helper does not set conditions on his or her acceptance of a client;
- there is an attempt by the helper to view reality from the internal frame of reference of the client; and
- the helper displays an attitude of *genuineness* towards a client, and does not erect any façade between herself and the client.

All of these guiding principles would seem to be very apposite to the area of HIV. The acceptance from others that many people with HIV infection receive is conditional and problematic. Some people with HIV infection may also have received a barrage of advice, of prescriptions, as to how they should act. It is important that these actions of stigmatizing and directing HIV antibody positive individuals are not present within a helping relationship, that acceptance is not made conditional.

Trying to see matters from the client's own frame of reference is a challenging task and one which calls for considerable personal engagement on the part of a helper. In explaining what achieving the internal frame of reference of a client involves, Carl Rogers uses the metaphor of the helper as a companion to the client. He talks about how:

> as the client is genuinely exploring the unknown, the counselor becomes wholly engaged in trying to keep step with this puzzled and puzzling search. His attention is completely focused upon the attempt to perceive from the client's frame of reference, and thus it is no longer a technique in operation, but the implementation of an absorbing personal purpose (Rogers, 1951, p. 112).

Being assisted to explore in this way without having any agenda imposed on one by a helper can be a very valuable, empowering experience. However, in the area of HIV, there may be occasions where a helper may usefully interpret certain aspects of a client's experience while in general facilitating the type of 'undirected' self-exploration which Rogers describes. The self that Rogers is suggesting that we assist the client to explore has been constructed from experience, and is not solely a private construction. Stigmatizing ways of thinking about AIDS which are common in our society may powerfully influence the way in which HIV antibody positive individuals make sense of their own experience. As a later section of this chapter argues, it may be very useful to explore with some clients how their feelings and thoughts are being influenced by the way in which AIDS has been represented and to negotiate with the client new meanings for HIV.

Looking at patterns of thinking

It would clearly be irresponsible for helpers who have not received specific training in one of the cognitive therapies to apply cognitive-behavioural techniques in a piecemeal way within their day-to-day practice. However, ideas from the *cognitive* approaches to therapy can be very useful tools for understanding the ways in which a client is responding to illness, loss and difficult social situations. Within the cognitively-based therapies, the accent is on attempting to assess how an individual is constructing a view of the world. As a helper builds up a picture of the client's world-view, he or she will attempt to identify particular thoughts and patterns of thinking which may be the source of distress and difficulties in everyday living.

The particular techniques used vary somewhat between the main schools of cognitive therapy, but the emphasis remains on helping clients to identify patterns of thinking which may be causing them difficulties and to 'restructure' these patterns of thinking. In other words, clients are assisted to construct a somewhat different, less rigid and troubling world-view. Those aspects of cognitive therapy which are concerned with pointing out to clients the possibility of forming a new more positive construction of the world seem particularly appropriate for work in the area of HIV, given the need to 'deconstruct' negative representations of HIV and to replace them with less threatening views of the disease.

People who are suddenly faced with loss or with situations of uncertainty may also demonstrate patterns of thinking which cognitive therapists have identified as a source of distress. These particular patterns of thinking are also commonly associated with depression. Among the types of reasoning which have been identified as creating difficulties and distress, are thinking about the world in somewhat black-and-white terms, assuming that things are either all good or all bad, overgeneralizing ('If my partner leaves me, I'll be completely alone') and greatly magnifying the nature of any difficulties which are experienced (Beck, 1972).

Assisting a depressed HIV antibody positive client to explore his or her construction of the world, to identify thoughts which may be the source of great pain, and to reshape these thoughts to some extent can be a very valuable set of therapeutic actions. As a caveat, however, a later section of the chapter examines how the source of much of the distress faced by an HIV antibody positive individual may be interpersonal in nature rather than simply the result of the individual's own construction of the world.

Problem-solving work

In addition to helping clients to 'deconstruct' troublesome thoughts and find new ways of looking at the world, helpers can give very valuable assistance to clients who wish to tackle particular problems that they are facing. Focused discussion with a helper can assist a client to clarify the exact nature of the problem that he or she is facing and to look carefully at how this problem is related to the general context of the client's life.

Once the problem has been identified in reasonably clear terms, the client and helper can work on coming up with a number of different possible solutions. The advantages and disadvantages of the solutions which have been identified can then be considered. This can be done either informally or in a more structured way by writing out a list of solutions and attaching advantages and disadvantages to each solution. It is important that this work of deciding on the most appropriate solution is not carried out in too mechanistic a fashion. The client needs plenty of time to explore the emotions that are associated with particular solutions, to be sure that particular solutions feel comfortable. He or she also needs to be sure that a solution does in fact meet his or her goals.

The next stage in a structured approach to problem solving involves identifying a comfortable set of tactics, or particular actions, to put the chosen solution or solutions into practice. At this stage, it is also useful to think in very concrete terms about how the solution is to be implemented. Helpers can also role-play with a client implementing certain solutions such as those which involve the client being assertive with a partner. The possible difficulties that a client may experience in putting a solution into practice can be previewed and ways of dealing with these difficulties considered.

At subsequent meetings, a helper and client can review how the process of solving a particular problem, or set of problems, has been working out in practice. Helpers can play an important role in encouraging and validating a client's attempts to find solutions to problems and in encouraging a fairly flexible approach to problem solving. If a chosen solution is not working out well in practice, alternative solutions can be considered. As circumstances change, the problems faced by a client are also likely to change and new solutions will have to be found.

'Positive asset' search

Successful problem solving requires that the client is able to identify clearly and appreciate his or her strengths, and does not focus exclusively on problems and difficulties. Within helping in the area of HIV, it may be important to explore positive aspects of the client's life, and sometimes to remind the client of assets that he or she possesses. Helping can seek to accentuate these more positive aspects of a client's life, as well as dealing with difficult, distressing aspects.

Enabling change through the acquisition of new skills

Helping which is concerned with enabling clients to exercise more control over their lives and to gain a greater element of choice as to how to live needs to concern itself with the passing on of techniques and skills. For example, a helper can assist a client to learn to solve problems in a more structured way, techniques of how to cope with anxiety or panic attacks, to relax, or use a variety of means to maintain health. Although it is appropriate that the accent is on ways of maintaining health and developing a positive outlook on life, attention also needs to be given to helping people to develop effective strategies for coping with illness and depression.

The helping relationship in HIV, therefore, can be thought about partly in terms of learning and teaching, in terms of enabling change to happen by the passing on of skills. It is crucial, however, that such skills are handed over, or knowledge passed on, in a sensitive manner. An attempt to push people to acquire skills which will enable them to be autonomous is likely to be self-defeating.

Although the accent in a helping relationship which aims to be as democratic as possible needs to be on the active transfer of skills, it is important to recognize the barriers to change which some clients experience. The daily life of a considerable number of clients may be very difficult and constraining, providing them with few opportunities for gaining greater control and choice. Such clients clearly may benefit considerably from developing confidence in themselves and from learning new ways of coping, but disappointment may follow if helper and/or client make unrealistic assumptions about the amount of change that can be achieved.

Ensuring that the ground rules of good practice are observed

Earlier sections of this chapter established that an initial training course for work in HIV infection needs to cover a large number of different content areas, ensure that helpers possess a sufficiently wide repertoire of skills which they can use in a flexible manner and provide sufficient opportunities for experiential learning and realistic preview of difficult situations. Such a course also needs to give participants a very concrete sense of how the standard ground rules for the conduct of helping relationships apply in the area of HIV infection. These ground rules exist to prevent abuses of power by helpers and to ensure that they act in a responsible manner.

Being alert to the vulnerability of some clients

Trainees or established helpers in the area of HIV infection may be more conscientious about applying the rules of good practice if they are reminded of the vulnerable position which clients place themselves in when they come for help or advice. Throughout this chapter, implicitly as well as explicitly, it is suggested that helpers should attempt to set up a relationship with a client which is democratic in nature and tries to minimize any inequalities in power. At the same time, though, it is necessary to recognize that there are likely to be a number of inequalities present within that relationship.

Within helping relationships in general, the client is frequently in an emotionally vulnerable condition and may be fairly desperate to find ways of coping with distress or particular problems. The client may have fairly high expectations of the benefits to be gained from counselling and commonly is prepared to accept interpretations of problems and advice which the helper gives. In the context of HIV, there also may be an important inequality in power which arises from the fact that the helper has a wider knowledge base concerning HIV infection and associated matters than the client.

Ways of reducing this inequality of power which comes from a difference in levels of knowledge are suggested in Chapter 6. It is important, though, that any inequalities which do exist in the relationship between a helper and an HIV antibody positive client are recognized, as a first step in ensuring that these inequalities are not, consciously or unconsciously, exploited by the helper. Helpers also need to be alert to the possibility that they may misuse power by becoming very involved in a client's problems in a way which is principally meeting their own emotional needs rather than those of the client.

Respecting confidentiality

One of the most important ground rules of good helping practice is that of respecting confidentiality. Any limitations on the maintenance of confidentiality, such as the sharing of information among a multidisciplinary team of workers, need to be made explicit before a client proceeds to make any disclosures about his or her personal life and feelings.

Normally, the practice of voluntary and professional helpers in HIV is guided by a strong belief in the importance of maintaining confidentiality. However, there may be instances where working assumptions established among a group of workers about what may or may not be construed as a breach of confidentiality can come into conflict with a more formal and strict definition of the client's right to confidentiality. A regular critical examination of practice in respecting clients' disclosures on the part of individual helpers, groups of workers and agencies is required if strict standards of confidentiality are to be maintained.

Obtaining consent

It is recognized within the literature on the ethics of counselling that gaining fully informed consent to counselling is a much more difficult business than, for example, gaining consent for medical procedures (Lakin, 1988; Holmes and Lindley, 1989). However, if a helping relationship is to be conducted in a responsible manner, it is important that clients are presented with sufficient information to make a rational choice about whether they wish to receive long-term counselling or not. In practice, consent on the part of the client may often be taken for granted, rather than be regarded as a matter which requires clarification and negotiation.

It may be almost impossible to provide clients with an exact sense of what is involved in the type of helping that is on offer, but it is at least possible to give a general description of the nature of the type of helping that will be provided. The way in which the helper sees his or her role can be described. Any boundaries that the helper is placing on the range of helping actions, and on the nature of the relationship itself, can be described. Any possible risks as well as benefits that may be associated with the type of helping that is on offer need to be mentioned. Initial helping sessions can also be offered in a tentative way as a sample of what is available, and the nature of the helping relationship gradually established and its terms deepened by a process of negotiation between client and helper (Holmes and Lindley, 1989, p. 156). This negotiation can take place either in a very informal way, or involve the agreement of a somewhat more formal 'contract' between client and helper.

Acknowledging personal limitations

Helpers may find that they lack the expertise or personal resources to meet the needs of a particular client. When this occurs, they need to acknowledge their own limitations as helpers and attempt to ensure that the client receives appropriate care from someone else who possesses the necessary expertise or personal qualities. One aspect of acknowledging their own limitations concerns helpers considering when their clients' interests would be served best by involving professionals such as clinical psychologists and psychiatrists. Neuropsychiatric problems are one of the wide range of possible sources of distress and disturbance in thoughts and feelings for an HIV-infected person (see Chapter 4). Clearly, the involvement of the appropriate professionals needs to be suggested by any responsible helper who suspects that there is an organic basis for some of the difficulties which a client is experiencing.

Acting with 'due care'

In addition to acknowledging their own limitations, responsible helpers are also required to take 'due care' in applying techniques to bring about change in a client. The following simple, working definition indicates what is involved in taking 'due care' not to harm a client in any way. It is suggested that acting with due care requires helpers to use their formal knowledge about counselling and associated disciplines and the experience which they have gained in helping situations to ensure that as far as possible individual clients are not exposed to therapeutic techniques which may have a damaging effect. As a second part of the definition of acting with due care, it is suggested that helpers need to allow for the possibility that the use of any therapeutic technique might lead to unintended harmful consequences, and to be alert for any signs that harm may have been inflicted. In cases where helpers suspect that some harm might have been done to the client, appropriate actions need to be taken to support the client and to correct the harm that has been inflicted.

Acting with due care in the conduct of intensive workshops

One of the areas in the field of HIV helping work where there appears to be a particular need to be alert to the requirement to act with due care is in the conduct of intensive workshops for people who are affected in some way or other by HIV. In these workshops, the participants explore their hurts, ventilate their feelings and, it is hoped, free themselves of much distress and develop a new, more positive approach to the challenges posed by HIV infection.

Such intensive workshops and short courses are very valuable for many participants, and the following remarks are not meant to be critical of the overall purpose of workshops of this type. However, if such workshops are to be conducted in a responsible, ethical way, quite a number of safeguards need to be observed. If informed consent is to be achieved, it would seem necessary to alert prospective participants to the fact that as well as offering positive benefits, such workshops may involve risks, such as being more acutely aware of one's pain and distress, at least for a time.

Within the workshops themselves, it is important that participants are given the opportunity to explore painful feelings at their own pace rather than being forced to explore more deeply and at a faster pace than they find comfortable. A sudden intensive exploration of feelings might not be appropriate to the current situation of some participants. Bringing feelings to awareness may often be a necessary first step in dealing with problems and reducing distress. However, it does not necessarily follow that being open to experience and encouraging the catharsis of negative feelings will automatically bring the relief of distress and a more vital way of being. An individual may need to spend a fairly long period of time working through and resolving difficult feelings that have been brought into awareness.

The responsible conduct of workshops also requires the establishment of a system for providing support to participants *after* the workshop. Some participants may find that, after a workshop, feelings have emerged which they find difficult to bear, or be aware of problems which they must now address. They may be in a more vulnerable position for some time after the workshop and in need of considerable support.

Respecting an individual's coping mechanisms

It is also important, within intensive workshops or in day-to-day helping, that an individual's personal ways of dealing with distress are respected, and that 'defences' are not seen as simply obstacles to personal growth. The protective function of defensive coping mechanisms needs to be acknowledged. It can be irresponsible to force individuals to confront too much reality, all at once. Experienced counsellors within the field of HIV, such as Miller and Bor, emphasize this point. They describe how 'The counsellor should be guarded against confronting patients who use denial as a coping mechanism as the patient might become very anxious, depressed and possibly suicidal, or totally dependent on the counsellor' (Miller and Bor, 1988, p. 11).

Ensuring that 'due care' is taken in the facilitation of self-help groups

Self-help groups have provided a very valuable service for people who are affected in some way or other by HIV. They have allowed individuals to have their experiences validated by others and to develop a sense of solidarity which is a source of strength and power. The success of self-help groups, however, depends in large part on the provision of responsible facilitation and the creation of a climate where the needs and vulnerabilities of individual members are respected. Groups need to be facilitated in a way which allows individual members to feel 'safe' and accepted. If the group is to function as a safe and secure base for all its members, certain ground rules are required. In particular, there is a need for rules which stress the requirements to respect each others' beliefs, to avoid being judgemental, and to avoid imposing a particular interpretation of a problem on another member of the group. Members also may need to be asked to avoid making demands for personal disclosures or expressions of feeling which individual participants may find invasive and distressing.

Setting helping efforts within a social context

Mention of the valuable contribution that self-help groups make to some individuals with HIV infection, serves as a reminder that help and support can come from many sources – from friends, partners, family, self-help groups, voluntary agencies and professional helpers in statutory services. At the same time, the social network of an HIV antibody positive individual, or the reactions of the wider society, may be the source of great distress.

The nature and purposes of the helping relationship offered to an individual with HIV infection will be very powerfully influenced by the extent to which the helper is alert to the social context of the individual's problems. It is possible that a helper may view the sources of distress experienced by a client in a somewhat asocial way and place emphasis on assisting the client to 'adjust' to a difficult reality. When this happens, responsibility for change is very much placed on the individual who is expected to assimilate to the world around him or her. The ways in which the people around an HIV positive individual, and society in general, may need to change to accommodate his or her needs are left unexamined.

It is regrettable when helpers view the situation of an HIV positive client from such a narrow 'individualistic' perspective. Many of the problems faced by people with HIV infection are the result of real hurts sustained in the social world, and are not simply a matter of internal adjustment to a new, difficult situation. Discrimination in housing, employment and the need to cope with a stigmatized condition are all problems that are imposed on people with HIV infection from outside. It makes sense, therefore, to see the origin of much of the distress that people who live with HIV infection experience as interpersonal in nature, rather than as a matter only of individual adjustment.

Some HIV positive individuals may have a style of thinking which leads them to attribute difficulties that they may be experiencing to factors within themselves or to their own actions. Such individuals may need to be reminded that many of the problems which they face are definitely not to be seen as 'their fault'. They may need to be given a different perspective on their life and informed that they are coping as well as they can with problems which are not of their own making, but have been imposed upon them.

The social representations of AIDS, images and metaphors

Within the media and in public discussion, frightening images have been used to represent AIDS, and stigmatizing metaphors have been used to describe people with HIV infection. AIDS has been represented as a condition which marks its 'victims' as socially different, and people with AIDS have sometimes been represented as a source of moral and social contamination and danger. Some of the distress or discomfort faced by an HIV positive individual, may derive from the ways in which HIV and AIDS have been socially constructed and from the images and metaphors which have been used to represent AIDS (Markova and Wilkie, 1987). It may be necessary to explore with clients how they see the nature of HIV and its effects, and to strip harmful metaphors that have been used to describe the disease of their power. While maintaining an attitude of respect for the client's world-view, a helper can suggest how some of his or her ways of thinking about HIV have been constructed by others and negotiate with the client a new set of meanings. The accent, though, needs to be on negotiation and assisting the client to reconstruct his or her view of the meaning of HIV, rather than on a surface imposition of an alternative, more positive perspective.

Providing helping which is appropriate to the client's cultural background

How an individual responds to an HIV antibody positive diagnosis may be shaped not only by the way in which AIDS has been represented in the media, but also by the beliefs held about how one should respond to illness in the culture to which he or she belongs. It is recognized, for example, that a willingness to report symptoms of illness varies considerably across cultures. The nature of illness and its causation is also explained in different ways in different cultures.

It is important, therefore, to gain a sense of how a person from another culture thinks about the nature of illness and how one should respond to illness. Any information given about HIV needs to be tailored to take account of the individual's culturally formed framework of beliefs for interpreting illness and the world in general. Helpers in the area of HIV who wish to provide counselling which is culturally appropriate also need to educate themselves concerning matters such as the expectations concerning family obligations and the role of the family in cultures different from their own. This general attempt to educate oneself about – and to listen carefully to a client's account of – a different set of cultural values and way of structuring the world, will probably need to include gaining knowledge about the sexual mores of the particular culture.

Throughout this chapter, and the book as a whole, much emphasis is placed on enabling clients with HIV infection to exercise more control over their lives. However, *control* may be perceived very differently in different cultures. Bart Aoki, writing about 'cross-cultural counseling' in the area of HIV, has noted that self-assertion and exercising control over events in the world is particularly valued in Western cultures (Aoki, 1989). Valuing of this type of control is linked with community efforts to gain better health education and care, and with an assertive attitude on the part of individuals concerning their rights to receive appropriate care. Aoki contrasts this Western valuing of control over external events and other people, with the values of some other cultures which 'place primary value upon the exercise of control over the self as opposed to the imposition of control over others' (Aoki, 1989, p. 26). Individuals who are influenced by such a cultural construct of control will prefer to rely on 'internal' mechanisms for coping with difficult situations, to attempt to control feelings and thoughts.

Aoki goes on to identify the way in which this culturally valued reliance on 'internal' coping mechanisms may affect the relationship with helpers. He describes how:

> patients who prefer to maintain self-control in the face of highly emotional issues may, despite being frustrated or confused, be hesitant to assert themselves with providers. Others, having experienced years of powerlessness in an oppressive system, may prefer as protection to devote their psychological resources to self-control rather than risking exposure to further frustration. Thus what may appear to be an attitude of fatalism among those with AIDS who are culturally different can have multiple underpinnings related to culture as well as to minority group status (op. cit.).

The quote from Aoki also highlights the real problems which many individuals in ethnic minorities face as a result of racial discrimination. It may sometimes be difficult for helpers to appreciate the way in which the discrimination faced by members of particular ethnic minority groups has shaped their experience of the world and narrowed their view of what can be expected from life.

The need to make very careful efforts to understand and respond appropriately to the world-view and customary style of coping with difficulties of an individual who is from a different culture would, one trusts, be generally recognized. However, less attention might be paid sometimes to the very different ways in which both formal and informal relationships are structured in different cultures. Helpers need to respond appropriately to the signals that they receive from a client who belongs to another culture as to what is an appropriate physical distance during a conversation and what quantity of eye contact should be made. They also need to show some sensitivity to clients' culturally formed expectations concerning how formal or informal the nature of the helping relationship should be; and their wishes to have either a very direct form of communication or to discuss difficult issues in an indirect, cautious fashion.

Recognizing barriers to change, and identifying sources of support

As preceding sections of this chapter have argued, whatever the cultural background of a client, the social world experienced by HIV positive individuals may place considerable limitations on their abilities to change and to make a 'positive' adjustment to a diagnosis of HIV infection. In the counselling of people with HIV infection, as in much health education concerning HIV (see Chapter 6), unrealistic assumptions can be made about the extent to which change can be brought about by an act of will without considering the wider constraints that exist on an individual's actions. These assumptions need to be resisted.

An attempt needs to be made by a helper to work with a client to identify sources of support and ways in which the client can make best use of the sources of support that are available. The approach to counselling advocated by Miller and Bor (1988) in their book *AIDS: A Guide to Clinical Counselling*, sets out to locate helping efforts firmly within an individual's wider pattern of social relationships. Their approach, which they describe as a 'systemic view', focuses on the reciprocity of relationships and their effects, on identifying a client's support network, and on relating the discussion of concerns or difficult issues to the client's social context. Taking a wider perspective on a client's situation, in the manner suggested by Miller and Bor, is likely to reduce the possibility of inappropriate solutions being suggested to the client and of dependence on the counsellor.

The helper as an agent or advocate of the client

Taking a wider perspective on a client's situation also brings into sharper focus the question of the extent to which a helper is prepared to act on behalf of a client. Voluntary helpers may often find themselves in the position of acting as an agent for the client, as an advocate on his or her behalf in dealings with various professionals and providers of money and services. For example, a helper may assist a client to communicate with a doctor, or be involved in advancing a client's case for particular welfare rights. There are occasions where the interests of a client may need to be defended or promoted with vigour and tenacity. At the same time, this vigorous promotion of a client's interests will require to be conducted with considerable social skill and intelligence. Pursuing a client's interests in a way which is likely to lead to antagonism and a lack of cooperation on the part of professionals or service providers clearly may be self-defeating.

Professional helpers in the area of HIV frequently may need to consider and make moral decisions about the extent to which they should engage themselves on a client's behalf. Some principled decisions by professional helpers to act as an advocate for a client may on occasion set them somewhat at odds with other colleagues or force them to battle with the policy of their employing organization.

For example, one difficult situation which might arise, is when a helper working in a hospital context finds her clients angry about a lack of monitoring of their health or a lack of availability of drug treatments which can be got at other hospitals. In such a scenario, helpers might respond by feeling that they had to 'manage' the client's responses and secure compliance to whatever treatment regime was available. Such a response would seem to give force to the characterization of counselling by some critics that it merely serves as a subtle means of bringing people to accept an unjust reality. Alternatively, a helper might indicate to a client that her frustration and anger was a reasonable response to an unjust situation, and attempt to act as an advocate for the client. Acting as an advocate for a client may on occasion involve some personal cost to the helper and call for considerable strength of will.

Interpretation and its dangers

As well as thinking carefully about the extent to which they can act as an agent for a client, helpers in the area of HIV need to consider how the interpretive framework that they are using to understand a client's problems is influencing their helping actions. Helpers who have a genuine wish to develop as demo-cratic a relationship as possible with a client need to avoid the danger of imposing an interpretation on a client which may not fit well with his or her felt experience.

Helpers can take a number of actions to ensure that they make responsible use of the power that comes from the ability to change a client's life by presenting him or her with an alternative interpretation of reality. They need, for example, to be alert to the limitations of the everyday assumptions, or the more formal ideas derived from psychology, that they are using to understand the situation of a person who is HIV antibody positive.

Ideas derived from psychological research that attempt to give a structured description of the reactions of individuals to situations of stress and uncertainty are necessary tools for a helper trying to understand the situation of a person who is HIV antibody positive. At the same time, the limitations on the descriptive range and the predictive power of particular ideas, or general theories, needs to be acknowledged. Using such ideas will only assist the helper to construct a reasonably valid account of *certain* aspects of a client's experience. Relying heavily on a *few* psychological concepts as tools for un-derstanding, also risks reducing the focus of a helper's interpretive efforts to a narrow range of aspects of the client's life.

The need to avoid using descriptive categories in a prescriptive way

A number of different concepts and descriptive theories have been formed which try to explain how most people react to situations of uncertainty and loss. There is a danger that some helpers may use these *descriptive* theories in a *prescriptive* fashion.

There is also a need for all helpers to be alert to the fact that some of these descriptive theories contain *implicit* prescriptions for helping practice. To illustrate this point, the well-known stage model of reactions to loss and death provided by Kübler-Ross (1970) gives a description of the sequence of reactions to loss and death that, it is claimed, can be observed in a dying patient. She identifies five stages that individuals pass through as they adjust to the prospect of death: denial, anger, bargaining, depression and acceptance. At the same time, however, her theory recommends that people working with dying patients see the last stage of reactions to death which she identifies (i.e. acceptance) as a goal of therapy (Kamerman, 1988).

There is a danger that helpers guided by such a theory might 'construct' a client in the image of the theory rather than respond to the person's own needs. They might attempt to move a client towards Kübler-Ross's descriptions of *acceptance*, towards conformity with an ideal type description of how one should cope with loss.

In the context of HIV, John Green and Lorraine Sherr have written on the dangers of using theoretical accounts of how people react to death and loss in a prescriptive way. They describe how helpers have sometimes:

> come to feel that unless people experience certain feelings or deal with these feelings in certain ways they will suffer psychological or even physical harm. Trying to force what happens to real people into rigid prescriptive theoretical models is at best unhelpful, at worst it prevents counsellors seeing what is really happening and makes them see only what they *expect* to see (Green and Sherr, 1989, p. 207).

Strategies for understanding the situation of a client

The need to avoid using particular descriptive theories in a prescriptive manner leads on to a consideration of the general strategies that helpers use to understand, to interpret, a client's life. A helper may adopt a strategy which tends to impose a definition of reality on a client, or one which remains sensitive to the context of the client's own meaning and experience.

For example, some helpers might use what could be described as a *top-down* strategy to understand the situation of an individual who is affected in some way or other by HIV. Someone using such a top-down strategy would take a predefined set of concepts and informal assumptions about what constitutes 'good adjustment' to understand a client's situation. The use of such a strategy does not allow a helper to capture a client's own intentions and meanings accurately and sensitively.

Alternatively, a helper may choose to use a more *bottom-up* strategy. This means that the helper will try to stay close to the client's own stated experience. The helper will choose to think about the client's situation in terms – of formal theories or less formal ideas – which seem to fit well with the emerging picture that the client presents of his or her experience. Any interpretations of the client's situation which emerge from this process of accurate, sensitive listening can be checked and modified to stay true to the client's experience. Any new perspective that a helper wishes to present to a client will also be advanced in a tentative way and be subject to negotiation, rather than being presented as a 'true version' of reality which the client must accept.

Avoiding a 'dualistic' view of a client's situation

Another matter which needs to be considered in a general review by helpers in the area of HIV of how they are interpreting the experiences of their clients, is the sort of division that they make between 'psychological' and 'bodily' problems. A potentially damaging narrowing of the helper's view of the client's life can occur if anxiety and stress are thought about as purely 'psychological' problems that require to be managed and controlled. The very real connection between anxiety and actual bodily distress, or anticipated bodily distress, needs to be recognized. Helpers need to avoid the 'dualistic' view that distressing psychological states can be thought about and dealt with independently of bodily conditions.

'Good adjustment'?

An earlier section of this chapter discussed in detail the danger of using descriptive theories in a prescriptive manner. This danger of prescribing to a client how he or she should cope with uncertainty and loss may arise also from the less formal assumptions which a helper holds concerning what constitutes 'good adjustment' to difficult situations and to illness.

The conceptions that an individual helper holds of what constitutes 'good adjustment' to difficult situations, loss and death may have been formed from a number of different sources. One powerful influence on the formation of their conceptions of 'good adjustment' will be their deeply held personal values – their beliefs concerning how life should be lived and the aims that people should be pursuing. Other formative influences on their conception of 'good adjustment' may be the values embedded in the particular approach to counselling in which they have been trained and the value system of the agency to which they belong.

In addition to the moral values that are guiding their view of what constitutes good adjustment to a diagnosis of HIV infection, or HIV-related illness, helpers are likely to be strongly influenced by the social construction of illness and health. We all tend to share a set of assumptions about the duties that ill people may need to perform. These assumptions are usually tacit, taken for granted, and never subject to scrutiny. As an example of such an assumption, we commonly require that patients must be seen to be making a conscious effort to regain health.

Individual helpers, and indeed whole groups of workers, may often be unaware of the extent to which their own conceptions of 'good adjustment' may be subtly influencing them to guide clients towards particular goals or actions. There can exist a fair degree of consensus of opinion among a group of workers in a voluntary or statutory agency concerning what constitutes 'successful' adjustment to a diagnosis of HIV infection or HIV-related illness. This agreement in opinion may have the result that many of the values and assumptions which form this conception of 'successful' adjustment remain unexamined. Clients who have a very different view of the world and goals from those espoused by a particular agency may find helping an uncomfortable and confusing experience, rather than empowering. As was argued earlier, there is a particular need for helpers to be aware of how the responses to difficult situations and to illness of clients from certain ethnic groups may be shaped by sets of cultural values which differ from their own values and everyday assumptions.

Supervision

This chapter has argued for an approach to helping in the area of HIV which attempts to avoid imposing models of adjustment or particular interpretations on a client, and one where the helper is responsive to the client's own expressed needs and goals. To achieve the aim of working from the client's own frame of reference, it was suggested that helpers need to take a very hard and long look at how they are interpreting a client's situation and how they see the sources of the distress that he or she may be experiencing. The need for a helper to be able to make flexible use of a wide repertoire of skills was highlighted. Importance was also attached to the passing on of skills to clients to allow them to gain greater control over their lives and to have more choices.

In the area of HIV, as in any other area of helping, careful supervision and review of a helper's actions is required to ensure that the commitment to follow a certain approach is in fact being carried out in practice. The guidelines that a voluntary or statutory agency adopts for the conduct of supervision could direct attention to matters which have been identified in this chapter as central to effective helping. In particular, such guidelines could emphasize the need to examine the extent to which a helper is working from the client's own frame of reference, and the extent to which a helper is working to share skills and to pass on relevant information. Providing clear criteria for regular assessment by peers, or self-assessment, can help to ensure that the stated commitment of an agency to work in a client-centred manner and to enable people with HIV infection to gain greater control over their lives is maintained in everyday practice.

References

Anderson, C. and Lockley, P. (1990). 'Issues in the training of volunteers'. Paper presented at the Royal College of Nursing International Conference, *AIDS: The Challenge for the Community*, Cardiff, April 1990.

Aoki, B.K. (1989). 'Cross-cultural counseling: The extra dimension'. In J.W. Dilley *et al.* (eds), *Face to Face: A Guide to AIDS Counselling*. San Francisco, AIDS Health Project, pp. 26–33.

Beck, A. (1972). *Depression: Causes and Treatment*. Philadelphia, University of Philadelphia Press.

Green, J. and Sherr, L. (1989). 'Dying, bereavement and loss'. In J. Green and A. McCreaner (eds), *Counselling in HIV Infection and AIDS*. Oxford, Blackwell Scientific Publications, pp. 207–23.

Holmes, J. and Lindley, R. (1989). *The Values of Psychotherapy*. Oxford, Oxford University Press.

Kamerman, J.B. (1988). *DEATH in the Midst of Life: Social and Cultural Influences on Death, Grief and Mourning*. Englewood Cliffs, N.J., Prentice Hall.

Kübler-Ross, E. (1970). *On Death and Dying*. London, Tavistock Publications.

Lakin, M. (1988). *Ethical Issues in the Psychotherapies*. Oxford, Oxford University Press.

Markova, I. and Wilkie, P. (1987). 'Concepts, representations and social change: The phenomenon of AIDS'. *Journal for the Theory of Social Behaviour*, **17**, 389–409.

Miller, R. and Bor, R. (1988). *AIDS: A Guide to Clinical Counselling*. London, Science Press.

Robinson, V. and Halliday, J. (1987). 'A critique of the microcounselling approach to problem understanding'. *British Journal of Guidance and Counselling*, **15**, 113–24.

Rogers, C. (1951). *Client-centered Therapy*. London, Constable.

Medical, psychiatric and epidemiological aspects of HIV

TWO

The Human Immunodeficiency Virus

ALEXANDER McMILLAN

Introduction

This chapter provides a brief historical background to the discovery of the HIV virus, looks at the nature of the HIV virus, its effects on the body, how it is transmitted, and tests to detect antibodies to HIV and virus material. The following chapter goes on to look at what is known about the natural history of HIV infection, HIV-related illnesses, AIDS and the treatment of HIV-related illnesses.

Historical background

In the 5 June 1981 edition of *Morbidity and Mortality Weekly,* the publication of the Centers for Communicable Diseases in the USA, five cases of what was later to be known as Acquired Immune Deficiency Syndrome (AIDS) were described. All the patients in these reported cases had been treated for 'opportunistic infections' – infections which occur very rarely, apart from in people whose immune system has been damaged or weakened in some manner. Doctors in Los Angeles, San Francisco and New York City noted that these infections occurred in young, previously healthy, gay men. Later in 1981, the Centers for Communicable Diseases were notified of the occurrence of these unusual infections; and a search for common factors linking the cases began.

By the autumn of 1981, the occurrence of opportunistic infections among male and female intravenous drug users and hameophiliacs had been observed. In these cases, the common element appeared to be the transmission of infection through blood. By 1982, the condition had also been identified among people from certain African countries.

In 1983, the cause of AIDS was attributed to a virus by a team of French scientists, and this was confirmed by a US team in 1984. The virus was initially given different names by the different research teams; but in May 1986, the international committee on the taxonomy of viruses adopted the name Human Immunodeficiency Virus (HIV). In 1986, a similar, but not identical virus, HIV-2 was identified among people with AIDS of West African origin. So far, there have been comparatively few instances of infection with HIV-2 in Europe and the USA. It is possible that other types of human immuno-deficiency viruses may exist.

In 1984, a test which was capable of detecting antibodies to HIV was developed; and in 1985, when a commercial HIV antibody test became available, the UK Blood Transfusion Service introduced the testing of all blood donations to protect the recipients of blood transfusions. In 1985, the heat treatment of blood products used in the treatment of patients with haemophilia was also introduced in the UK.

In 1985, the first international conference on AIDS was held in the USA. By that time, it was clear that HIV was not restricted to the previously identified 'risk groups', but was a sexually transmitted disease that could affect all sexually active people, as well as being an infection which could be transmitted from mother to baby.

By 1986, the drug zidovudine, AZT, had become available, though its effectiveness was still to be measured. Since 1986, the spread of HIV to most countries of the world has been observed and is discussed in Chapter 5.

As the decade of the 1980s advanced, it became clear to researchers that the effects of HIV infection were variable and not necessarily confined to the life-threatening conditions identified in the official definitions of AIDS. People with HIV infection may remain well and show no troubling symptoms for many years. Later in the course of infection, harmful changes to their immune system may be observed, and they may develop some HIV-related health problems. People with HIV infection may also in time go on to develop opportunistic infections and cancers which can be life-threatening. The variability in the effects of HIV infection has led some clinicians in recent years to prefer to think in terms of a range of HIV-related illnesses and conditions, rather than in terms of sharply defined stages of illness. The categories, i.e. medical definitions, used to describe the effects of HIV infection are discussed at somewhat greater length in Chapter 3.

Over the last decade, the prognosis for people who are diagnosed as having AIDS has also improved considerably. As a result of earlier detection of HIV infection, the availability of antiviral drugs such as zidovudine, and greater expertise in the detection and treatment of opportunistic infections, people with AIDS are living considerably longer than they did in the early stages of the epidemic. They are also likely to be admitted to hospital only for short periods during acute episodes of illness.

Viruses

To understand the way in which the human immunodeficiency virus replicates itself inside human cells and the nature of the tests which diagnose the presence of HIV infection, it is necessary to look first at the structure and nature of viruses in general.

Viruses are the smallest disease-causing agents that have been identified. They can only reproduce themselves by acting in a parasitic way. A virus particle 'invades' a single living cell of some other living organism and uses the material of that cell to create other virus particles, i.e. to multiply. Many different kinds of virus have been identified; and usually an individual virus is able to reproduce only within a very specific type of living organism. In other words, a specific virus will infect only a particular species of animal, plant or bacterium.

Examples of viruses which cause disease in humans include the polio-myelitis virus, hepatitis virus, influenza virus, herpes virus and the common cold viruses. The viruses which cause disease in humans do not multiply simply by invading any type of human cell. Individual viruses multiply only within certain specific types of cells. For example, the hepatitis virus reproduces itself within liver cells, and common cold viruses multiply within some of the cells of the respiratory tract. The human immunodeficiency virus reproduces itself principally within particular cells in the immune system which protects the body against infection.

How cells are replicated

The genetic information of all cellular organisms which allows them to build copies of themselves, i.e. to reproduce themselves exactly, is contained principally in a complex protein called DNA. When a cell comes to reproduce itself, the information stored in its DNA is passed to another protein of similar structure contained in the cell, called RNA. The genetic information which is now present in RNA is then translated into the creation of a new cell. The set of instructions for creating individual proteins which make up the cell and for organizing these individual proteins into an integrated unit are put into effect.

The structure of viruses

Viruses have a much simpler structure than other disease-causing agents. The basic structure of a virus consists of the parts shown in Fig. 2.1. At the centre of the virus is a core of genetic material in the form of either DNA or RNA. This core is surrounded by a protein shell, known as the *capsid*, and some viruses, including HIV, also possess an outer protective envelope, in addition to the capsid.

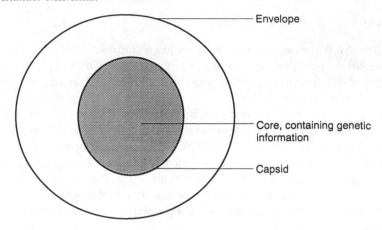

Figure 2.1 The basic structure of a virus

How viruses replicate

To reproduce itself, a virus first enters a cell and then 'takes control' of the cell's own metabolic processes to produce many copies of itself. These new virus particles are released from the cell and each of them can go on to infect another cell in the organism.

As a first stage in replication, the virus is absorbed to the surface of the particular type of cell which it infects. There is an interaction between certain molecules on the outer surface of the virus and molecules on the surface of the target cell which act as *receptor sites*. In the case of HIV, the first step of viral entry into a cell occurs when a protein on the viral envelope, known as gp120, binds to a molecule on the surface of the cell known as CD4. CD4 receptor sites are present in considerable quantity in certain cells of the immune system called T–helper lymphocytes, which are the principal target of the human immunodeficiency virus. (The function that T–helper cells play in the body's system of defence against infection is described in the section on 'The body's defences against infection'). There are some CD4 receptor sites on the surface of other cells of the body, such as monocytes and macrophages, and in micoglial cells within the brain. It is possible, therefore, for the human immunodeficiency virus to gain entry into cells of these types.

After a virus particle has gained entry into a host cell, the genetic material stored in the core of the virus becomes integrated into the DNA of the cell. In other words, the genetic information that contains instructions for the creation of new virus particles forms one segment of the cell's own genetic information. This means that the virus 'has access to' the cell's own machinery for reproduction; and that it will persist during the lifetime of the cell. If the cell itself reproduces, the virus will be present in its new copies.

A virus which has become integrated into a cell's own genetic material may remain *latent* in the cell; that is, it does not actively reproduce itself, but it remains viable. It is also possible that some new virus particles may be created, but the cell itself is not destroyed. Infection of a cell by a virus can, however, result in the creation of many new virus particles and the destruction of the cell.

Retroviruses

The process by which HIV replicates itself is somewhat more complicated than that of most other viruses. It was mentioned earlier that the genetic material present in the core of a virus consists of either DNA or RNA. In most viruses, genetic information is coded in the form of DNA. However, the genetic information of a group of viruses, called *retroviruses*, is coded in the form of RNA.

The first retroviruses to be identified by scientists were a number which cause disease in animals, including disorders of the immune system, such as the feline leukaemia virus. In humans, two retroviruses had been identified which cause certain types of leukaemia, prior to the discovery that HIV belonged to the class of retroviruses.

The genetic information contained in the RNA of a retrovirus, such as HIV, needs to be changed into the form of DNA before it can be incorporated into the genetic blueprint of the host cell. This translation of the genetic information in the retroviral RNA into DNA is brought about by the action of an enzyme contained within the HIV virus, known as reverse transcriptase. Once the retroviral RNA has been converted to DNA, it can be integrated into the cell's own genetic information and the cell's own process can then be used to create new virus particles. The most effective current therapy against HIV, zidovudine, (Retrovir™, AZT), acts by inhibiting the action of the reverse transcriptase enzyme.

The principal features of the structure of HIV are now quite clearly understood and are represented in Fig. 2.2. The viral RNA and reverse transcriptase are covered by two coats of core protein, called p18 and p24. These protein coats, in particular p24, are of importance in laboratory testing for the presence of the virus, a subject which is discussed later in this chapter. The lipid membrane that makes up the outer envelope of the virus and the gp120 protein together with another protein gp41, to which it is anchored, are also indicated in Fig. 2.2. Important parts of the genetic information contained in the viral RNA have also been identified and much is now known about the action of individual HIV genes.

This increase in detailed knowledge of the structure of the HIV virus and of the manner in which it replicates has allowed researchers to search for antiviral therapies which act by blocking the replication of the virus at one or other of the crucial steps in its cycle of replication.

Although there is a basic similarity of structure in the virus particles found in all HIV–infected individuals, it is also clear that there is some genetic variability in the coding of certain parts of the virus, i.e. somewhat different strains of the virus can be, and are, found. This genetic variability in the virus is one of the many factors which makes the production of a vaccine against HIV such a difficult and challenging task.

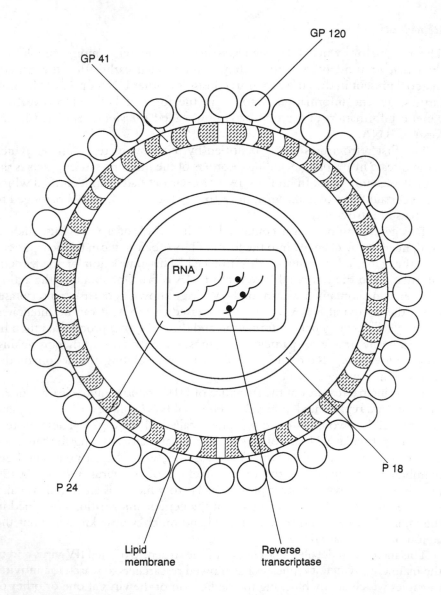

Figure 2.2 The basic structure of the HIV virus

The body's defences against infection

The immune system of the body which provides protection from disease is a very complex system. It identifies and deals with the very large number of potentially harmful microorganisms which exist within our environment. The microorganisms, or pathogens, which may infect the body fall into four main classes: viruses, bacteria, protozoa and fungi.

The nature of viruses was discussed in the previous section of this chapter. Bacteria are single-celled organisms, and very many different types of bacteria exist. Most sore throats and chest infections are caused by bacteria, and conditions such as tuberculosis, salmonella infection and gonorrhoea are caused by specific bacterial agents. Protozoa are single-celled parasites which can cause diseases such as amoebic dysentery. Fungi are very simple plants. Common fungal infections found in people with HIV infection are oral thrush (candidiasis) and athlete's foot (tinea pedis).

Aside from physical barriers to infection such as the skin and the mucous membranes, the body possesses a wide array of chemical agents and specific types of cells which can detect and destroy the microorganisms discussed in the preceding paragraph. Within this system of protection against infection, a broad distinction is often made between *non-specific defences* against disease and *specific body defences*.

Non-specific defences

Looking first at a few of the most important elements of the body's non-specific defences. There are a large number of cells within the body which are known as *phagocytes*. Individual types of phagocytes, such as macrophages and neutrophils, can act against a wide range of bacteria, viruses and other harmful agents. They act by detecting a foreign particle, binding to it and engulfing it. As was stated earlier, HIV can gain entry to macrophages. Another important component of the body's non-specific cellular defences are the *natural killer cells*, which are capable of directly attacking and killing virus-infected, or cancerous, body cells.

The classes of antimicrobial substances known as *interferons* and *complement* form a significant part of the body's general chemical defences against disease. Interferons are a class of small proteins which are released by virus-infected cells. These interferons assist in protecting uninfected cells from viral entry and in mobilizing the immune system. Genetic engineering techniques now make it possible to produce interferons in sufficient quantities to use in treatment, including treatment for HIV-infected individuals. A number of trials are in progress to establish how effective interferon itself, or in combination with other drugs, may be in stimulating the immune system and reducing the problems experienced by individuals with symptomatic HIV infection. The term *complement* refers to a group of different plasma proteins which act to kill bacteria and certain other types of cells, enable macrophages and neutrophils to adhere to and engulf microorganisms more rapidly, and intensify the body's inflammatory response to infection.

Specific defences

There are a considerable number of types of cells within the immune system which are concerned with producing a defence which is precisely targeted against *specific* microorganisms. The immune system is able to recognize specific antigens (molecules foreign to the body) and then to destroy or neutralize them. Initial exposure to a particular antigen, to an infectious agent, customarily leads to a series of changes in the immune system which allows the body to react more quickly and vigorously on subsequent encounters with this antigen.

Antibody production and antibodies

B-cells within the immune system are involved in the production of *antibodies* when an infectious agent is encountered. Antibodies are made up of different types of *immunoglobulin* (Ig). They are able to 'recognize' foreign proteins or sugars on the surface of a particular antigen, and to bind specifically with that antigen. At the same time, 'memory cells' are produced which are capable of being activated on subsequent encounters with a specific infectious agent, and of generating responses to this infectious agent. Antibodies circulate within the blood and the lymph where they can bind to bacteria, to toxins created by bacteria and to free viruses.

Antibodies act against infectious agents in a number of different ways, e.g. by marking them for destruction by phagocytes or complement or activated T-cells, by neutralizing toxic chemicals secreted by bacteria, by binding to specific sites on viruses that prevent the viruses in turn from binding to receptor sites on tissue cells.

T-cells

Antibodies, then, play an important part in the destruction of microorganisms that are circulating freely in body fluids. However, they cannot penetrate living cells and thus have a much more limited role to play in preventing the replication of a virus, or other infectious agent, *within* the body's own cells.

In contrast, T-cells can, under specific circumstances, recognize antigens which are attached to, or displayed on, surfaces of the body's own cells. One of the main groups of T-cells, known as *cytotoxic T-cells* or *killer T-cells*, can be activated to recognize cells which are displaying particular antigens, and to destroy these cells.

These cytotoxic T-cells, which are capable of destroying cells which have been infected by viruses, or certain other infectious agents, form one of the four main types of T-cells:

- cytotoxic T-cells (killer T-cells);
- delayed hypersensitivity T-cells (memory cells);
- helper T-cells; and
- suppressor T-cells.

When delayed hypersensitivity T-cells (memory cells) meet the same antigen again, they release chemicals which enhance the body's defence against the antigen.

T-cells play a very important part in regulating the overall activity of the immune system. The regulatory functions carried out by T-cells are very complex, and some aspects of their regulatory role are not yet altogether clearly understood. The helper T-cells play an essential role in activating and co-ordinating immune response. Once they themselves are activated, they stimulate the production of other T-cells, including cytotoxic cells, and of B-cells which are beginning the process of producing antibodies.

Suppressor T-cells, as their name suggests, slow or stop the activity of B- and T-cells once an infection has been dealt with. In other words, they play an important part in bringing an end to immune responses that are no longer needed.

The effects of HIV on the immune system

A description has already been given of how, although HIV can infect quite a number of different cells in the body, a chief target of the virus is helper T-cells. The virus can bind to CD4 receptor sites which are present on helper T-cells.

The principal way in which HIV causes the functioning of the immune system to be compromised is by the damage which it causes to helper T-cells. Later in the course of HIV infection, the absolute number of helper T-cells declines markedly, and the normal ratio of helper to suppressor cells is disturbed. Infection with HIV can interfere with the ability of helper T-cells to recognize antigen and to activate other components of the immune system. Given the central role that helper T-cells play in stimulating and co-ordinating the body's defences against infection, this interference with their functioning can lead to considerable problems in the functioning of the whole immune system. It appears that HIV can also have considerable, albeit less severely, damaging effects on other cells which form part of the body's defences against infection, such as macrophages. Cumulative damage as a result of HIV infection can reduce the body's ability to defend itself against infection.

This decline in the ability of the immune system to defend the body against infection – what is sometimes described as immunocompromise – means that people with advanced HIV infection may be subject to a range of 'opportunistic' infections: rare infections which rarely trouble people with a normally functioning immune system. A description of the opportunistic infections which are most commonly met with in individuals with a high level of immunosuppression as a result of HIV infection is presented in the following chapter.

Use of the terms CD4 and CD8 cells

The presence of CD4 receptor sites on helper T-cells, also serves as a chemical 'marker' which serves to distinguish them from other types of T-cells. For this reason, helper T-cells are often referred to in the context of HIV infection as CD4 cells or T4 cells. Similarly, cytotoxic/suppressor cells which can be detected by the presence of a CD8 marker on their surface, are often referred to as CD8 or T8 cells.

Tests to detect the presence of HIV infection

HIV antibody tests

In adults, the detection of the presence of HIV infection is normally achieved by taking a sample of blood and detecting *antibodies* to HIV in the serum. The two most commonly used methods for testing for the presence of antibodies to HIV are the ELISA (enzyme-linked immunoabsorbent assay) and the Western Blot. A number of other systems for detecting the presence of antibodies in serum, such as radioimmunoprecipitation (RIP), are available, but are used principally for research purposes. There is also a test which can detect the presence of antibodies to HIV in saliva.

A range of psychological and social issues surrounding HIV antibody testing are discussed in Chapter 7, and guidelines for the provision of appropriate pretest counselling are presented.

If a laboratory detects the presence of antibodies to HIV in a sample of serum, this finding is confirmed by using another testing system on another sample of serum. When antibodies are found in an individual's serum, that person is described as being HIV antibody positive (sometimes written as +HIV) or as having seroconverted. An HIV antibody positive test result reveals that an individual has been exposed to HIV infection at some time in the past, and potentially may infect others with HIV. In itself, however, the HIV antibody test cannot predict whether, or at what rate, an individual may develop HIV-related illnesses.

The systems of HIV antibody testing described above have a very high degree of accuracy in discerning if antibodies are present in the serum; and confirmatory tests are made when a positive result is found. 'False positive' tests may occasionally occur, but they are unlikely.

There is one important limitation on the ability of HIV antibody tests to detect the presence of HIV infection. A negative HIV antibody test means that antibodies to the virus have not been detected. This may mean that the individual is not infected with HIV. There is also the possibility, however, that the individual may have been infected in the recent past, but has not yet developed antibodies to HIV.

It takes between 3 and 6 months for antibodies to be produced after infection with HIV. This period between infection and the production of antibodies is often referred to as the 'window period'. For this reason, individuals who believe that they may have been exposed to a risk of infection in the recent past are advised of the need to take a repeat test. There are individuals with HIV infection, particularly infants who have been infected in the womb, who do not develop antibodies to HIV but are shown to be infected by the use of molecular biological methods.

HIV antigen tests

HIV antigen tests establish infection with HIV by directly detecting 'antigen', parts of the viral material itself. There are a number of different systems which can be used to establish the presence of HIV antigen in the serum. The tests which at the moment are used in clinical settings are those which can identify the p24 protein found in the core of the virus.

Testing for the presence of the p24 protein can play some part in the detection of HIV infection in the period shortly after infection occurs. Soon after infection with HIV, but prior to the development of antibodies to HIV, circulating viral material, including HIV p24, can be detected in the serum.

In most individuals, however, HIV p24 antigen declines to undetectable quantities as the body begins to produce specific antibodies to HIV. HIV p24 antigen may remain undetectable for a long period after seroconversion (i.e. the production of antibodies to HIV), while the individual remains free of symptoms. Later in the course of HIV infection, the level of antibodies to HIV in the serum falls, and generally p24 antigen reappears in the serum. This reappearance of p24 antigen in the serum is often associated with evidence of a decline in the functioning of the immune system and the appearance of HIV-related symptoms.

The PCR (polymerase chain reaction a 'gene amplification' technique) to detect the presence of HIV RNA and DNA is used principally for research purposes rather than as a clinical diagnostic test.

Tests which can monitor the effects of HIV infection

A close monitoring of the functioning of the immune system in individuals with HIV infection is an important part of their health care. Such monitoring assists the early detection of HIV-related problems, and can serve as a guide as to when it is appropriate to begin treatment with antiviral drugs, such as zidovudine, and prophylactic treatment against specific opportunistic infections. This monitoring of the degree of immunosuppression also indicates the effects of any antiviral treatment which is being administered.

A number of laboratory tests are available which can serve as 'markers' of the degree of immunosuppression in an HIV-infected individual. The diagnostic and predictive power of individual 'marker' tests is limited. However, when the results from several of these different tests are looked at together, a reasonably clear picture can be gained of the current state of immunosuppression, and predictions made which can guide treatment decisions.

An important test for monitoring the functioning of the immune system is the CD4 (T4) lymphocyte count. The normal range of the CD4 count is 500 –1500 per mm³. Individuals who have a CD4 count of under 200 may possibly face a more rapid development of symptoms.

One of the group of tests commonly used to monitor the functioning of the immune system is the *p24 antigen test*. As was indicated in the last section of this chapter, reappearance of p24 in the serum of HIV-infected individuals is often indicative of a decline in the functioning of the immune system and associated with a more rapid progression towards the development of symptoms.

Another test which is useful in monitoring the functioning of the immune system is one which measures the level of beta-2 microglobulin, a protein associated with some cells in the immune system. The level of this protein is greater than normal in immunocompromised people.

Care needs to be taken over how the results of regular monitoring with laboratory tests are communicated to patients. It is important that individuals with HIV infection understand the purposes that these 'marker' tests serve in monitoring health and guiding treatment decisions. The limitations on the predictive power of these tests also need to be made clear. It is also vital that the results from individual sets of tests are communicated to the person with HIV infection in a careful and sensitive manner. A lack of care and sensitivity in communicating a set of results which indicate the possibility of some decline in immune function may lead the HIV-infected person to interpret them in an unnecessarily fatalistic fashion.

Transmission of HIV

It is important to distinguish between how HIV can be transmitted from one person to another and where, i.e. in which body fluids and tissues HIV has been isolated in laboratory situations. A lack of clarity and understanding about these two situations has caused much confusion. In the laboratory, HIV has been isolated from body fluids and organs including blood, semen, vaginal and cervical secretions, cerebrospinal fluid, breast milk and tears. HIV has also been found in most organs and tissues of the body, including the skin.

For transmission of HIV from one person to another to take place, a *sufficient* amount of viral material must pass from the infected person to another by certain *specific* routes. A large number of studies have established that there is no evidence of the spread of the virus through social contact, through actions such as touch, hugging, kissing, sneezing or drinking from the same cup (Fischl *et al.*, 1987; Friedland *et al.*, 1990; Gershon *et al.*, 1990). Similarly, transmission does not seem to result from the bites of insects such as mosquitoes or bed bugs. HIV can only be transmitted by the routes which are identified in the following sections.

Transmission of HIV through blood, blood products and organ transplants

Studies have shown unequivocally that HIV can be transmitted by an injection of blood from an HIV-infected individual to another person. This has happened through blood transfusion, through the use of blood products such as the clotting factors Factor VIII and Factor IX used by haemophiliacs, and through the sharing of injecting equipment in intravenous drug use. Issues related to assisting intravenous drug users to move to safer injecting practices are discussed in Chapter 12. There have also been a very limited number of cases of medical and nursing staff becoming infected with HIV through needle stick injuries. Guidelines and instructions for staff have been introduced to prevent such injuries.

There have been a number of cases where HIV was transmitted by organ transplants. The donors of organs are now tested for HIV antibodies, so it is very unlikely that HIV will be transmitted by this route in the future.

The knowledge that HIV can be transmitted via blood and blood products has led to fears about the safety of receiving a blood transfusion or blood products. Blood products used in the UK, such as the clotting factors VIII and IX, are now heat-treated to ensure their safety. A more detailed discussion of the issues faced by haemophiliacs as a result of the transmission of HIV through blood products is provided in Chapter 13.

In the UK, the screening of all blood donations for antibodies to HIV was introduced in 1985. This screening has been very effective in ensuring the safety of blood transfusions. Because of the 'window period' (discussed earlier in this chapter), the Blood Transfusion Service has introduced a system where prospective blood donors are recommended not to donate blood if they think that they are, or have been, at risk of contracting HIV. As a result of the use of these screening methods, the possibility of contracting HIV from a blood transfusion in the UK is now *extremely* unlikely. However, there are some countries in the world where the screening of blood transfusions for HIV is still not routine and where, as a result, there may continue to be transmission of HIV via transfused blood.

Transmission of HIV from mother to child

With the recognition of AIDS in children, it became clear that HIV can be transmitted from mother to child. There are a number of ways in which the infection may be transmitted from mother to child. Before birth, HIV may pass across the placenta to the developing foetus. The virus has been found in organs taken from foetuses as early as 13 weeks of gestation, and therefore it is clear that infection can take place early in pregnancy. HIV may also be transmitted during birth from infected vaginal secretions as the baby passes down the birth canal, or from the mother's infected blood.

The risk of an infected mother having an infected child is difficult to estimate. Early studies of women who had already had a child with AIDS estimated that about 50% of these women would go on to infect further infants in subsequent pregnancies. It is now understood that these women had advanced disease and that the same risk does not necessarily apply to all HIV-infected women. In particular, HIV-infected women who have no HIV-related symptoms at the time of conception may not have the same risk of infecting their baby as those with more advanced disease (Mok, 1988). The European Collaborative Study, which is following up a large number of children born to HIV-infected mothers in eight European centres, have estimated the risk of transmission from mother to child to be about 24% (The European Collaborative Study, 1988).

The detection of antibodies to HIV in an adult or in an older child is a specific indicator of HIV infection. However, the presence of HIV maternal antibodies in the newborn child limits the usefulness of the HIV antibody test in this group. Evidence shows that all infants born to mothers who are HIV antibody positive will themselves be HIV antibody positive at birth, because they have inherited maternal antibodies. However, this does not necessarily mean that they are infected with HIV. Some studies have shown that most of these infants loose maternal antibodies from 9 to 12 months of age, while other studies have reported the persistence of maternal antibodies up to 15 months of age.

It was mentioned earlier that HIV has been isolated from breast milk. A case has been reported where the mother received an HIV-infected blood transfusion after delivery of a child, who subsequently became HIV-infected and is presumed to have been infected via breast milk (Ziegler *et al.*, 1985). Two other cases where there is evidence that transmission may have taken place via breast milk have also been reported (LePage *et al.*, 1987). Given that there may be a risk of transmitting HIV in breast milk, HIV antibody positive mothers are advised not to breastfeed their infants. There has been controversy over the degree of risk which breast milk may pose for the transmission of HIV from mother to child (Baumslag, 1987; Senturia *et al.*, 1987); and it is certainly a much lower risk than intrauterine or perinatal transmission.

Sexual transmission of HIV

HIV can be transmitted via semen, and vaginal and cervical secretions in penetrative intercourse without a condom. Virus in semen and vaginal secretions can enter the bloodstream through the sensitive linings of the vagina, the rectum or the urethra. Virus in these body fluids can also get into the bloodstream through an open wound.

The virus can be transmitted from a man to a woman, from a man to a man, and from a woman to a man. Transmission from a woman to a woman has been reported (Greenhouse, 1987; Monzon and Capellan, 1987), but so far this appears to have occurred rarely.

The risk of infection from a single sexual contact is highly variable. Transmission of HIV can take place as the result of a single sexual contact; but there have also been documented cases where many episodes of sexual contact with an infected partner have not led to transmission of the virus. At present, the factors which may affect both the infectivity of someone with HIV infection and the susceptibility to infection of the sexual contacts of such a person are not very clearly understood. However, there is evidence which suggests that the presence of another sexually transmitted disease at the time of exposure to HIV may facilitate the transmission of infection. This is particularly so when that disease is associated with ulceration, such as syphilis, chancroid and genital herpes (Kreiss *et al.*, 1988).

The stage that an infected person is at in their illness may also affect their ability to transmit infection to their sexual partner. Studies among haemophiliacs who are HIV antibody positive and their female partners have shown that the risk of the female becoming infected increases as the infected male partner becomes sick and as the CD4 (T4) cell count in the peripheral blood of the male partner decreases (Goedert *et al.*, 1987).

The findings of some studies suggest that the transmission of HIV infection from women to men may be somewhat less efficient than from men to women. However, there is a need to deal with certain methodological problems, and to have more evidence from new studies before any definite statement can be made about the relative efficiency of transmission from female to male compared with transmission from male to female (Johnson and Laga, 1988; Johnson *et al.*, 1989).

A number of studies suggest that for both men and women, receptive anal intercourse where a condom is not used is the form of sexual contact which carries the greatest risk of transmitting the virus. However, the fact that a somewhat greater risk is attached to the practice of unprotected anal intercourse does not mean that the risk posed by unprotected vaginal intercourse should be downgraded. Johnson *et al.* (1989), in reporting the results of a study on the transmission of HIV to heterosexual partners and their review of the literature on this subject, conclude that:

it is important to maintain the essential Public Health message for heterosexual couples that unprotected vaginal intercourse with a sero-positive person is a high risk activity for transmission of HIV, and that one episode of vaginal intercourse is sufficient for transmission to occur.

References

Baumslag, N. (1987). 'Breast-feeding and HIV infection'. *Lancet*, **ii**, 401.

The European Collaborative Study (1988). 'Mother to child transmission of HIV infection'. *Lancet*, **ii**, 1039–43.

Fischl, M.A. *et al.* (1987). 'Evaluation of heterosexual partners, children, and household contacts of adults with AIDS'. *Journal of the American Medical Association*, **257**, 640–44.

Friedland, G. *et al.* (1990). 'Additional evidence for lack of transmission of HIV infection by close interpersonal (casual) contact'. *AIDS*, **4**, 639–44.

Gershon, R.R.M. *et al.* (1990). 'The risk of transmission of HIV-1 through non-percutaneous, non-sexual modes – a review'. *AIDS*, **4**, 645–50.

Goedert, J.J. *et al* (1987). 'Heterosexual transmission of human immunodeficiency virus: Association with severe depletion of T-helper lymphocytes in men with hemophilia'. *AIDS Res Human Retroviruses*, **3**, 355–60.

Greenhouse, P. (1987). 'Female to female transmission of HIV', *Lancet*, **ii**, 401–2.

Johnson, A.M. and Laga, M. (1988). 'Heterosexual transmission of HIV'. *AIDS*, **2**, Suppl. 1, 549–56.

Johnson, A.M. *et al.* (1989). 'Transmission of HIV to heterosexual partners of infected men and women'. *AIDS*, **3**, 367–72.

Kreiss, J. *et al.* (1988). 'Role of sexually transmitted diseases in transmitting human immunodeficiency virus'. *Genitourinary Medicine*, **64**, 1–2.

LePage, P. *et al.* (1987). 'Postnatal transmission of HIV from mother to child'. *Lancet*, **ii**, 400.

Mok, J. (1988). 'Children born to women with HIV infection'. *The AIDS Letter*, Royal Society of Medicine, No. 7, June/July 1988.

Monzon, O.T. and Capellan, J.M.B. (1987). 'Female-to-female transmission of HIV'. *Lancet*, **ii**, 40–41.

Senturia, Y.D. *et al.* (1987). 'Breast-feeding and HIV infection'. *Lancet*, **ii**, 400–1.

Ziegler, J.B. *et al.* (1985). 'Postnatal transmission of AIDS-associated retrovirus from mother to infant'. *Lancet*, **i**, 896–8.

THREE

HIV-related illnesses and AIDS

ALEXANDER McMILLAN

Illness immediately after infection with HIV

Many people who are HIV-infected have no symptoms and show no signs of their infection until some unknown period after coming into contact with HIV. The only way these people can be identified is by serological testing for HIV (see Chapter 2). However, a small proportion of individuals develop glandular fever-like illnesses within a few weeks of becoming infected with HIV and before antibodies become detectable in the serum. These individuals may develop a temperature, complain of headache, tiredness, aching pains in the joints and muscles (arthralgia and myalgia), sore throat, diarrhoea, skin rashes and swollen lymph glands in different parts of the body. A type of inflammation of the brain (meningoencephalitis) may also be a feature at this early stage of infection. The majority of these symptoms usually disappear after 2–3 weeks, although enlargement of the lymph glands tends to persist.

These glandular symptoms are very similar to, and may be confused with, glandular fever (infective mononucleosis), which is caused by the Epstein Barr virus. This similarity of glandular symptoms can at times delay the prompt diagnosis of HIV.

After any early infection with HIV, the person usually makes a complete recovery and feels well. It may be some considerable time, several or many years, before the person develops HIV-related infections. This period of time is very variable and it is impossible to say in individual cases how long it will be between becoming HIV antibody positive and developing some HIV-related symptoms. Earlier, less serious symptoms include lymphadenopathy (which is described later in the chapter), various skin disorders and some fungal infections, affecting in particular the mouth.

The natural history of HIV infection

The natural history of HIV infection has neither been clearly nor definitively described. There are individual variations in the length of time that a person takes to develop HIV-related infections and which infections they develop and the severity of illnesses. It is, therefore, impossible to predict what will be the course of illness in an individual patient. People with HIV may have long illness-free periods. During these periods, they may suffer from minor infections associated with HIV – infections which are discussed later in the chapter.

The importance that co-factors may play in the progression of the illness is still very uncertain. Some workers, however, have identified a clear effect of age on progression of the illness. For example, Moss *et al.* (1988), studying a cohort of men in San Francisco, have suggested that infection is more likely to progress in men over the age of 35 than in those of a younger age group. Blaxhult *et al.* (1990), studying a group of people infected with HIV through blood transfusion, also found a relationship between belonging to an older age group at the time of transfusion and a more rapid progression to AIDS. Infection with mycoplasmas, a somewhat atypical bacteria, may also be an important co-factor in disease progression (*Lancet*, 1991).

Progression from HIV to AIDS

Work in San Francisco suggests that approximately 50% of patients have developed AIDS within 10 years of contracting HIV (Moss and Bacchetti, 1989), and this evidence is supported by other studies. When a person with HIV infection develops particular secondary infections such as *Pneumocystis carinii* pneumonia, certain cancers, including Kaposi's sarcoma and non-Hodgkin's lymphoma, or neurological conditions including dementia, myelopathy and peripheral neuropathy, the person is said to have AIDS. At the beginning of the AIDS epidemic, there was a tendency to describe the progression from initial infection with HIV to AIDS in clearly defined stages.

Two major systems for classifying the effects of HIV infection have been devised, the Walter Reed system of classification, and the much more commonly used CDC (Centers for Disease Control, USA) classification of HIV disease. The CDC classification distinguishes the following stages:

Group 1: Acute infection. This stage identifies the problems which are observed in some individuals a few days to a few weeks after infection with HIV, and are described in the first section in this chapter.

Group 2: Asymptomatic infection. This identifies those individuals who have HIV infection and no symptoms.

Group 3: Persistent generalized lymphadenopathy. Some individuals with HIV infection develop what is known as persistent generalized lymphadenopathy (PGL), which means that they have a continuing enlargement (i.e. swelling) of the lymph nodes at several sites in the body. At one time it was believed that the existence of PGL in itself indicated the existence of a greater amount of immune damage than would be present in Group 2, and the possibility of a more rapid progression to AIDS. However, this is no longer believed to be true, and the presence of PGL in itself is not seen as an indicator of a more rapid progress in immune dysfunction.

Group 4: Other disease. This general category identifies individuals who have symptoms related to HIV infection. The group is broken up into a number of subgroups, and the following categories of problems are recognized:

- constitutional disease;
- neurological disease;
- secondary infectious diseases;
- secondary cancers; and
- other conditions resulting from HIV infection.

Each of the subgroups identified above might include individuals who have more minor symptoms, as well as individuals who are very ill.

The category *constitutional disease*, defined by the presence of at least one of the following – weight loss greater than 10%, fever longer than 1 month, diarrhoea longer than one month – used to be known as ARC.

Many of the specific diseases and conditions identified in the categories *secondary infectious diseases* and *secondary cancers* are discussed later in this chapter, and a description of some of the illnesses in the category *neurological disease* is provided in Chapter 4.

Certain of the infections and cancers identified within the different subgroups of Group 4 are regarded as 'indicators' of a case of AIDS and are listed in the CDC definition of AIDS. For example, as was indicated earlier in the chapter, a person with HIV infection who develops a secondary infection such as *Pneumocystis carinii* pneumonia, or a cancer, such as Kaposi's sarcoma, is defined as having AIDS. The CDC paediatric definition of AIDS, the specific diseases which are regarded as 'indicators' of AIDS in infants and children, is somewhat different from the definition used for adults.

It has already been stated that there is great variation in both how the illness progresses and the speed at which it progresses, and as a result many clinicians prefer now to talk about a range of HIV–related illnesses rather than a series of distinct stages. Certain symptoms in people who have been infected with HIV for a number of years usually indicate a deterioration in the immune function and a lowering of the CD4 (T4) cell count. These symptoms include the development of fatigue, fever lasting for more than 3 months, night sweats, significant weight loss (usually described as more than 10% of total body weight), persistent diarrhoea and the mouth infections oral candidiasis and oral hairy leukoplakia. The person may have very severe episodes of illness followed by periods of well-being.

Later in the course of HIV illness, secondary infections occur. The most common sites for these secondary infections in HIV-infected persons with AIDS (or late HIV illness) are the lungs, throat, oesophagus, the bowel and colon, the bloodstream, the nervous system and the eye.

These infections may be caused by viruses, fungi, protozoa or bacteria. Some of the more common agents and the nature of the infection they cause are described in the following sections under the headings: respiratory infections; illnesses of the mouth, throat and oesophagus; gastrointestinal illnesses, cancers (neoplasms); HIV infection and the eye; skin conditions.

It should be noted that the conditions and infections described are those that are found in people with HIV disease who live predominantly in the UK, Europe and the USA. Similar symptoms may be apparent in people with HIV disease in Africa; but there are also differences between Africa, Europe and the USA in the types of infections found in those with HIV disease and in the prevalence of these infections.

Respiratory infections

The most common respiratory infections in people with HIV and AIDS are pneumonia and tuberculosis. *Pneumocystis carinii* pneumonia (PCP) is the most common cause of pneumonia. The signs of the illness are fever, difficulty in breathing (dyspnoea), a productive cough, and chest pain or tightness in the chest.

PCP

Diagnosis
The diagnosis of PCP is usually confirmed by detecting the organism in sputum induced by inhalation of strong saline.

Treatment
Treatment of PCP is usually with a high dose of *co-trimoxazole* given intravenously, or in less severe cases by mouth. Sometimes there are side-effects of fever, rash, nausea and vomiting. An alternative treatment is *pentamidine*, also given intravenously. Pentamidine can have quite severe side-effects, including low blood pressure (hypotension) and low sugar content in the blood (hypoglycaemia).

Once people have recovered from PCP, it is now recommended that they commence prophylactic co-trimoxazole or pentamidine, both of which can be administered by a nebulizer. Use of a nebulizer allows an individual to breathe in a spray of the drug directly to the lungs. Smaller doses of pentamidine are given in this method of administering the drug and, consequently, there are far fewer and less troublesome side-effects from the drug. The course of treatment is also given prophylactically to people who have not had PCP, but whose immune system has been seriously weakened.

A pneumonia very similar to PCP, but caused by cytomegalovirus (CMV), is also common in AIDS. Frequently, there is dual infection of the lungs with *Pneumocystis carinii* and cytomegalovirus. Treatment for CMV pneumonitis is with *focarnet* or *ganciclovir*.

Tuberculosis

People with AIDS may be infected with *Mycobacterium tuberculosis*. The symptoms of this infection are fever, a cough which may or may not produce blood-stained spit, and difficulty in breathing on exertion.

Diagnosis
Diagnosis is made by finding the organism in smears of clinical material and by culture.

Treatment
Treatment is by the drugs which are normally used in the treatment of tuberculosis, i.e. a combination of three or more antibiotics. The most commonly used drugs are *isoniazid, rifampicin, pyrazinamide, ethambutol* and *streptomycin*. Isoniazid may cause peripheral neuropathy, damage to the peripheral nerves of the hands and feet with resulting pain. To protect against this problem, the drug *pyridoxine* is prescribed along with isoniazid. A very long course of treatment is necessary for people with HIV infection who have tuberculosis.

Pneumonias caused by other bacteria such as *Streptococcus pneumoniae* or *Haemophilus influenzae* are not uncommon. Diagnosis is by culturing the organism from the sputum, and treatment is with an appropriate antibiotic.

Illnesses of the mouth, throat and oesophagus

Illnesses of the mouth, throat and oesophagus are common in people with HIV and AIDS. Dentists are in a unique position to recognize early lesions of the mouth during routine dental examinations.

Candidiasis

Candidiasis, or oral thrush, is a fungal disease most frequently caused by the species *Candida albicans*. It is characterized by the presence of creamy white plaques on the mucosa of the mouth. The mucosa may look red where the plaque is visible. The white plaques may be removed by scraping, which leaves a bleeding surface.

A number of factors can predispose people to develop candidiasis. These include antibiotic therapy, steroid and other immunosuppressive drugs, and primary and acquired immunodeficiency. A variety of symptoms are associated with candidiasis, including complaints of a burning sensation in the mouth, changes in taste and problems in eating spicy food. A severe attack of candidiasis can cause considerable difficulty in eating and drinking and can result in weight loss. It is therefore important that an accurate diagnosis is made quickly so that treatment can begin.

Diagnosis
Candidiasis is a common organism in the mouth and is diagnosed by its clinical appearance and by the detection of organisms on smears and cultures.

Treatment
The response to treatment is often very good with both symptoms and lesions disappearing within 2–5 days. However, relapses are often common because of the underlying immunodeficiency. Oral candidiasis may be treated either topically or systemically. Treatment is usually with *nystatin* pastilles or *amphotericin* lozenges. The effectiveness of such topical treatment depends on the patient taking all of the course of lozenges in the way prescribed by his or her doctor. *Ketoconazole* or *fluconazole* are given by mouth if the infection has spread to the oesophagus.

   It is important that good dental hygiene is maintained. If treatments containing sweetening agents are used for long periods, daily fluoride rinses should be considered as concurrent treatment. Cleaning the teeth with soft brushes which should be changed frequently and the regular use of dental floss will help to keep a clean and comfortable mouth. Antiseptic mouthwashes, e.g. *corsodyl* (Chlorhexidene), are also recommended.

Angular Cheilitis

This cracking at the angle of the lips is often due to candida, and can be treated with *canesten* (1% Clotrimazole cream).

Oral Hairy Leukoplakia

This condition appears to be uniquely associated with HIV infection. It is an infection of the mucous membranes of the mouth, identified by fuzzy white patches or plaques on the tongue. These patches cannot be rubbed off. Treatment of symptomatic disease is with *acyclovir* in high dosage.

Gingivitis (inflammation of the gums)

Inflammation of the gums and dental abscesses are common in HIV, and are an indication of the decline in the effectiveness of the immune system.

Treatment

The treatment of gingivitis is with oral *metronidazole* and/or oral *penicillin*. The use of antibiotics may disrupt the normal flora of the mouth causing candidiasis. For this reason, treatment with antibiotics should be accompanied by prophylactic antifungal therapy. Antiseptic mouthwashes may prevent the occurrence or the recurrence of these conditions.

The treatment of dental abscesses is immediate referral to the dentist for assessment and antibiotics if considered appropriate.

Ulcers of the mouth and oesophagus

Ulcers of the mouth can be caused by herpes simplex and cytomegalovirus (CMV). The ulcers can be on the lips, in the mouth and in the oesophagus. It is most common to find these ulcers on the lips. People with oesophogeal ulcers complain of pain behind the breast bone and behind the sternum as well as experiencing difficulty in swallowing. The pain is often of a burning nature.

Diagnosis

The diagnosis of oesophogeal ulcers can be made by oesophagoscopy (passing a tube into the oesophagus and removing some tissue for culture).

Treatment

The treatment of oesophogeal herpes is by intravenous *acyclovir*. Long-term acyclovir is sometimes necessary to control herpes and to prevent recurrence. Treatment of oral herpes is with oral *acyclovir*.

Gastrointestinal illnesses

Gastrointestinal problems, in particular diarrhoea, abdominal discomfort and nausea, are very common in people with advanced HIV-related infections and AIDS. Diarrhoea is often accompanied by weight loss and malabsorption of nutrients.

Diagnosis

It is often possible to identify the organism causing the diarrhoea. Investigations include stool culture, endoscopy and biopsy.

Treatment

Initially, treatment is of the symptoms of diarrhoea and will include nutritional, fluid and electrolyte replacement and anti-diarrhoeal drugs. It is necessary to replace fluid. In acute diarrhoea, this can be with intravenous infusion of glucose and an infusion which will replace electrolyte imbalance. It may be necessary to feed some very ill patients by passing a gastrointestinal tube into the stomach.

People who can tolerate food by mouth can be given nutritional supplements such as Build Up Vitamin, and mineral supplements should be given and should possibly be taken prophylactically by all people with AIDS.

There are several different anti-diarrhoeal drugs, which include kaolin and other absorbents and the morphine derivatives such as *imodium, lomotil, codeine* and *morphine*. Morphine, codeine and lomotil have some side-effects, including dizziness and drowsiness.

Diarrhoea in people with AIDS may be caused by several different organisms, including:

Cryptosporidium
This intestinal parasite can cause diarrhoea in individuals with a normal immune system. In people with AIDS, it can be associated with chronic and extremely severe diarrhoea. The diagnosis is made by the detection of the organism in the faeces or by biopsy. Although there is no effective drug treatment, symptoms may decline after the initiation of treatment with *zidovudine*.

Isospora belli
This parasite is a not very common cause of diarrhoea in people with AIDS. Diagnosis is by the detection of the organism in the stool. Treatment with *co-trimoxazole (septrin)* may be effective.

Giardia intestinalis
This parasite has often been found in gay men and is common in the tropics. It can cause persistent diarrhoea, abdominal discomfort and weight loss. Diagnosis is made by detecting the organism in the stools and treatment is with *metronidazole (flagyl)*.

Shigellae species
Shigellae, particularly *S. flexneri*, may be a cause of diarrhoea in a person whose immune system is severely weakened. The symptoms are nausea, cramps, blood-stained diarrhoea and fever. Diagnosis is by culture of the organism in the stools and treatment is by antibiotics, although recurrent infection is common.

Salmonella species
Salmonella enteritidis or *Salmonella typhimurium* are the most common forms of salmonella found in people with AIDS. Persistent or recurrent diarrhoea is a common symptom, with some people passing a considerable amount of watery diarrhoea. Diagnosis is by culture of the organism in the stools.

Treatment is with antibiotics. As recurrent infection is common, life-long prophylactic treatment with antibiotics may be recommended. People with salmonella infection should be given dietary information about what is appropriate to eat and what will cause least aggravation to the digestive tract. It is possibly wise for people with salmonella infection to avoid eating foods such as lightly cooked eggs and undercooked or reheated poultry, which may be sources of further infection.

Cytomegalovirus (CMV)

Cytomegalovirus in the gut can cause colitis. The symptoms are profuse watery diarrhoea, weight loss, abdominal discomfort and distention, and fever. Diagnosis is by culture of the organism in the stools and by biopsy, and treatment is with *foscarnet* and *ganciclovir*.

Atypical mycobacteria

Many atypical mycobacteria can produce infection in the immunosuppressed person. In people with AIDS, the most common are *Mycobacteria avium-intracellulare* and *Mycobacteria kansasii*, and they are all usually found in the later stages of the infection. The most common symptoms are night sweats, high fever, weight loss and diarrhoea. Atypical mycobacteria can also cause lung disease. Diagnosis is made by culturing the organism in the stools or blood. Treatment is generally ineffective.

Campylobacter Species

Campylobacter species are frequently a cause of diarrhoea in people with AIDS. Diarrhoea is often preceded by fever, headache, pains in the joints and cramps in the lower abdomen. Diagnosis is by sigmoidoscopy.

Treatment is with *erythromycin* or *tetracycline*. As in the case of gastrointestinal infections caused by salmonella, patients should be given dietary advice about appropriate non-aggravating food, as well as advised about the possible source of further infection in lightly cooked eggs and undercooked or reheated poultry.

Herpes Simplex Virus

This is a common viral infection that causes 'cold sores' of the lips as well as genital herpes. An earlier section of the chapter described how herpes simplex may cause ulcers on the lips, in the mouth and in the oesophagus. Herpes simplex may also cause ulcers in the perianal area. The ulcers are painful and tender and will persist if left untreated.

Treatment with *acyclovir*, given intravenously if the person is very ill and otherwise given orally, is very effective. As the virus is not eliminated from the body, treatment with acyclovir is used to prevent recurrence. Prophylactic treatment is one tablet of acyclovir four times a day. Acyclovir is safe and has very few side-effects.

Cancers (neoplasms)

Kaposi's Sarcoma

Kaposi's sarcoma (KS) was considered a rare form of sarcoma and was first described by a Hungarian doctor in the late nineteenth century as a slow-growing tumour. It appeared as purple nodules and plaques on the feet and lower legs of elderly Italian and Eastern European men of Jewish background. Since then, it has been seen in the context of HIV and AIDS as a tumour of blood or lymph vessel (endothelial) cells, most frequently among homosexual men. The reasons for its prominence among gay men and its insignificance in the haemophilia and intravenous drug-using populations is still unclear. As KS has been described in HIV seronegative gay men, it has been suggested that this neoplasm is caused by another sexually transmissible organism.

Kaposi's sarcoma skin lesions can appear almost anywhere on the body, but especially on the head and neck (behind the ears and at the tip of the nose). The tumours are reddish blue skin lumps. The diameter varies from a few millimetres to several centimetres. Generally, the lumps are symptomless. However, Kaposi's sarcoma of the face can be cosmetically unacceptable and very distressing for the affected person.

Tumours of the feet may be associated with swelling of the feet and inflammation of the skin of the legs.

Kaposi's sarcoma of the mouth is common. Tumours are most frequently found in the hard and the soft palate. Tumours in the mouth can cause a very noticeable bad breath (halitosis). KS tumours of the gastrointestinal tract are very common. Kaposi's sarcoma are also found in the perianal region and resemble anal abscesses.

Treatment

The major reason for treating Kaposi's sarcoma in people with AIDS is for cosmetic reasons and the relief of locally troublesome, painful and distressing lesions. The aim is to keep the skin as normal as possible and reduce distress, e.g. when someone has facial lesions.

Lesions of the face may respond to localized chemotherapy and radiotherapy. It is also important that people have the opportunity to use camouflage make-up to help cover unsightly marks. Kaposi's sarcoma of the feet should be treated by radiotherapy and lesions in the mouth may be helped by chemotherapy. When Kaposi's sarcoma is widespread in the body, treatment by *vinblastine* and *bleomycin* may be used. Small localized tumours may be surgically excised and it is unlikely that they will reappear in that site.

People rarely die of Kaposi's sarcoma. However, it is often followed by opportunistic infections. When an individual with KS is being treated with *zidovudine*, the occurrence of opportunistic infections and other problems will most probably be delayed.

Lymphomas

Lymphomas are cancers of lymphatic tissue. They may become apparent because of sudden painful enlargement of the lymph nodes. Most commonly, they affect the central nervous system or the gut.

Diagnosis is made by using the appropriate radiological investigations (e.g. barium enema) or a biopsy. Lymphomas of the brain are usually diagnosed by CT scanning (CAT scan). Treatment is by chemotherapy. If lymphomas occur early in the course of HIV-related illness, full remission may occur. However, many of these tumours respond poorly to treatment and result in an increase in morbidity and mortality.

Carcinomas

Cancers (carcinomas) of the anal region and of the mouth have been described in HIV-infected gay men. In one study, pre-cancerous changes have been found in the cervix of a high proportion of HIV-infected women. However, other workers have not noticed this. Annual cervical cytology is recommended for HIV-infected women.

HIV infection and the Eye

The majority of people with more severe HIV infection and with AIDS have some eye problems. The most common of these eye problems are *retinal cotton wool spots*, *Kaposi's sarcoma* and *cytomegalovirus retinitis*.

Retinal cotton wool spots

Cotton wool spots in the retina are the most common abnormality of the eye found in people with HIV. The spots are white, fluffy in appearance and feather edged. Diagnosis is by examination by an ophthalmologist (eye specialist). There is no treatment for retinal cotton wool spots, which seldom cause difficulties with sight. Individual cotton wool spots may disappear after about 2 months, but new ones may then appear.

Kaposi's sarcoma of the conjunctiva and eyelids

Kaposi's sarcoma of the conjunctiva and/or the eyelids is the second most common lesion of the eye seen in people with severe HIV infections or AIDS. Kaposi's sarcoma lesions on the conjunctiva appear as bright red spots of different sizes. These spots are painless. KS lesions of the eyelids appear as purple, firm lumps.

Diagnosis of Kaposi's sarcoma of the conjunctiva or the eyelids is almost always confirmed by biopsy of lesions elsewhere in the body. It is unusual to biopsy KS lesions of the conjunctiva or the eyelids.

Kaposi's sarcoma of the eye rarely requires treatment. The lumps are not painful. However, in some circumstances, when the lesions have begun to interfere with vision, surgery may be necesssary. In other cases, surgery may be requested for cosmetic reasons.

Cytomegalovirus Retinitis

Cytomegalovirus (CMV) retinitis is the most serious complication of the eye affecting people with AIDS. In some patients, CMV may be asymptomatic, but many patients complain of decreased visual acuity, photophobia (intolerance to light), flashes of light, redness and pain.

Diagnosis is by examination of the retina with an ophthalmoscope. *Ganciclovir* and *foscarnet* appear to stop or slow down CMV retinitis.

Skin conditions

Skin problems are very common early symptoms of HIV. Skin disorders are many and varied and include such conditions as athlete's foot, shingles, warts and cold sores. Most skin conditions are not necessarily painful, but they are often very distressing with itchiness and tenderness being common symptoms. Some skin problems are visible to others and even disfiguring, affecting the face, the scalp and other parts of the body that are normally exposed. This adds to the distress of the person and even adds to their isolation should the person be unwilling to go out.

Skin conditions can be caused by a virus (e.g. herpes simplex) and by fungal agents (e.g. athlete's foot – tinea pedis), as well as by bacterial infections due to some failure in the immune system. Skin conditions that appear as an early symptom of HIV may also be present when a person has AIDS.

Although many individuals with PGL do not have other symptoms related to immune dysfunction, some develop skin conditions. The more common skin conditions found in people with HIV-related illnesses or AIDS are:

- severe athlete's foot (tinea pedis);
- extensive reddening, scaliness or weeping of the groin area (tinea cruris) as a result of fungal infection;
- pityriasis versicolor, a fungal infection of the skin, resulting in extensive areas of brown discolouration and scaling;
- severe dandruff or greasy red-brown spots on the face, chest and arm (seborrhoeic dermatitis);
- multiple small abscesses of the hair follicles (folliculitis);
- troublesome and persistent warts of the genital and anal regions;
- recurrent herpes of the lips or genitals;

- shingles (herpes zoster);
- dry scaly skin (ichthyosis); and
- extensive bruising because of a low number of platelets in the blood (thrombocytopoenia).

Special considerations in the treatment of HIV and HIV-related illnesses

As yet there is no cure for HIV infection itself, but there are increasingly effective treatments for people with HIV-related illness. Many of the clinical problems encountered in daily care are treatable, and in many situations both the quality of life and the life expectancy of people infected with HIV have been improved.

Substantial problems still remain. HIV is biologically very complex, designing and testing effective vaccines and antiviral drug therapy is problematic, the secondary infections associated with HIV are often unusual, treatment regimes are toxic and often unfamiliar, and the complex psychological, social and emotional needs of the patient are not always met. In all clinical situations associated with HIV, early diagnosis and commencement of treatment enhances the possibility of a favourable outcome.

Infections and HIV-related complications are often subtle in their onset, yet more severe in their clinical manifestations than in non-HIV people. In addition, these infections often respond more slowly to specific therapies. People infected with HIV have a high frequency of adverse drug reactions, and many of the drugs themselves are toxic and difficult to administer.

Some secondary infections do tend to recur. Therefore, in addition to effective treatment for an acute episode, long-term (often life-long) therapy or prophylaxis against these infections is often desirable. It is also now realized that although there is a similarity in the clinical manifestations of HIV infections common to all infected with HIV, there are considerable variations in the incidence and degree of complications.

The earlier sections of this chapter have indicated the often very effective treatments which are available for the specific opportunistic infections which HIV-infected individuals may experience. Considerable progress has also been made in the last few years in the development of antiviral drug therapies, agents which inhibit the replication of HIV at some points in its life-cycle. The next section of the chapter describes a few of the best-known, and most commonly used, of the antiretroviral therapies.

Antiviral agents

Zidovudine (3'azido-3'deoxythymidine, AZT, Retrovir™) is the first antiviral agent which has been shown to be clinically effective and is licensed for use in the treatment of HIV infections. The way in which zidovudine acts to inhibit the replication of HIV is described in Chapter 2.

Initially, the drug was given to individuals who had been treated for opportunistic infections or who had had major symptoms of HIV infection, including encephalopathy. Double-blind placebo controlled trials demonstrated convincingly that zidovudine reduced the mortality and frequency of opportunistic infections significantly in individuals with HIV-related illnesses, including individuals classified as having AIDS.

Since September 1989, the use of zidovudine for asymptomatic patients has become more widespread. Generally, the drug is given orally in a dosage of 250 mg every 6 hours. Patients begin to feel much better within a few weeks of commencing treatment, with in some cases weight gain and a decrease in fatigue. There is evidence that there is a decrease in the frequency of opportunistic infections in patients on zidovudine and improvement in neurological symptoms associated with HIV infection.

The number of CD4 cells (T4 helper cells) in the peripheral blood increases during the first month of beginning treatment, but in the majority of patients they then decrease to the pre-treatment levels. During treatment, HIV can be cultivated from peripheral blood lymphocytes more easily than before treatment started. In some patients in whom serum antigen was detected before the start of treatment, serum antigen becomes undetectable. In other patients, serum antigen persists. The significance of these findings is still unknown.

Studies have shown that although very small concentrations of zidovudine inhibit the growth of the virus in certain cells that bear the antigen on their surface, larger concentrations are required to inhibit viral replication in macrophages. This suggests that zidovudine may not react at all the sites of viral replication and may explain why clinical deterioration may occur even during treatment.

There are side-effects of zidovudine, including nausea, headache and skin rash, which are all common during the first few weeks of treatment and which generally go away. During the first month of treatment of people with severe HIV infection, severe depression in the production of red cells may necessitate a blood transfusion and even cessation of treatment. Another type of anaemia (called macrocytic anaemia because the red cells are larger than usual) often occurs as treatment progresses and can be sufficiently severe to require a reduction in the dose or to stop treatment. Zidovudine treatment may also cause leucopoenia (a severe depletion in the number of white cells), and treatment may have to be stopped or the dosage reduced.

Certain problems may arise, during the second year of treatment, including a rapidly progressive inflammation of the muscles. An acute inflammation may follow a reduction in the dose.

It has been reported that *paracetamol* (panadol) can interact with zidovudine and the use of paracetamol on a long-term basis in conjunction with zidovudine should be avoided.

It is not yet possible to draw firm conclusions about the long-term efficacy of zidovudine, as it has so recently been introduced into clinical practice and research and data collection are continuing. Trials in which zidovudine is administered in combination with another antiviral drug or immunostimulant agent are in progress. Preliminary data have suggested that a combined treatment of zidovudine and *acyclovir* has a beneficial effect. There also appears to be a beneficial interaction between zidovudine and *phosphonoformate* (Foscarnet).

2'3'-Dideoxycytidine (ddC) is another drug that acts in a similar way to zidovudine, as it appears to break the viral DNA chain and is also known to kill HIV in the test tube. Studies of its use are in progress. It is known to have as a side-effect peripheral neuropathy, a condition of the nerve endings which can be very painful. *Dideoxinosine* (DDI) is at present undergoing clinical trials to determine its efficacy. Early clinical studies appear promising. The side-effects are different from those of zidovudine, the most common being pancreatitis.

Other drugs

Scientists are continuously looking at other pharmaceutical ways in which HIV can be attacked and have considered that the cell membranes of the virus would be a good target for an antiviral agent. The drug *interferon* inhibits the binding of animal retroviruses and its use in the treatment of HIV is being investigated to be prescribed alone or in combination with other drugs. Certain substances inhibit the growth of HIV *in vitro*. Such substances include protein kinase inhibitors such as *dextran sulphate*. What is not known is whether the virus continues to remain viable in cells within a living person treated with such substances, and further studies are in progress.

Although there is at present no single ideal treatment against HIV, it has already been discovered that over 100 different agents inhibit the growth of the virus and their application to clinical medicine is being studied in many centres throughout the world.

Treatment: The holistic approach

So far, the focus on treatment for HIV and AIDS has been on drug therapy. It is believed that an holistic approach to the care of the individual with HIV is important and that drug treatment is part of such an approach. In such an approach, some of the following therapies may be considered along with conventional therapy: acupuncture, acupressure, herbalism, hypnotherapy, spiritual healing, meditation, yoga, visualization and massage. Both conventional therapy and alternative therapies suggest that attention should be paid to diet, exercise and rest, and to psychological and emotional well-being.

It may suit some people with HIV and AIDS to take drug treatment as required, but not to use alternative therapies. Others will wish to explore complementary therapies and will benefit from their use. It is important that the choices are given and that the information is available.

Nutrition

The action of the immune system can be inhibited by drugs, tobacco, alcohol, poor nutrition, obesity, a sedentary lifestyle and stress. People living with HIV who are asymptomatic should have a varied and well-balanced diet. People with HIV-related illnesses and AIDS frequently suffer from problems in absorbing nutrients, and considerable weight loss. Some dieticians recommend the addition of such vitamins and nutrients as vitamins A, C, B6, E, and zinc, selenium and arginine, but also stress the importance of moderation. Other dieticians have recommended an aggressive approach to both maintaining and improving the nutritional status of the patient. Nutrition, however, does not provide all the answers to HIV-related illnesses, and physicians and counsellors may need to help individuals gain a balanced approach to dietary care.

Specific symptoms can be alleviated by appropriate nutrition. When the person is suffering from infections or lesions of the mouth or oesophagus, changing the acidity, the temperature and the amount of seasoning in food may make it easier to swallow. Modifying the diet may reduce the volume and frequency of bowel movements in those with diarrhoea. Meals should be small and taken frequently.

It is important that people living with HIV are aware that some opportunistic infections, such as salmonella, can originate from improperly cooked food. Meat, in particular chicken, but also other types of poultry and pork, needs to be well cooked, as do eggs. Soft cheeses may also pose a certain risk to people with severe HIV infection. Care should also be taken in observing good hygiene in the kitchen. Pre-cooked meals need to be reheated thoroughly to guard against the risk of infection. When microwaves are used, the manufacturer's instructions should be followed carefully to ensure that food is thoroughly cooked.

Dental treatment

Regular dental examination and good oral hygiene are necessary for people with HIV-related illnesses so as to prevent oral infection and for their own comfort. It is advisable that people with HIV inform their dentist of their HIV status. Some dentists are unhappy about treating people with HIV and some are inexperienced in this work. Counsellors can assist by finding out what is the attitude of the patient's dentist to those who are HIV antibody positive.

Dentists and hygienists protect themselves from infection by routinely wearing gloves. For some procedures, it may be necessary for the dentist to protect him- or herself from blood spatter and splash by wearing a mask, gown and goggles. It is important that the need for these procedures is explained to patients beforehand. This is particularly crucial in the case of children and younger patients.

HIV-related illnesses and AIDS in children

HIV-related illnesses and AIDS create similar problems for children as are found in adults; but there are also specific issues peculiar to children and infants.

It is essential to establish a diagnosis of paediatric HIV infection before the onset of opportunistic infections if the complications of AIDS are to be prevented, and if an improved long-term prognosis is to be achieved. Therefore, children and infants suspected of having paediatric AIDS should be evaluated with laboratory studies to demonstrate immunodeficiency, to isolate the virus, and in the case of infants to exclude other congenital and acquired immunodeficiency disorders.

Prospective studies have shown that infants at risk for developing AIDS may be both clinically and immunologically normal at birth. T-cell abnormalities usually develop before the onset of symptoms. Infants may become symptomatic as early as 1 month. In general, infants who have developed AIDS from blood transfusion have had a shorter incubation period than those infected from maternal transmission. The explanation for this may be that most infants requiring blood transfusion in the first days of life are either critically ill or premature and both of these factors can result in immunodeficiency.

Many of the clinical manifestations of paediatric HIV-related illnesses and AIDS are similar to those of adults. An impaired immune system and almost all the opportunistic infections described in adults have been observed in children. Failure to thrive, weight loss, mild to severe developmental delay and gradual neurological deterioration are common. As in adults, the range of abnormalities in affected children varies greatly from no abnormalities to abnormalities involving several systems of the body.

Diagnosis of paediatric AIDS

The progression from asymptomatic HIV infection to AIDS, as officially defined, in infants can be very rapid. A diagnosis of AIDS in children can be established on the basis of (1) the presence of a risk factor associated with HIV, (2) detection of HIV antibody in infants over the age of 6 months and (3) the presence of immunodeficiency established by laboratory tests.

General treatment of a child with AIDS

Treating an infant or a child with AIDS is especially challenging because of the complications of the disease superimposed on the need of the child to thrive and grow. The complications of diarrhoea, fever and feeding problems can all contribute to malnutrition. This creates a further problem, as once a child is suffering from malnutrition it is more prone to infections. Nutrition presents particular problems in paediatric AIDS, as children require a high amount of calories in order to maintain their rate of growth. High protein, high calorie feeds and vitamin supplements may be required.

Prophylactic therapy is an important part of the treatment in paediatric AIDS. Children with HIV infection who have impaired immunity (e.g. abnormal T4/T8 cell ratios) may benefit from monthly intravenous gamma-globulin treatment. Children with damaged immune systems risk suffering from severe complications from infections such as chickenpox, measles and mumps that are commonly contracted in school or nursery schools. The risk of the child contracting such infections should be evaluated. The risk of the child being severely infected following exposure to chickenpox may be reduced by administration of specific immunoglobulin.

Immunization
There has been considerable discussion about the appropriateness of vaccination and immunization for HIV-infected children. Earlier studies on the immunization of HIV-infected children recommended vaccinating children asymptomatic for HIV but not those with symptoms. Following reports of severe measles in symptomatic HIV children and in the absence of reports of serious adverse effects of MMR (the vaccine for measles, mumps and rubella), paediatricians are now considering MMR vaccine for all HIV-infected children regardless of symptoms. As studies of the effect of live vaccine on symptomatic HIV-infected children are still inconclusive, many paediatricians are still reluctant to offer vaccinations to these children.

Effect on the family
HIV-related illnesses and AIDS in children, and the treatment of these illnesses, can create very severe emotional problems for the child and the family. Families need to be kept fully informed of the nature of their children's treatment, and when possible become actively involved in their children's health care.

References

Blaxhult, A. *et al.* (1990). 'The influence of age on the latency period to AIDS in people infected by HIV through blood transfusion'. *AIDS*, **4**, 125–9.

Lancet Editorial (1991). 'Mycoplasma and AIDS – what connection'. *Lancet*, **337**, 20–21.

Moss, A.R. and Bacchetti, P. (1989). 'Editorial review: Natural history of HIV infection'. *AIDS*, **3**, 55–61.

Moss, A.R. *et al.* (1988). 'Seropositivity for HIV and the development of AIDS or AIDS related condition: Three year follow up of the San Francisco General Hospital cohort'. *British Medical Journal*, **296**, 745–50.

FOUR

Psychiatric and neuropsychological aspects of HIV infection

ALISON RICHARDSON

It is now well recognized that there are profound psychological, psychiatric and neurological consequences of HIV infection and AIDS. These have not always been well differentiated, partly because a diagnosis can be difficult to establish. Anxiety, depression and obsessional states are not unusual in those who are infected, but neither are they in those who fear HIV infection, those who are often referred to as 'the worried well'. This category itself covers a wide variety of problems which may be encountered. There are those who are truly worried and well and who may be easily reassured by information alone or information together with a negative test result. Others may be more psychologically disturbed and may not be effectively helped by information alone or even by repeated negative tests in the absence of risk behaviours (King, 1990). There is little reason to view the latter as any different from individuals who suffer from other illness phobias, such as of cancer or of obsessional behaviours involving fear of contamination. It is likely, however, that individuals who are predisposed to such psychological problems may be precipitated into illness because of the existence of the disease in society, with all its attendant media exposure.

The problems which develop in those who *are* infected with HIV fall broadly into two categories; those which primarily involve psychological and psychiatric problems of varying severity and those which are more directly concerned with organic brain function. The distinction between these categories is often difficult to make and it is important for those working with individuals who are infected to be aware of the diagnostic problems within the area.

Psychological problems and neurotic states

Anxiety, depressive reactions and other neurotic states may develop in response to many of the stresses associated with a diagnosis of HIV infection.

They may involve a reaction to the initial diagnosis, to the development of any illness or to the diagnosis of AIDS. These problems may occur in infected individuals, regardless of their HIV status, and it should not always be assumed that the *cause* of such states is HIV, though it is likely to be of some relevance in most cases. A diagnosis of this kind is likely to bring many difficulties to the fore, not least problems in relationships or in general adjustment to family or other problems. Concerns about personal health, about infectivity and about sexual practices are often present and it can be difficult to differentiate between 'normal' and 'abnormal' concerns.

In the majority of such people, such reactions are readily understandable and, ironically, those who suffer in this way may be considerably easier to help than those who are *not* infected but who suffer from similar problems. Acute anxiety, depression or a preoccupation with infection and illness following a life event of such severity should not necessarily be regarded as a psychological problem at all, but rather as a normal reaction to a potential or actual life-threatening diagnosis.

In some cases, those who are living with HIV may suffer from more severe states of depression and anxiety which may require psychological or psychiatric intervention. It is important for the caring professions to distinguish between those whose reactions can be considered normal and those who may be more severely disabled. Dilley *et al.* (1985) found that 13 out of 40 HIV-infected patients seen at San Francisco General Hospital had been given a psychiatric diagnosis, most frequently of depression. Thoughts of suicide appear common, though it is uncertain how many may actually make an attempt. In the USA, Marzuk *et al.* (1988) have reported a much increased risk of suicide among men with AIDS. Within this area of work, the intention to commit suicide can be a decision made rationally, the individual having evaluated the future as one which holds little but continued illness and loss. Others may kill themselves impulsively, precipitated by depression, by illness or perceived illness or by other life events. Depressive illness may be often accompanied by suicidal ideation, which can be alleviated by appropriate treatment and it is therefore of major importance that those in the field evaluate such problems very carefully.

Drug users may be particularly at risk, often having access to controlled drugs, either prescribed or illicit. Many are regarded as attention seeking and difficult and suicidal threats may not be given the attention that they would in others who are living with HIV. In Edinburgh and the surrounding area, which has a very high rate of infection among drug users, there have already been a number of deaths from overdoses. It is difficult to determine whether these have been accidental or intentional.

Biological symptoms of clinical depression include early morning wakening, loss of appetite and weight loss, variations in mood during the day and loss of libido. Some of these are recognized as physical symptoms of HIV disease itself and/or psychological sequelae so that diagnosis may be very difficult. This is elaborated further below.

Symptoms of anxiety are also frequently misinterpreted as physical symptoms of HIV disease. In acute states of anxiety, people may suffer from chest pain, sweating, trembling, diarrhoea and a myriad of other physical symptoms. Education about anxiety, including explanations about adrenalin effects, may help to alleviate some of the fear which such symptoms engender, but specific anxiety management techniques may be of great benefit when anxiety is acute and debilitating. Medication to reduce anxiety, in the form of minor tranquillizers such as diazepam, may be helpful in symptom relief, particularly at times of crisis, giving time out from acute anxiety to tackle underlying problems, though these should generally only be prescribed for short periods of time.

Issues of control are often very important in managing anxiety. Many individuals report that they feel that their lives have been taken over by the virus; repeated hospital visits, blood tests, counselling and even attendance at support or self-help groups may contribute to, rather than alleviate, anxiety if they keep the individual focusing on their position in life as a person 'who has the virus'. Physical symptoms of anxiety are real and frightening and it can be immensely helpful for people to find that they can exert control over them.

Obsessional behaviour, thoughts and hypochondriacal fears also arise in the context of infection. These may take the form of repeated checking of the body for blemishes or rashes, thoughts of death, or of trying to recall how and from whom the virus was contracted or repeated visits to the doctor for check-ups, in the absence of any symptoms. In severe forms, reassurance is rarely helpful for more than hours or days and more specific psychiatric or psychological treatment may be necessary.

Psychotic illness

There have been a number of reports of severe psychotic illnesses in those with HIV disease (e.g. Gabel *et al.*, 1986; Rundell *et al.*, 1986; Thomas, 1987 Buhrich *et al.*, 1988; Schmidt and Miller, 1988). The psychoses are generally characterized by thoughts, fears, worries or suspicions which have no basis in reality and may appear in the form of mania, schizophrenic types of illness or depression. In mania, there may be ideas of grandeur, such as a belief that the individual has found a cure for AIDS or has been miraculously cured. In paranoid schizophrenia, the person may believe that he is being persecuted in a way that is not reality based, such as in hearing voices. Depressive illness may also be of a severity that the hopelessness experienced is out of proportion to reality and the person may suffer from delusions or hallucinations. All of these have been documented in those who have serious HIV-related illnesses. In some cases, it has been reported that such episodes precede the appearance of intellectual deficits indicative of HIV encephalopathy (HIV encephalopathy is discussed later). However, in a review of psychiatric disorder in individuals with HIV infection, King (1990) has suggested that the rate of psychiatric disorder is lower than originally predicted.

In those who are infected, an understandable anxiety about infectivity, publicity, illness, etc., may appear to elide from neurotic behaviour in to psychosis. In these states, the individual is also unable to distinguish between realistic and unrealistic fears. The development of severe psychiatric illness may be independent of HIV disease and it is often impossible to determine the aetiology of such illness, when it first presents. Psychiatric assessment should always be sought in such cases.

Fenton (1987) has pointed out that psychotic states are more likely when there is a previous history of such illness. In the present state of knowledge, it is difficult to distinguish between the following factors as aetiological events, when someone presents with psychotic illness.

1 An existing predisposition to such illness, regardless of HIV.
2 An existing predisposition, which is exacerbated by the stress of diagnosis.
3 An existing predisposition, which is exacerbated by the direct effects of the virus on the nervous system.
4 Direct effects of the virus on the nervous system.

Neurological problems

There are a number of organic neurological disorders which may be caused by infection, such as toxoplasmosis and malignancy (e.g. lymphoma), both of which may affect the brain, or through direct HIV infection of the nervous system which causes a dementia.

The most common infections and tumours which cause neurological complications are given in Table 4.1. All of these can be treated, though treatments may be less effective in those who are immunosuppressed through HIV infection than in those who are not. The occurrence of a dementia which appears

Table 4.1 Neurological complications in AIDS

Infections	*Neoplasms*
Toxoplasma gondii	Primary CNS lymphoma
Cytomegalovirus	Metastatic lymphomas
Cryptococcus neoformans	Kaposi's sarcoma
Mycobacterium tuberculosis	
Papova virus	
Herpes simplex	
Candida albicans	
Varicella zoster	
Epstein–Barr	

unrelated to the specific viral or bacterial infections in Table 4.1 is now well documented and is apparently the most common cause of neurological complaint (Lechtenberg and Sher, 1988).

Dementia as a result of HIV infection was first described by Snider *et al.* (1983) as subacute encephalitis. Navia *et al.* (1986) have reported that infection and malignancy account for only about 30% of neurological complications and they found that nearly two-thirds of their study group, examined at post-mortem, had signs of this dementia, which they referred to as the AIDS Dementia Complex. This has also been termed HIV encephalopathy. Studies have shown that this encephalopathy may be the sole manifestation of HIV infection and patients may present with such symptoms as the first sign of HIV disease, though this is comparatively rare. Once identified, it is now a criterion for the diagnosis of AIDS, in the same way as opportunistic infections such as *Pneumocystis carinii.* pneumonia.

Both early and later symptoms of this dementia are now well documented, but problems of diagnosis are particularly acute in the early stages where the distinction between psychological problems, psychiatric illness and neurological problems may be particularly difficult to make.

Many of the early symptoms of the AIDS Dementia Complex are indistinguishable from depression. Early presentation is characterized by complaints of forgetfulness, poor concentration and loss of interest; all recognizable as symptoms of depression. In some, there may also be weight loss, symptomatic both of progressing HIV disease and of depressive illness. Holland and Tross (1985) also reported loss of libido, blunted affect and psychomotor retardation as early symptoms of HIV encephalopathy; again, symptoms associated with depression.

Results of diagnostic tests often fail to provide definitive results. EEG (in which brain activity is measured through electrodes attached externally to the skull) and computerized tests, such as CAT scans and MRI scans (which provide kinds of X-rays of the brain), may show few, if any, changes. Lumbar puncture, which involves taking a specimen of the fluid which surrounds the brain and spinal cord, may reveal HIV antibodies in cerebrospinal fluid, but such positive results have been found in people with AIDS who do not have neurological problems (Hollander and Levy, 1987).

Neurophysiological assessment by evoked potential, may prove to be a useful, speedy and non-intrusive test indicating organic cognitive dysfunction (Egan *et al.*, 1989). In one study, neuropsychological assessment suggested that specific tests may be sensitive to HIV encephalopathy in its early stages. Grant *et al.* (1987) studied a group of 44 HIV positive individuals who were classified as follows: (a) HIV infected, without serious symptoms; (b) those with symptoms, without having been diagnosed as having AIDS; and (c) those with AIDS. None had obvious neurological abnormalities, but in comparison with HIV negative controls, there was evidence of increasing cognitive impairment with disease progression. Egan *et al.* (1990) investigated 80 people at different CDC stages of HIV infection (the CDC system for classifying the effects of

HIV infection is described in Chapter 3), who had been infected through drug use, and found evidence of cognitive impairment. However, with HIV negative controls, they concluded that the observed deficits were more likely due to drug use than to early symptoms of the AIDS Dementia Complex.

Overall, it seems more likely that cognitive impairment in those who are otherwise asymptomatic is rare and that complaints of loss of attention and memory are more likely due to psychological and psychiatric problems. Continuing prospective longitudinal studies of HIV positive asymptomatic individuals, using a variety of measures are underway in the UK, but it will be some time before these can be expected to provide results which may prove useful in clinical settings.

Later symptoms of HIV encephalopathy are more obvious. Progression of symptoms may be rapid, but more often decline occurs over a period of months. Later symptoms include motor disturbance, which may cause difficulty in walking, seizures, spasticity, incontinence and mutism. It is these features which many find such a terrifying prospect, so that they will present at hospital clinics complaining of memory or concentration difficulties which are more likely to be indicative of an acute anxiety state than of dementia. It is always important to take such reports seriously and to carry out further investigation.

By 1987, Faulstich reported that 30–40% of AIDS patients present signs of neurological dysfunction and that 80% show post-mortem results indicative of such abnormalities (Faulstich, 1987). Lechtenberg and Sher (1988) have suggested that even when there have been no neurological signs or symptoms, autopsy indicates neurological abnormalities in 80–90% of cases. It is important to remember that perhaps the majority of these will not be aware of significant difficulties in their day-to-day behaviours, thoughts, memories or emotions and that post-mortem results such as these are not necessarily reflected in the person's experience. Such statistics are frightening for those who are infected, who fear that there will be progressive deterioration in their mental functions and that they will suffer symptoms such as incontinence or blindness. The fact that many of those infected are highly knowledgeable about the disease and aware of possible illness is a factor which can have a profound psychological impact.

In practice, where neurological involvement is suspected, a variety of tests are carried out. The case report of Schmidt and Miller (1988) is typical of the kind of results found. Their patient presented with hypomania, a condition marked by over-excitability, and was assessed with lumbar puncture and EEG (both normal), and CAT scan which showed minor cortical changes. Neuropsychological assessment revealed impairments of concentration, memory and orientation, a finding which would not necessarily lead to a diagnosis of underlying organic impairment in one who was also psychotic. The patient responded to anti-psychotic medication but then rapidly became demented and died.

The following case history and discussion also illustrate the difficulty of diagnosis when psychological factors, psychiatric illness and neurological problems must be considered.

Case study 1

Mr X, a 37-year-old gay man, presented at a hospital clinic in 1987. He complained of depressed mood, loss of energy, weight loss and was particularly concerned about his work performance. He had become increasingly aware of difficulties with his concentration and memory and felt that this was becoming evident to colleagues. Although he had not been tested for HIV, he was well aware that he might be HIV antibody positive and that these symptoms might be related. He was clearly distressed and anxious but reacted relatively calmly to his positive result. Because there was concern about his reported symptoms, he was asked to attend on a regular basis for a variety of tests, including neuropsychological assessment. He cooperated fully, though this caused him some inconvenience, due to his working and home circumstances. Over a period of 3 months, Mr X attended the hospital regularly during which time he remained reasonably well but was naturally concerned about his health. None of the tests carried out were interpreted as indicative of the AIDS Dementia Complex or other neurological complaints. At that time, he suddenly developed pneumonia and was admitted to hospital with a presumptive diagnosis of *Pneumocystis carinii* pneumonia.

On admission, he was extremely agitated but settled as his physical state improved. He remained worried about his work and the possibility of losing his job and expressed understandable concern that the diagnosis of AIDS would be discovered by colleagues, neighbours, etc. He received considerable support from relatives and friends whom he had told about the diagnosis. During the admission, however, he experienced increasing short-term memory problems so that he sometimes had difficulty in remembering names of staff, events and locations on the ward.

After a 4-week stay in hospital he was discharged, to stay with relatives, but a few days later he was readmitted in a confused and agitated state. He had become increasingly fearful, not only for himself but for those close to him, about the possibility of public disclosure of his condition. He was worried about his own infectivity and could not cope with the medication regime. After readmission these concerns did not abate and he became convinced that there were reporters after him, that staff would lose their jobs and friends be ostracized because of their association with him. The initial impression of an anxiety state was replaced by a diagnosis of paranoid psychosis, since his fears and suspicions were not related to actual events, and he was treated with antipsychotic medication. At the same time, his memory problems were clearly worse and he reported having difficulty in remembering how to dress himself. Neuropsychological assessment showed significant cognitive deterioration.

He was also started on zidovudine (AZT), and given anti-depressant drugs during admission and gradually showed an improvement both physically and mentally. He was discharged again 3 months after the original admission, with clear signs on testing that his memory had shown improvement. He was no longer paranoid and his anxiety was appropriate considering his circumstances.

Three months later and a full year after his original presentation, Mr X was back at work full time and reported no further problems of either a psychological or neurological kind. Neuropsychological assessment indicated that his cognitive state had shown further improvement after discharge.

In this man's case, there is neither a satisfactory explanation for his psychological and intellectual deterioration nor for the dramatic improvement which was subsequently demonstrated. The following are all possible factors:

1 He may have been suffering from early signs of HIV encephalopathy with associated psychosis. In this case, he has made a remarkable recovery, which may or may not be sustained.
2 The diagnosis of HIV infection, perhaps exacerbated by the stressful months of hospital tests, precipitated the psychotic state, although complaints of cognitive change preceded that state.
3 The psychosis may have been entirely unrelated to his HIV status.
4 He may have had an existing predisposition towards mental illness which was precipitated directly by HIV effects on the brain.
5 His rapid deterioration following initial discharge from in-patient care may also indicate that he was neither psychologically nor physically ready to leave the relatively safe environment of the hospital. This may also have been a precipitating factor.
6 The co-existence of concurrent pneumonia and neuropsychiatric problems has been poorly investigated, but it is possible that there is a causative relationship.

His recovery may similarly be ascribed to a variety of factors. There are other reports of patients improving on anti-psychotic drugs. However, within a short period of time, he was prescribed antibiotics for his pneumonia, anti-psychotic drugs, anti-depressants and zidovudine. It is therefore impossible to tease out which, if any, had a helpful effect. There are some case reports of improvement in cognitive function with zidovudine in high doses.

The diagnostic picture may be further confused with those who are former or current drug users, since there is little evidence about the kind of cognitive impairment that drug use may engender. The following case indicates further the multiplicity of factors which may have to be considered in making a diagnosis.

Case study 2

Mr Y is in his mid-20s and is a former intravenous drug user. He probably became infected with HIV in 1983 or 1984, but gave up intravenous drug use in 1985 following a head injury sustained in a road traffic accident. It was discovered that he was HIV antibody positive in 1987. Although he had made a good recovery from the accident, he continued to suffer from problems in walking and had some difficulty with speech. In 1988, he presented at the hospital clinic maintaining that he had discovered a cure for AIDS. He became angry when this assertion was questioned and demanded payment for revealing the name of the cure. At the same time, he became convinced that he was immune from police prosecution and smoked cannabis resin publicly, a habit which he had previously confined to the privacy of his home. This resulted in his prosecution by the authorities.

He was entirely unwilling to take any other form of medication, since he was already taking 'the cure', though he was finally persuaded to take small amounts of anti-psychotic medication. Although this calmed him down to a large extent, he continued to believe in 'the cure' and that he was no longer seropositive. He is now highly suspicious of professional input, asserting that he knows that they think that he is mad.

In addition to the factors mentioned in Case 1, the previous drug use, current cannabis intake and effects of brain injury may be of significance. There is also a family history of schizophrenia which complicates the picture. Physical investigations were unrevealing, as was neuropsychological assessment, because of lack of cooperation ('You are trying to prove that I'm stupid'). Current management is to try to get him to take anti-psychotic medication and to try to draw him back into a therapeutic relationship with his doctor, psychologist and psychiatrist. The main obstacle to this lies in the ethical ground of deciding whether or not to collude in his delusions, in particular, that he has found the cure for AIDS. Such collusion *might* result in greater cooperation with the treatment regime, but might equally make him feel that he was being humoured and therefore feed his paranoia about those who are trying to help him, including family and friends as well as professionals.

These cases give some indication of the difficulties in diagnosing and responding to neuropsychiatric problems which present in the context of HIV infection. The lines between understandable anxiety or depression following diagnosis or progression of the disease, psychiatric illness and organic neurological dysfunction continue to be blurred. As it has become clear that neuropsychiatric dysfunction is a highly prevalent aspect of HIV disease, there have been increasing research efforts in this direction. It is likely that it will be some time yet before we have any definitive means of distinguishing between the different aspects of the problem.

References

Buhrich, N. *et al.* (1988). 'HIV infection associated with symptoms indistinguishable from functional psychosis'. *British Journal of Psychiatry*, **152**, 649–53.

Dilley, J.W. *et al.* (1985). 'Findings in psychiatric consultations with patients with AIDS'. *American Journal of Psychiatry,* **142**, 82–6.

Egan, V.G. *et al.* (1989). *Abstract P300 Correlates with Neuro-Psychological Testing in HIV Positive Drug Users at CDC Stages 2 and 3.* Presented at the Neurological and Neuropsychological Complications of HIV Infection Conference. Quebec City, Canada, 31 May–3 June. Abstract NP6.

Egan, V.G. *et al.* (1990). 'The Edinburgh cohort of HIV-positive drug users: Current intellectual function is impaired, but not due to early AIDS dementia complex'. *AIDS,* **4**, 651–6.

Faulstich, M.E. (1987). 'Psychiatric aspects of AIDS'. *American Journal of Psychiatry,* **144**, 551–6.

Fenton, T.W. (1987). 'AIDS related psychiatric disorder'. *British Journal of Psychiatry,* **151**, 579–88.

Gabel, R.H. *et al.* (1986). 'AIDS presenting as mania'. *Comprehensive Psychiatry,* **27**, 251–4.

Grant, I. *et al.* (1987). 'Evidence for early central nervous system involvement in AIDS and other HIV infections'. *Annals of Internal Medicine,* **107**, 828–36.

Holland, J.C. and Tross, S. (1985). 'The psychosocial and neuropsychiatric sequelae of AIDS and related disorders'. *Annals of Internal Medicine,* **103**, 760–64.

Hollander, H.R. and Levy, J.A. (1987). 'Neurologic abnormalities and recovery of HIV from cerebrospinal fluid'. *Annals of Internal Medicine,* **106**, 692–5.

King, M.B. (1990). 'Psychological aspects of HIV Infection and AIDS: What have we learned?'. *British Journal of Psychiatry,* **156**, 151–6.

Lechtenberg, R. and Sher, J.H. (1988). *AIDS in the Nervous System.* New York, Churchill Livingstone.

Marzuk, P.M. *et al.* (1988). 'Increased risk of suicide in persons with AIDS'. *Journal of the American Medical Association,* **259**, 1333–7.

Navia, B.A. *et al.* (1986). 'The AIDS dementia complex: 1. Clinical features'. *Annals of Neurology,* **19**, 517–24.

Rundell, J.R. *et al.* (1986). 'Three cases of AIDS related psychiatric disorders'. *American Journal of Psychiatry,* **143**, 777–8.

Schmidt, U. and Miller, D. (1988). 'Two cases of hypomania in AIDS'. *British Journal of Psychiatry,* **152**, 839–42.

Snider, W.D. *et al.* (1983). 'Neurological complications of AIDS: Analysis of 50 patients'. *Annals of Neurology,* **14**, 403–18.

Thomas, C.S. (1987). HIV and schizophrenia (letter to the editor). *Lancet,* **ii**, 101.

FIVE

The current epidemiology of HIV infection and AIDS

DAVID WILKIE

An inevitable problem about preparing a statistical chapter for a book on a subject such as HIV and AIDS is that the statistical facts are changing so rapidly that they may be out of date by the time the book is published, let alone read. Here, however, the information is as up-to-date as possible at the date of writing, January 1991.

In this chapter the current statistics about AIDS and HIV infection in the UK are discussed first, followed by sections about the numbers of AIDS cases in the USA, the world position and the rest of Europe. (Published information about the numbers of reported HIV positive individuals in countries other than the UK is not readily available.) There follows some discussion about suitable ways of forecasting the likely number of future cases of AIDS and the number of people infected with HIV. Reference is then made to two reports on forecasting AIDS and HIV infection in England and Wales, the Cox Report (1988) and the Day Report (1990).

It should be noted that, although medical opinion now considers that there is not necessarily a clear-cut distinction between someone with AIDS and an individual with HIV-related illness who is not classified as having AIDS, for statistical purposes a clear, if arbitrary, distinction is made according to a definition of AIDS put out by the Centers for Disease Control in the USA.

The way that AIDS has spread differs in different countries. The World Health Organization (WHO) has described three patterns: in Pattern I countries the main spread is among homosexual men, and a secondary spread is among injecting drug users; in Pattern II countries, the main spread is among heterosexuals; in Pattern III countries, there has so far been very little spread at all. North America and Western Europe, including the UK, have followed Pattern I; parts of Africa and the Caribbean have followed Pattern II; Eastern Europe, Asia and the Near East have so far followed Pattern III. These are not precise categories, but they give some indication of the variations.

United Kingdom

In the UK, statistics about AIDS are recorded separately for England, Wales and Northern Ireland by the Communicable Diseases Surveillance Centre (CDSC), which is part of the Public Health Laboratory Service (PHLS), and for Scotland by the Communicable Diseases (Scotland) Unit [CD(S)U]. Although reporting of cases of AIDS, and of deaths from AIDS, is done voluntarily by doctors, it is believed that most identified AIDS cases are reported. Microbiologists at public and private laboratories also report the number of persons found to be HIV antibody positive when tested. Reports of tests carried out are fairly complete, but it is possible that there are a great many more HIV antibody positive persons than have ever been tested.

A total of 4098 cases of AIDS had been reported in the UK up to the end of December 1990. Of these, 2256 (55%) are known to have died.

The number of newly reported cases of AIDS, and newly reported deaths from AIDS, in each year from 1982 to 1990 is shown in Table 5.1, along with the percentage increase in these numbers in each year. From 1983 to 1987 the number of newly reported cases roughly doubled each year. In 1988 and 1989, the percentage increases were 16 and 12% respectively. In 1990 the percentage increase rose to 50%.

Table 5.1   Reported cases of AIDS and deaths from AIDS in the UK

Year	Cases	% increase	Deaths	% increase
To 1982	3		0	
1983	26		15	
1984	77	196	40	167
1985	160	108	85	112
1986	305	91	153	80
1987	653	114	404	164
1988	758	16	362	−10
1989	848	12	553	53
1990	1268	50	644	16
Totals	4098		2256	

The number of newly reported deaths also doubled each year from 1983 to 1987. There was then a fall in the new deaths reported in 1988, probably caused by time-lags in reporting, followed by a 53% increase in 1989, which reflects a catch-up of reporting, and a 16% increase in 1990.

Reporting delays

There may be a considerable delay between the date that a case of AIDS is diagnosed and the date that it is reported to CDSC. Some of this delay occurs because the paperwork necessarily takes a little time to complete, but some may occur because reporting hospitals and doctors leave reports to accumulate until there is sufficient time to deal with them. It is less easy to explain why some cases are first reported to PHLS as much as 4 years after the apparent date of diagnosis!

A table in the Day Report (1990) shows that, in England and Wales, excluding visitors, of 217 cases diagnosed in 1985 and reported by the end of September 1989, only 114 (53%) had been reported by the end of 1985, with a further 63 (29%) reported in 1986, 36 (17%) in 1987 and 4 more in 1988 and the first 9 months of 1989. Of the 415 cases diagnosed in 1986 only 209 (50%) had been reported in 1986, with 164 (40%) reported in 1987, a further 39 (9%) in 1988, and 3 in the first 3 months of 1989. Thus, whatever the numbers reported by any date, there are almost certainly a considerable number of cases already diagnosed, not yet reported, but 'in the reporting pipeline'. Similar delays in reporting must occur for deaths, but the data published by PHLS do not allow the delays to be estimated.

There are further problems when figures for different countries are compared, as in the statistics published by WHO. There is a delay between the national reporting body preparing its figures, and WHO receiving them. In some cases the delays are very great.

Distribution by 'risk category' and by sex

Reported AIDS cases are classified by 'risk category' and the distribution of cases in the UK reported up to 31 December 1990 classified in this way is given in Table 5.2, together with the percentage of the total in each risk category. It can be seen that over 79% of cases (3234 cases) had occurred among homosexual and bisexual men, with quite small numbers in other risk categories. The next largest group was heterosexual contact cases (268 cases,

Table 5.2 Distribution of cases of AIDS reported by 31 December 1990 in the UK

Risk category	Cases	%
Homosexual or bisexual men	3234	79
Injecting drug users	161	4
Homo/bisexual and IDU	61	1
Haemophiliac	228	6
Blood transfusion recipient	67	2
Heterosexual partner	268	6
Mother to child	36	1
Other and undetermined	43	1
Totals	4098	100

6% of the total), followed by 228 haemophiliacs, and 161 cases among injecting drug users (222 if the 61 cases who were both drug users and homosexual
or bisexual are included).

In Table 5.3 the same figures are shown, further subdivided, with the
numbers for males and females, and the numbers of deaths and the percentage
of cases whose deaths had been reported. The overall percentage dead so far of
55% is typical of most groups, with a few exceptions. However, among
haemophiliacs 68% had died, and among transfusion cases 67%; this may
reflect the early dates when these cases occurred, or may reflect poorer survival prospects for such cases. It is possible that some of those in need of blood
transfusions had some disability other than AIDS that caused their death.

Table 5.3   Distribution of cases of AIDS reported by 31 December 1990 in the UK

Risk category	Males	Females	Total	Dead	% dead
Homosexual or bisexual men	3234	—	3234	1789	55
Injecting drug users	123	38	161	70	43
Homo/bisexual and IDU	61	—	61	32	52
Haemophiliac	225	3	228	156	68
Blood transfusion recipient					
abroad	13	24	37	23	62
UK	16	14	30	22	73
Heterosexual contact					
partner(s) with above risk factor	11	23	34	19	56
others					
known exposure abroad	145	63	208	93	49
no evidence of exposure abroad	13	13	26	9	35
Mother to child	15	21	36	15	42
Other and undetermined	39	4	43	28	65
Totals	3895	203	4098	2256	55

Of the total 4098 cases, only 203 (5%) had occurred among females, of
whom 99 (49%) had died. The largest group among females were those with
heterosexual contact, 99 cases (49%). Other significant groups were injecting
drug users (38 cases) and those who had received blood transfusions (38 cases).

During 1990, there were 123 new cases of AIDS among those with hetero-sexual contact, as compared with 69 in 1989 – an increase of 78%. Among injecting drug users, there were 81 new cases in 1990, as compared with 41 in 1989 – an increase of 98%. The numbers of cases in these two groups have increased much more than the numbers among other groups.

It may be noted that 30 out of the 67 blood transfusion cases (of both sexes) had received blood abroad, and that 208 out of the 268 heterosexual cases had 'exposure abroad'. Contact abroad may seem to be a significant route for the transmission of HIV infection. However, the total figures include a number of visitors who have perhaps come to the UK for treatment, and this may confuse the picture. This is also the case in Belgium, where a high proportion of the early reported cases had apparently come from Zaïre (the former Belgian Congo) for treatment.

HIV antibody positive reports

Reports of persons testing HIV antibody positive are collected by PHLS from public and private laboratories in the UK. A total of 15 166 such reports had been received by the end of December 1990. The numbers of reports in successive years, in England and Wales plus the Channel Islands, from 1985 to 1990 are shown in Table 5.4. After an initial spate in 1985 and 1986, the numbers fell in 1987 and 1988, rising slightly in 1989. The large number of reports during 1990 is partly attributed by PHLS to 'backlog being cleared as the reporting system is refined and streamlined'. This makes it very difficult to see what the true trend is.

Table 5.4   New HIV antibody positive reports in England and Wales and the Channel Islands

Year	No.
Up to 1985	1 872
1986	2 338
1987	2 212
1988	1 680
1989	1 780
1990	3 128
Totals	13 010

It is not clear what proportion of HIV antibody positive persons in the UK population those numbers represent. Earlier estimates, such as those made in the Cox Report (1988), suggested that the number of persons in fact HIV antibody positive was much larger than the number of HIV positive tests reported. But because (a) the number of new HIV positive tests each year has not been rising (at least until 1990) and (b) the number of new AIDS cases has risen much more slowly than previously expected, it now seems likely that the number of individuals infected with HIV in the UK population is not as great as had been thought a few years ago, and hence is lower now than was forecast at that time.

On the other hand, it is possible that many people, particularly heterosexuals, are carrying HIV infection unsuspectingly, and it is also possible that some who might suspect that they may be infected prefer to avoid being tested, because of the possible adverse consequences of the knowledge that one is HIV antibody positive. The position is not clear.

One plausible way of obtaining more information about the numbers of individuals infected with HIV in the population would be widespread systematic testing of the population for HIV infection. This, however, has practical as well as ethical difficulties. It is not easy to find unbiased representative samples of people to test; and when the proportion in the total population who are HIV positive is very low, it would be necessary to test very large numbers of people in order to discover what the proportion was, or to measure the extent to which that proportion was changing.

Distribution of cases of AIDS by region

The reports of AIDS cases and of HIV antibody positive tests in England are classified by PHLS according to the Health Board Region in which the case or the test is reported. The numbers by country and by region within England are shown in Table 5.5, along with rates per 100 000 population (estimated by the author).

About 68% of cases come from the three out of the four Thames regions which cover London and the South East of England (North West, North East and South East Thames). In these three regions, the number of cases has been 25.9 per 100 000 population, as compared with 2.8 per 100 000 in the rest of the UK. Over the rest of the country (including South West Thames), the number of cases per 100 000 population is reasonably level, with a band of rather lower incidence stretching from East Anglia through the Midlands to Merseyside, Wales and Northern Ireland, and areas of rather higher incidence north and south of this.

The region from which the report comes, however, may not be where the person lives, since it is possible that a number of people with AIDS seek treatment in London where facilities may be thought to be better, and anonymity may be easier to protect.

HIV antibody positive reports

The numbers of HIV antibody positive reports in each country and in each Health Board Region in England and the estimated numbers per 100 000

Table 5.5 Distribution by country within the UK and by Health Board Region within England of cases of AIDS and of HIV antibody positive reports reported by 31 December 1990

Country/region	Cases	Deaths	HIV reports	Per 100 000 population Cases	Per 100 000 population HIV reports
Northern	83	46	357	2.7	11.6
Yorkshire	112	67	395	3.1	11.0
Trent	80	43	394	1.7	8.5
East Anglia	42	30	203	2.1	10.2
NW Thames	1621	797	4682	47.0	135.8
NE Thames	733	395	2507	19.5	66.7
SE Thames	453	275	1640	12.5	45.3
SW Thames	141	100	425	4.8	14.3
Wessex	94	62	318	3.3	11.1
Oxford	83	48	388	3.4	15.7
South Western	76	51	310	2.4	9.8
West Midlands	91	54	496	1.8	9.6
Mersey	52	37	190	2.2	7.9
North Western	156	95	680	3.9	17.0
England	3817	2100	12985	8.1	27.5
Wales	64	44	229	2.3	8.1
Scotland	195	93	1874	3.8	36.6
Northern Ireland	22	19	78	1.4	5.0
Channel Islands (CI)	4	4	25	—	—
Total UK + CI	4102	2260	15191	7.2	26.7

population are also shown in Table 5.5. The same contrast is evident between the same three Thames regions (where the number of reports per 100 000 is 81.5) and the rest of the country (11.0 per 100 000), excluding Scotland where a high number of HIV antibody positive reports have been made (36.6 per 100 000).

The reason for the particularly high number of HIV antibody positive reports from Scotland is known to be that a high proportion of injecting drug users in Edinburgh were infected through sharing needles, and that this group has been extensively tested. Detailed figures, however, are not published by PHLS to identify this.

USA

The first cases of AIDS officially identified were found in the USA in 1981. The epidemic first grew large in the USA and the number of cases reported there is almost as many as in the rest of the world put together. Statistics are published by the Centers for Disease Control (CDC), part of the US Department of Health and Human Services. The figures include US overseas territories such as Puerto Rico (where there is a considerable number of cases) and small Pacific islands (where there are very few).

It is worth considering the position in the USA in some detail, because there are so many cases of AIDS, the numbers in many subgroups are sufficiently large to be significant, and it is possible that the epidemic in other similar countries may develop in the same sort of way. However, the number of HIV infections reported in the USA are not published by CDC, and are not discussed here.

The total number of cases of AIDS reported in the USA by the end of November 1990 was 157 525, of whom 98 530 (63%) had been reported as dead. The number of cases diagnosed (*note:* cases are recorded by date of diagnosis rather than by date of report) in successive years from 1981 to 1990 (first 11 months) among these reported cases is shown in Table 5.6. It can be seen that the numbers in the early years of the epidemic roughly doubled each year, but since 1986 there has been a slowing in the rate of increase. It must be remembered, however, that there are delays in reporting in the USA as in the UK, and that the number of cases that will eventually be reported as having been diagnosed in 1989 and 1990 will be larger than the numbers shown in the table.

Table 5.6   Cases of AIDS and deaths reported by 30 November 1990 in the USA, classified by year of diagnosis and by year of death

Year	Cases diagnosed	Deaths occurred
Up to 1980	84	31
1981	305	131
1982	1 110	449
1983	2 967	1 461
1984	5 992	3 346
1985	11 223	6 610
1986	18 210	11 308
1987	27 016	15 191
1988	32 339	19 240
1989	35 198	24 264
1990 (to Nov.)	23 081	16 338
Date of death unknown	—	161
Totals	157 525	98 530

The numbers actually reported in the 12 months ending November 1990 were 42 442, which was 19% higher than the numbers reported during the previous 12 months (35 614).

USA distribution by 'risk category' and by sex

The distribution of cases of AIDS in the USA by 'risk category' and by sex, as at 30 November 1990, is shown in Table 5.7. As in the UK, homosexual and bisexual men form the largest risk category (58%), but injecting drug users form a much larger proportion than in the UK, at 21%. There is a further 7% that falls into both these categories. The other groups form small proportions, but (relative to the UK) large enough numbers to be significant. The proportion of heterosexual contact cases is much larger than in the UK, at 5%; about half of these are recorded as having had sex with an intravenous (IV) drug user.

Table 5.7 Distribution of cases of AIDS reported by 30 November 1990 in the USA

Risk category	Males	Females	Children[a]	Total	%
Homosexual or bisexual men	92 049	—	—	92 049	58
Injecting drug users	25 995	7 699	—	33 694	21
Homo/bisexual and IDU	10 356	—	—	10 356	7
Haemophiliac	1 327	33	138	1 498	1
Blood transfusion recipient	2 222	1 402	250	3 874	3
Heterosexual contact partner(s) with above risk factors	1 282	3 762	—	5 044	3
others known exposure abroad	1 544	600	—	2 144	1
no evidence of exposure abroad	434	582	—	1 016	1
Mother to child	—	—	2 280	2 280	1
Other and undetermined	4 449	1 055	66	5 570	4
Totals	139 658	15 133	2 734	157 525	100

[a] 'Children' are those less than 13 years old.

There have been over 15 000 cases of AIDS among adult and adolescent females (aged 13 and over), which is 10% of the total adult and adolescent cases. Over half these cases have been found among IV drug users (7699 cases or 51%). A further 33% (4944 cases) are recorded as coming from heterosexual contact, of which 76% (3762 cases) are attributed to sex with a partner in one of the primary risk groups. A further number (600 cases) are attributed to persons born in a 'Pattern II' country (roughly Africa and the Caribbean) or who had sex with a person born in a Pattern II country. Only 582 women (4% of the females) had been infected sexually from a person not in one of those risk groups. This is greater than the number of men so infected (434, or 0.3% of the males).

Paediatric cases

In the USA, paediatric cases of AIDS are defined as those among children less than 13 years old. Up to 30 November 1990, there had been 2734 such cases reported. Apart from 138 cases among those with haemophilia or other coagulation disorders, who were mostly boys, the cases appear to be roughly equally divided among boys and girls. About 9% (250 cases) were in receipt of blood transfusions, blood components or tissues.

The majority of paediatric cases (2280 or 83%) acquired HIV from a mother who was infected with HIV herself. The distribution of the mothers among risk categories is quite similar to that of females with AIDS. More than half of them were IV drug users and a further 21% had had sex with an IV drug user.

Around the world

Statistics of the total number of cases of AIDS recorded in each country in the world are collected and published by WHO. The figures published by WHO at any given date are those which have been reported to WHO by that date and may well not be the numbers reported in the country concerned by that date. For example, the number of cases reported from the UK as at 31 December 1990 was 3884, which was the number reported to PHLS by 31 October 1990. There is always a lag of 1–2 months, such as this one, but the reporting authorities in some countries have at times been many months behind in their reporting to WHO; so the figures, and in particular changes in the figures, must be treated with caution.

Table 5.8 shows the number of cases of AIDS reported to WHO by 31 December 1990 (in general, therefore, those cases reported nationally by 31 October or 30 November 1990) in the 27 countries for which more than 1000 cases have been reported. The USA is well ahead with 154791 cases. Uganda, Brazil and Zaïre have reported over 10000 cases, France nearly 10000, Kenya over 9000, and several over 7000. The UK is fifteenth on the list. Of these 27 countries, 10 are 'developed', 12 are in Africa, 2 (Haiti and the Dominican Republic) are in the Caribbean, and the remaining 3 are Brazil, Mexico and Romania.

Table 5.8 also shows the estimated populations of those countries as at 31 May 1990 and the number of cases per 100000 population (provided by C.D. Daykin, personal communication). There is a considerable variation in these rates, from 96.1 per 100000 in Congo to 4.5 per 100000 in Romania.

It is not surprising that countries with larger populations report a greater number of cases, so Table 5.9 shows selected countries ranked according to the number of cases per 100000 population, including all those with more

Table 5.8   WHO reports: Countries with more than 1000 cases of AIDS reported to WHO by 31 December 1990

Rank	Country	No. of AIDS cases reported	Estimated population (millions)	Cases per 100 000 population
1	USA	154 791	250.0	61.9
2	Uganda	17 422	18.7	93.0
3	Brazil	12 405	151.6	8.2
4	Zaïre	11 732	36.5	32.1
5	France	9 718	56.3	17.3
6	Kenya	9 139	25.6	35.7
7	Italy	7 576	57.3	13.2
8	Malawi	7 160	8.6	83.7
9	Tanzania	7 128	27.8	25.6
10	Spain	7 047	39.4	17.9
11	Germany	5 500	77.2	7.1
12	Zimbabwe	5 249	9.9	53.3
13	Mexico	5 113	89.4	5.7
14	Canada	4 427	26.6	16.6
15	UK	3 884	57.0	6.8
16	Ivory Coast	3 647	12.8	28.4
17	Zambia	3 494	8.6	40.6
18	Rwanda	3 407	7.3	46.4
19	Burundi	3 305	5.5	59.9
20	Haiti	2 456	6.6	37.5
21	Australia	2 295	16.8	13.6
22	Congo	1 940	2.0	96.1
23	Ghana	1 732	15.2	11.4
24	Switzerland	1 548	6.5	23.7
25	Netherlands	1 487	14.8	10.1
26	Dominican Republic	1 423	7.2	19.7
27	Romania	1 055	23.3	4.5

than 20.0 cases per 100 000 (of which there are also 27), as well as all those in the first list.

Of the top 27 in the second list, only two (the USA and Switzerland) are 'developed', 12 are in Africa and 13 are in the Caribbean. Most of the developed countries drop down the list, with the UK falling to 57th. The very small numbers recorded from some Caribbean countries make the rates unreliable, but the accumulation of Caribbean countries in the list is significant. Most of the African countries in the lists are in Central and East Africa. West Africa is represented only by Ghana and the Ivory Coast. Rates in southern Africa, except in Zimbabwe, are low, and rates in North Africa almost zero.

The reported numbers of cases of AIDS and rates per 100 000 population

Table 5.9   WHO reports: Selected countries ranked by number of AIDS cases per 100 000 population reported to WHO by 31 December 1990

Rank	Country	No. of AIDS cases reported	Estimated population (thousands)	Cases per 100 000 population
1	Bermuda	147	58	252.7
2	French Guiana	232	94	246.2
3	Bahamas	554	251	220.9
4	Turks and Caicos	8	8	100.0
5	Congo	1 940	2 019	96.1
6	Uganda	17 422	18 740	93.0
7	Malawi	7 160	8 555	83.7
8	USA	154 791	249 982	61.9
9	Burundi	3 305	5 522	59.9
10	Guadelope	195	341	57.3
11	Anguilla	4	7	57.1
12	Barbados	145	262	55.4
13	Trinidad and Tobago	693	1 292	53.7
14	Zimbabwe	5 249	9 857	53.3
15	Rwanda	3 407	7 345	46.4
16	Martinique	142	332	42.8
17	Zambia	3 494	8 599	40.6
18	Haiti	2 456	6 558	37.5
19	St Christopher	18	48	37.4
20	Kenya	9 139	25 606	35.7
21	Zaïre	11 732	36 512	32.1
22	Ivory Coast	3 647	12 823	28.4
23	Cayman Islands	6	22	27.2
24	Tanzania	7 128	27 792	25.6
25	Switzerland	1 548	6 524	23.7
26	St Vincent	26	110	23.5
27	Central African Republic	662	2 946	22.5
28	Dominican Republic	1 423	7 232	19.7
31	Spain	7 047	39 394	17.9
32	France	9 718	56 258	17.3
33	Canada	4 427	26 612	16.6
40	Australia	2 295	16 825	13.6
41	Italy	7 576	57 344	13.2
44	Ghana	1 732	15 230	11.4
47	Netherlands	1 487	14 773	10.1
52	Brazil	12 405	151 594	8.2
56	Germany	5 500	77 157	7.1
57	UK	3 884	56 955	6.8
66	Mexico	5 113	89 379	5.7
73	Romania	1 055	23 317	4.5

are low throughout Eastern Europe (except in Romania), the Near East and Asia, and in South America other than in Brazil and the Guianas (French Guiana, Surinam and Guyana). It was discovered during 1990 that quite large numbers of children had been infected with HIV in Romania (see below), and recent press reports suggest that the incidence of HIV infection among prostitutes in Thailand is rising quite rapidly. It may be the case that HIV infection has not yet reached many countries, rather than that they will escape it.

The published WHO figures do not identify the distribution of cases by transmission category or by sex, but it is suggested that in most of the African and Caribbean countries approximately equal numbers of males and females are affected, and the transmission is presumed to be mainly heterosexual. It has also been suggested that the presence of other genital infections may facilitate the transmission of HIV in these countries, but one cannot conclude this from the WHO figures.

Europe

AIDS statistics for Europe are collected by the European Centre for the Epidemiological Monitoring of AIDS (ECEMA) in Paris. The health authorities of 32 countries assist by contributing data, and a report is published quarterly. For this chapter, the data for 30 September 1990 are available. By that date, a total of 41 549 cases of AIDS had been reported – 35 610 (86%) males and 5939 (14%) females – which included 1873 (4.5%) paediatric cases (aged less than 13 years).

The countries of Western Europe fall into the WHO Pattern I description, with infection being predominantly among homosexuals and IV drug users; the countries of Eastern Europe fall mostly into Pattern III, with rather few cases so far, except in Romania. Table 5.10 shows the total number of cases reported to ECEMA by 30 September 1990 for the 18 countries for which more than 100 cases had been reported, together with the rate per 100 000 population, the number of cases reported in 1989, and the percentage increase in the number of new cases reported in 1988. It can be seen that the number of cases per 100 000 population is greatest in Switzerland, Spain, France, Italy and Denmark, and that the rate of increase in 1989 was highest in Spain (79% increase year over year), Norway (50%) and Italy (44%). The UK had the lowest rate of increase in 1989 (12%), along with Yugoslavia (13%) and Belgium (17%).

Table 5.11 shows the percentage distribution of reported cases by transmission group. There is a clear northern European cluster, including Norway, Sweden, Denmark, the Netherlands, Germany and the UK, in which over 70% of cases have been among homosexual and bisexual men, leaving rather few in any other group. At the other extreme, in Spain and Italy over 60% of cases are reported to be among IV drug users, while Switzerland, Yugoslavia and Ireland have over 30% in this group.

Table 5.10   Cases of AIDS and rates per 100 000 population for European countries with more than 100 cases reported to ECEMA by 30 September 1990. Also numbers of new cases reported in 1989 and percentage increase over 1988

Country	Total AIDS cases reported	Cases per 100 000 population	New AIDS cases reported, 1989	% increase over new cases, 1988
Switzerland	1 497	22.5	457	31.7
Spain	7 047	18.1	2 468	79.4
France[a]	9 718	17.3	3 228	25.0
Italy	7 576	13.2	2 299	44.0
Denmark	663	12.9	160	23.1
Netherlands	1 443	9.7	380	38.7
West Germany	5 266	8.5	1 527	37.6
Belgium	764	7.7	172	17.0
UK	3 798	6.6	848	12.3
Austria	474	6.2	133	37.1
Yugoslavia	147	6.2	44	12.8
Sweden	487	5.7	124	33.3
Portugal	481	4.7	149	36.7
Ireland	161	4.6	50	22.0
Romania[b]	999	4.3	—	—
Norway	176	4.2	45	50.0
Greece	375	3.7	107	30.4
Israel	125	2.7	—	—

[a] France up to 31 March 1990.

[b] The definition of AIDS used in Romania differs from that in other countries; most of these cases were not reported until 1990.

Belgium is exceptional, in that 44% of cases are attributed to heterosexual transmission, but it has been suggested that many of these cases are among people from Zaïre who have sought treatment in Belgium. In Greece and Portugal over 20% of cases are reported to be among heterosexuals; this is not associated with a particularly high proportion of drug users.

The proportion of cases among haemophiliacs, those suffering from other coagulative disorders and transfusion recipients is highest in those countries in which the total prevalence of AIDS is low. This is just a consequence of low numbers in other groups in these countries.

The ECEMA reports do not subdivide cases for individual countries by sex, but an indication of the numbers of women with AIDS can be obtained from the proportions of mother-to-child cases reported. The numbers of such cases are highest in France (194 cases), Spain (181 cases) and Italy (164 cases), with smaller numbers in Belgium (45 cases), Germany (34 cases), the UK (28 cases), Romania (28 cases) and Switzerland (26 cases). These are mostly still small numbers.

Table 5.11 Percentage of AIDS cases in selected transmission groups for European countries with more than 100 cases reported to ECEMA by 30 September 1990

Country	% cases in transmission group						
	Homo/bi-sexual	IDU	Homo/bi-+ IDU	Hetero-sexual	Haemo + Trans	Mother to child	Others, unknown
Switzerland	46	34	2	12	2	2	2
Spain	17	63	3	4	5	3	5
France[a]	52	19	2	11	9	2	6
Italy	15	66	3	6	3	2	5
Denmark	78	4	1	8	4	1	4
Netherlands	80	8	1	5	3	0	2
West Germany	70	13	1	3	7	1	6
Belgium[b]	35	3	1	44	9	6	3
UK	79	4	2	6	8	1	1
Austria	45	28	1	7	10	2	8
Yugoslavia	22	36	0	12	21	1	6
Sweden	72	3	1	12	12	1	1
Portugal	45	11	1	28	10	0	5
Ireland	40	34	4	4	11	4	2
Romania[c]	1	0	0	5	41	3	51
Norway	70	9	1	9	10	1	2
Greece	50	3	1	22	17	1	6
Israel	50	10	4	6	22	2	6

[a] France at 31 March 1990.
[b] Many cases in Belgium are ascribed to non-residents, possibly people from Zaïre seeking treatment.
[c] 94% of the cases in Romania (935 out of 999) are paediatric.

The position in Romania is exceptional. Most of the 999 cases reported so far were reported in 1990. Of the total, 935 are paediatric cases, many discovered just after the revolution of Christmas 1989. Many of these are attributed directly to infected transfusions, but the reason for more than half of them has not yet been identified. Further, the definition of AIDS used in Romania (the Bangui definition which is a clinical definition developed for countries with limited diagnostic resources) is different from that used elsewhere in Europe.

It can be seen from these figures that the position in each country in Europe is, in general, particular to that country. There is still a rapid increase in Spain and Italy, where IV drug users form a large proportion; but there has also been a sharp upturn in Norway, which otherwise fits the northern, predominantly homosexual pattern; and the rate of increase in Yugoslavia, which has a relatively high IV drug user proportion, has recently been quite low. Ireland does not fit the northern European pattern. France, with the largest numbers of all, has no particularly high proportion in any transmission group, though still over half the cases are among homosexual men.

The age distribution of cases of AIDS

Figures are available for the USA, for all 32 European countries combined, and for the UK, showing the distribution of AIDS cases by age at diagnosis, for each sex separately. These are shown in Table 5.12. The percentage distribution in the main transmission groups, among adult and adolescent cases only, for each sex in the USA, and in the 32 European countries combined, is shown in Table 5.13.

Table 5.12   Percentage of AIDS cases in age groups, by sex, for USA (reported by 30 November 1990), for 32 European countries (reported by 30 September 1990) and for the UK (reported by 30 June 1990)

Age group (years)	USA		Europe (inc. UK)		UK	
	Males	Females	Males	Females	Males	Females
Under 5	1	7	3	13	0	1
5–12	0	1	0	1	0	2
13–19	0	1	1	1	1	3
20–24	4	6	7	16	5	17
25–29	16	19	22	31	16	23
30–34	24	25	21	17	21	19
35–39	22	19	16	7	21	15
40–49	22	13	19	5	26	14
50+	11	10	10	8	11	6
Totals	100	100	100	100	100	100
No. of cases	141 131	16 394	35 610	5 939	3 130	132

It can be seen that, in each territory, and for both sexes, the great majority of cases of AIDS have been at young adult ages, with smaller proportions of cases below age 20, and few above age 50. Within this general pattern, however, there are differences. The peak age group for females in Europe is 25–29, with 31% of cases, and the span from 20 to 34 covers 64% of all cases. For females in the USA, the peak ages are 5 years older, with 25% in the 30–34 group and 63% in the span from 25 to 39. The UK is intermediate between Europe and the USA.

Males with AIDS in the USA are a little older than the corresponding females, with a broader peak from 30 to 39, and over 84% in the span from 25 to 49. In Europe, males are younger than in the USA, but older than females in Europe, with a peak from 25 to 34. The UK is closer to the USA.

Table 5.13   Percentages of AIDS cases in main transmission groups among adults/adolescents, by sex, for USA (reported by 30 November 1990) and for 32 European countries (reported by 30 September 1990)

Risk group	USA		Europe (inc. UK)	
	Males	*Females*	*Males*	*Females*
Homo/bisexual	66	—	53	—
IDU	19	51	30	57
Homo/bi and IDU	7	—	2	—
Haemophiliac	1	0	3	0
Blood transfusion	2	9	2	11
Heterosexual	3	33	5	27
Other and undetermined	2	7	5	5
Totals	100	100	100	100
No. of cases	139 658	15 133	34 558	5 111

It is not surprising that the males with AIDS in Europe are younger than those in the USA, since the proportion of injecting drug users among the AIDS cases is higher in Europe than in the USA (30% as compared with 19%), and drug users appear to be younger than homosexual men. It is, however, surprising that females with AIDS in Europe are younger than those in the USA, since the proportion of drug users among them is rather closer (57% compared with 51%).

Forecasting the future of the AIDS epidemic

Various ways of forecasting the numbers of future cases of HIV infection, and of AIDS, have been developed by epidemiologists. Some of their 'forecasts' are better described as 'projections', since they purport to show what might happen if some particular set of circumstances persisted or occurred ('what if . . .' scenarios), rather than being forecasts of the most likely future development.

There are three main ways in which projections have been made. The first is by a simple (or perhaps complicated) mathematical projection of existing trends, perhaps taking account of plausible changes in the course of the epidemic, but not attempting to model the underlying nature of the epidemic. The crudest of these approaches is the 'constant doubling time' approach. In the early years of the epidemic, the numbers of new cases roughly doubled each year. The numbers in future years can easily be calculated if this trend is assumed to continue, but it is soon seen that the numbers escalate ridiculously, so that within a number of years the whole population is infected. This seems implausible, and other more suitable methods of this type, in which the compound rate of increase reduces as time goes by, are appropriate. While such methods may be useful for very short-term forecasts, they are not suitable for any long-term projections. They do not allow systematically for any particular changes in human behaviour, in the nature of the disease, or in the possible treatment of it.

A related method is the so-called 'back-casting' method. From reports of the numbers of cases of AIDS, and with further assumptions about the length of the incubation period, it is possible to make estimates of the numbers, who must have been infected with HIV in previous years from among whom the present new cases of AIDS have developed. From these estimates of those infected with HIV, it is possible to give a good forecast of the minimum number of new cases of AIDS in the next few years. However, since this method provides no estimates of the numbers of new HIV infections occurring now or in future years, it has limited long-term applicability.

The transmission dynamics of HIV infection

A more satisfactory method of making long-term projections, and of understanding the 'transmission dynamics' of HIV infection, is through an epidemiological transmission model. All such models have the same underlying principle, though they differ considerably in the amount of detail they attempt to represent. For example, some models consider only homosexual transmission, others only heterosexual. Each is suitable for use in certain countries, but neither represents the interaction of homosexual men, bisexual men, drug users of both sexes and their various heterosexual partners. Some models have included many of these features, but they then suffer from lack of good data about how different groups interact, either socially or sexually.

Some of the information that is required to construct a good transmission mdoel is reasonably readily available. In developed countries, there are good statistics about the numbers of the existing population, their distribution by age and by sex, and about the likely birth and death rates (in the absence of HIV infection) in future years.

For those who have developed AIDS, there are good records of the average period from diagnosis to death, and the distribution of survival times, subdivided by age and sex, by transmission category, and by the symptoms that first manifest themselves. The average survival time overall seems to be rather over a year; about half those who develop AIDS die within 1 year, about half the survivors die in the second year, and so on. There are still some survivors after 5, 6 or 7 years, but not more than would have been expected on this basis. This survival time pattern may have been lengthened but the evidence is not yet clear.

Much is known about the statistics of the period from becoming infected with HIV to being diagnosed with AIDS. However, because the disease was only identified relatively recently, only the pattern of the first 10 years or so of the 'incubation period' is understood. Surveys such as the San Francisco study (Rutherford *et al.*, 1990) show that about 54% of those infected with HIV have developed AIDS within 11 years of the infection, and the development has been at a steadily increasing rate during that period, with about 8% after 4 years, 20% after 6 years, 37% after 8 years and 51% after 10 years. What will happen to those who have reached 11 years, and who have not yet shown symptoms, is not known. Only time will show, but epidemiologists have had to make some sort of estimates, based usually on the continuation of a steadily increasing rate of development of AIDS.

The Cox Report projections

In March 1988, a group of epidemiological experts, under the chairmanship of Sir David Cox, was appointed to advise the Chief Medical Officers of England and Wales on the probable course over the next 2–5 years of the epidemic of AIDS and HIV infection. The group reported in December 1988.

The group estimated the number of those infected with HIV by direct assessment of HIV positive reports, rated up to allow for the estimated proportions of each sub-group of the population. They estimated that there were between 20000 and 50000 individuals infected with HIV in England and Wales at the end of 1987. This figure was found to be consistent with the results of some of the models of the transmission of the disease also considered by the group.

A number of different methods of forecasting the number of new cases of AIDS was used, including mathematical projection and transmission models. When different assumptions were used, it was possible to reproduce the first few years of the epidemic, for which figures were known reliably, and yet to produce very different forecasts for the future, even within a few years. Using mathematical models, the range of predictions of new AIDS cases to be diagnosed for 1992 ranged from an upper limit of 10700, resulting from the assumption of an unchanged doubling time, to a lower figure of 1590, assuming a particular type of mathematical function (a logistic function).

The range found by using transmission models was as great and depended critically on the assumptions made about the extent of changes in the behaviour of homosexual men and on when they might have taken place. One model (Wilkie A) looked at what might have happened if there had been no change in behaviour and gave a projection of 12097 new AIDS cases in 1992. Another (Wilkie E) assumed significant changes in behaviour from 1984 onwards, and gave a projection of 3490 new cases of AIDS in 1992. This projection also took account of the possible effectiveness of drugs such as AZT in delaying the deaths of those with AIDS.

The projections of new cases to be diagnosed in England and Wales in 1989 ranged from 1380 to 2577, with a range for 1990 of 1500–4417. Even the lowest of these now looks much too high, since the number of cases reported (*not* diagnosed) for the whole UK (not just England and Wales) for 1989 was only 848, and for 1990 was 1268 (see Table 5.1). The number eventually reported as having been diagnosed may turn out to be greater than this, but not considerably greater.

The fact that the numbers in the short term are much lower than predicted in the Cox Report does not necessarily mean that the epidemic will die away. The transmission models used for that report were based on homosexual men only, and did not take account of the separate (but interconnected) epidemics among drug users and heterosexuals. The authors of the report warned that a large-scale epidemic among drug users could lead to a rapid rise in the numbers of new cases, as has in fact occurred in Spain and Italy.

The Day Report projections

A working group with almost the same members as were involved with the Cox Report, but under the chairmanship of Professor Nicholas Day, reported in February 1990. Separate projections were made for different risk groups. The range for the total number of new cases of AIDS forecast for 1992 was narrower and lower than the Cox Report projections (1135–3275, with a preferred estimate of 2000 for 1992; and 1175–4825, with a preferred estimate of 2700 for 1993). However, the range for separate groups was very wide. Thus the estimate for injecting drug users for 1993 was from 50 to 1000, with a preferred estimate of 400, and for heterosexuals was from 50 to 1500, with a preferred estimate of 650.

One has to conclude that there is too little information available about the actual prevalence of HIV infection at present and about its rate of spread, particularly in what are at present 'smaller risk groups', for it to be possible to make any sort of reliable forecasts, even in the short term. However, the spread of HIV infection among the whole population in parts of Africa and in the Caribbean, the spread among drug users in parts of the USA, Spain and Italy, and the spread among women in the USA, should give one cause to think before assuming that the relatively low rate of increase of new cases in the UK means that the dangers of HIV infection have passed.

References and sources of information

Centres for Disease Control (CDC), US Department of Health and Human Services, *HIV/AIDS Surveillance*, monthly.

Cox, Sir David (Chairman) (1988). *Short-term Prediction of HIV Infections and AIDS in England and Wales*. Department of Health and Welsh Office, London, HMSO.

Day, Professor N.E. (Chairman) (1990). *Acquired Immune Deficiency Syndrome in England and Wales to end 1993: Projections Using Data to end September 1989*. PHLS, Communicable Diseases Report. London, HMSO.

Department of Health, Press release, *Quarterly (Monthly) AIDS Figures*.

European Centre for the Epidemiological Monitoring of AIDS, *AIDS Surveillance in Europe*, quarterly.

Rutherford, G.W. *et al.* (1990). 'Course of HIV-1 infection in a cohort of homosexual and bisexual men: An 11-year follow-up study'. *British Medical Journal*, **301**, 1183–8.

World Health Organization, *Update: AIDS Cases Reported to Surveillance, Forecasting and Impact Assessment Unit (SFI) Global Program on AIDS*, monthly.

Coping with HIV

SIX

Giving information, handling information

CHARLES ANDERSON

Introduction

This chapter focuses on information giving within the context of a one-to-one interview, although some of the discussion should also be of value to helpers and trainers who work with small groups or are involved in different types of outreach work within the community. At the end of the chapter, a set of guidelines is provided on the general areas that helpers need to be well informed about, but the chapter itself does not set out to be a compendium of all possible answers to common questions concerning HIV and AIDS. It is concerned rather with looking at general issues which apply across a whole range of enquiries. The emphasis is on looking at *how* best to communicate information about HIV and AIDS, and on the need for workers to achieve clarity concerning their personal goals in giving information about HIV.

The first general issue that I want to examine is an aspect of information giving that is often neglected – the need for helpers to use the power that comes from their possession of knowledge about HIV responsibly.

Using power responsibly

Exploring the effects of personal beliefs

Within the area of HIV, there is the possibility that there may be an important inequality in power between a helper and a client which arises from the fact that the helper has a wider knowledge base concerning HIV infection and associated matters than the client. Many writers on the social aspects of HIV have stressed that 'the facts about HIV and AIDS' do not represent some unquestionable reality, but are the products of complex processes of social construction. Helpers who wish to make responsible use of the power which comes from their knowledge concerning HIV, need to look carefully at the ways in which they themselves interpret 'the facts about HIV' and the ways in which they represent aspects of HIV to their clients.

In particular, helpers need to scrutinize their own practice to ensure that the information that they are providing to individuals is not being unduly affected by strongly held convictions of their own concerning certain HIV-related issues. It is possible that as a result of our own beliefs, concerning say the desirability or undesirability of being tested for HIV antibodies, or our advocacy of a particular experimental treatment for HIV infection, that we may be slanting information in a way which does not allow an enquirer to have a fair chance of making his or her own decisions on the matter.

Within a training group, prospective helpers can be provided with the opportunity to examine their own convictions concerning particular aspects of HIV and to consider how these convictions may influence the way in which they give information.

Looking at implicit, or explicit, beliefs about health education

It is a valuable exercise for any helpers beginning work in the area of HIV to examine their implicit theories about how best to give information. It is also helpful for established workers in the area of HIV to clarify the implicit beliefs which are guiding their practice, and to look at the relation between any explicitly held beliefs and day-to-day practice. Helpers may see themselves as 'experts' giving advice to enquirers. Alternatively, they may see themselves in the role of 'empowering' clients to make rational choices, as enabling clients to gain information, new skills and greater awareness of their own possibilities to make choices.

If a fairly democratic relationship is to be established between a helper and an enquirer, it would seem necessary for there to be a willingness to share knowledge about HIV in a full and open manner, if that is requested, rather than just answer individual questions. There also needs to be a willingness to hand over techniques and skills which may enable enquirers to exercise more control over their lives. When information is being given in a way which respects the enquirer's own capacity for decision making, he or she will not be 'told' how to act to protect his or her health. Rather sufficient information will be provided for people to be able to decide what are *realistic* choices, or changes of behaviour, for them personally.

The desire to reduce inequalities in power between helper and enquirer and to allow effective learning to take place also suggests the need for any enquirer to be given an active, participatory role in any information-giving exercise. Health education also needs to be tailored carefully to the personal experience and social and cultural background of individual clients, or groups of clients.

Although helpers may wish to enable enquirers to make rational choices, and to have the skills to protect themselves against HIV infection, they need at the same time to recognize that changing behaviour to avoid the risk of HIV infection may not be an easy matter. The next section of the chapter explores the barriers which some clients may face to making changes in their behaviour to protect themselves against HIV infection. It is also necessary to note that many of the enquiries about HIV and AIDS which a helper will encounter are not from people who are asking for information on how they may need to change their behaviour. Many enquiries are from people who wish a very specific piece of information, such as about travel restrictions to certain countries, or who have unfounded personal anxieties about AIDS that they wish to explore, or who wish to clear up uncertainties about some aspect of HIV infection.

Health education and behaviour change

Looking carefully at what constitutes 'rational' or 'irrational' behaviour

Providing people with sufficient information and helping them to develop new skills may very often enable them to make changes in their life which eliminate, or reduce, their chance of being exposed to HIV infection. However, it is recognized from long experience of work in areas of health promotion, such as stopping smoking and changing dietary habits, that individuals can find it very difficult to change health-related behaviours. There is no easy, direct correspondence between gaining information about a risk and implementing a change in behaviour. Helpers are required to be sensitive to the nature and the magnitude of changes in sexual behaviour that some clients may need to make to avoid the risk of HIV infection.

Given the serious, and potentially life-threatening, long-term consequences of HIV infection, it is tempting to label the feelings and motives which lead people to engage in 'unsafe' sexual or drug-using practices as 'irrational' or 'self-destructive'. Such a form of labelling may interfere with the provision of an appropriate helping response to people who are finding it difficult to change their behaviour to avoid the risk of HIV infection.

Viewed from the outside, actions which potentially may endanger life are likely to be seen as 'irrational' and as motivated by 'negative' forces, such as a lack of impulse control. However, effective helping requires that such actions are viewed from the perspective of the individual client's own world-view. Viewed in terms of an individual's own subjective experience, actions which carry a risk of HIV infection may be seen to have a rational motivation, albeit a rationality that is very different from that of the helper. 'Unsafe' sex may seem to offer the satisfaction of desire, and hold out the promise of security and love. The potential negative long-term consequences of 'risky' sexual behaviour may seem of lesser importance to an individual who perceives the future as anyway being a bit uncertain and unpromising.

A helper who wishes to assist an individual to change sexual or drug-taking behaviour to minimize the risk of HIV infection needs to appreciate the attractions that such behaviours may hold for the individual and the 'rational' motivations which may be guiding his or her actions. Unsafe sexual or drug-taking practices cannot simply be dismissed as acts motivated by irrational feelings and negative impulses. They must be seen in terms of the personal situation, motives and needs of the individual.

Factors which may influence changes in behaviour

Although much research is being conducted into people's beliefs concerning HIV, their understanding of HIV and its transmission, and changes in behaviour in response to HIV, we are still very far from being able to construct a satisfactory and sufficiently complex model of what motivates individuals to change their behaviour to avoid the risk of HIV infection.

A considerable number of studies on behaviour change in relation to HIV have been guided by the *health belief model* (Becker, 1974; Rosenstock, 1974). In attempting to account for individuals' readiness to act to change health-related behaviours, this model gives central importance to how individuals perceive both the *severity* of a possible health problem and their personal *susceptibility* to the health problem. The model also takes into account the effects on action of how people estimate the *costs* and *benefits* of adopting behaviours that will benefit their health. Another important element identi-fied in the model is the need for a *cue to action*, which signals the need to appraise and possibly change current behaviours.

The failure of the health belief model to give sufficient weight to the powerful emotional and social factors which influence behaviour change in the area of HIV limit its usefulness as an explanatory framework. However, it does point up some of the factors which may make changing behaviour difficult or unlikely. The preceding description of the model has indicated that it identifies perception of personal susceptibility as a key matter in deciding whether or not to make a change in health-related behaviour. The next section discusses how the particular ways in which HIV and AIDS have been presented in the media have led many individuals to see themselves as having very little susceptibility to HIV infection and, consequently, experience little need to change their behaviour.

The health belief model also draws attention to the perception of costs as well as the benefits which are involved in changing behaviour. It is important to note that even among individuals who have successfully changed their sexual behaviours to avoid the risk of HIV infection real psychological costs of change have been observed (Joseph *et al.*, 1989), and that change may involve actual as well as anticipated costs.

Even when individuals do see themselves as potentially susceptible to HIV infection, and are willing to shoulder the costs as well as receive the benefits which they perceive changes in behaviour will bring, change may not happen instantaneously. A number of researchers in the area of health promotion and change have drawn attention to the fact that individuals may need to pass through stages of changing attitudes and assimilating information before they make actual changes in their behaviour (see, for example, the discussion in Chapter 12).

Individuals who wish to make changes in their behaviour to eliminate, or reduce, the risk of HIV infection may need assistance in acquiring the social skills which will enable them to put the intention to protect themselves into practice. Acquiring new social skills may not be enough in itself, however, if the individuals do not possess a strong sense of self-efficacy, a firm belief in their own capacities to exercise personal control (Bandura, 1989). Individuals who do not possess a firm belief in their own capacity to exercise control in their everyday lives may require very careful counselling and considerable support to achieve a stronger sense of self-efficacy.

In much of the discussion of health education and behaviour changes in the are of HIV, attention is focused on how *individuals* perceive and respond to risk. It needs to be acknowledged that the perception of risk is to a very large degree determined by the individual's social and cultural context, and is not simply a matter of individual judgement. Risks are constructed in a complex fashion in terms of the values, beliefs, images and history of particular cultures; and sometimes 'risk' is defined more in terms of 'corruption', of the endangering of moral and social purity, than in terms of objective physical harm to individuals (Douglas and Wildavsky, 1982).

The ability of an individual to change behaviour to reduce the risk of HIV infection will be very much influenced by the general attitudes towards HIV and AIDS of the social and cultural group to which he or she belongs, and by the extent to which that group perceives HIV infection to be a threat. It is also well established that people pay much more attention to health education messages which they receive from lay or professional educators who share their social and cultural identity, educators with whom they can readily identify.

The rapid and very marked change towards safer sexual practices among gay men in large cities throughout the Western world was made possible not only by a generally high group perception of risk but also by energetic community-based health promotion initiatives and a supportive social environment. In contrast, when group perception of the risk of HIV infection is low and there is hostility to any changes in sexual behaviour, it may be very difficult for any one individual to attempt to make changes which will avoid the risk of HIV infection.

Power to influence events also tends to be unequally distributed among the individuals within a society. As Patricia Wilkie argues in Chapter 10, some women find themselves through no fault of their own in a position where it is very difficult for them to exercise personal control over their sex lives. It is important that helpers, who wish to provide appropriate information and assist clients to acquire the skills which will enable them to avoid the risk of HIV infection, do not underestimate the barriers to implementing and maintaining change which some clients may encounter. Helpers also need to be alert to the wide range of factors which may impede, or facilitate, changes in behaviour. One of these factors is the picture of HIV and AIDS which clients have gained from the media.

HIV, the media and lay beliefs concerning disease

Public health information campaigns

People who wish to become involved in a helping role in the area of HIV need to look carefully at how their work of giving information is affected by the way in which HIV and AIDS have been discussed and represented in health information campaigns and within the media in general. Looking first at government-sponsored health campaigns in the mass media, such campaigns as a side-effect may raise anxieties and the demand on professional and voluntary helpers for information.

The public health campaigns on HIV and AIDS that have been run in the UK have certainly served to heighten public awareness of HIV as an issue. However, these campaigns have been recognized to have a number of weaknesses. In particular, evaluations of those campaigns (such as the one with the slogan 'Don't die of ignorance'), which have relied on fear-inducing messages, have suggested that they had little effect on behaviour but may have brought about unnecessary fear and anxiety among the public (Nutbeam and Blakey, 1990). There has also been criticism of public health campaigns in general on the grounds that they have been too abstract to be meaningful, that they could have been more direct in their discussion of methods of transmission and ways of avoiding infection.

People have also encountered difficulties in dealing with what they see as conflicting accounts of the nature of HIV and its transmission between different health education campaigns and different media reports. For example, in their review of recent public health campaigns about HIV and AIDS in Scotland, Hastings *et al.* (1990) comment that: 'In Scotland, mass media campaigns from three different bodies have been run, each fulfilling different objectives. The result is that audiences are left with conflicting interpretations of the issues involved.' After a large-scale public health campaign, quite a lot of the work of information giving may be about correcting misconceptions, as much as providing a fuller, clearer account of the 'facts' about HIV and AIDS.

Representing and misrepresenting HIV in the media

The body of knowledge about HIV and AIDS is ever-changing, and some parts of it are somewhat complicated and not easy to interpret. As the last paragraph indicated, people may find it difficult to deal with conflicting statements about the nature of the disease and its transmission, and these difficulties may on occasion lead to scepticism about any public statements that are made about HIV, and a distrust of 'the experts'.

The difficulties that people may face in interpreting information about HIV have been greatly increased by the imprecise, or plain incorrect, use of terms in discussion of HIV within the media. For example, there is very often a failure to distinguish between *HIV*, as a transmissible infection, and *AIDS*, as a disease syndrome. Use of the term 'AIDS test' to describe HIV antibody testing is also common.

The use of the term 'risk groups' to distinguish constituencies where there is a higher risk of HIV infection than in the surrounding population is necessary within epidemiological studies of HIV infection and some other academic research. However, the widespread use of the term 'risk groups' within the press and television, and a concentration on the *social* identity of those at greatest risk of HIV infection, have had very undesirable consequences. This emphasis on risk groups rather than on practices which carry a risk of transmission of HIV has meant that individuals who do not see themselves as gay or as intravenous drug users can magnify their sense of invulnerability to HIV infection. When discussion is focused on 'risk groups' rather than 'risky practices', concern about HIV infection can on occasion serve as a front for the expression of homophobic or racist sentiments.

Chapter 1 drew attention to how the metaphors and images used to represent HIV and AIDS within the media can have a deeply damaging effect on people who are HIV antibody positive. The negative, highly charged images which have been used to represent AIDS and to stigmatize people with HIV infection have also made it more difficult to conduct a rational, humane public debate concerning the issues surrounding HIV infection. Similarly, the identification of 'innocent victims' of the disease, with the implied contrast with 'the guilty' who have 'brought it on themselves', has created difficulties for people with HIV infection and for achieving a rational public understanding of the nature of the transmission of the virus.

Allan M. Brandt has written in his study of the social history of venereal disease in the USA of how: 'AIDS, like other sexually transmitted diseases in the past, has been viewed as a fateful link between social deviance and the morally correct. Such fears have been exacerbated by an expectant media' (Brandt, 1987, p. 193). This association by some sections of the media of a fear-provoking medical problem with fears of moral disorder and social deviance has meant that health education work in this area needs to be concerned with combating prejudice, stigma and irrational fears as well as with providing information in a clear, appropriate manner.

Certain groups within the community have felt excluded from the public discussion of HIV and from official health education efforts. Lesbians, for example, have felt that they have been socially marginalized within the debate around issues concerning HIV and that their particular needs for education about safer sex have been ignored (see Chapter 10). It is also evident that ethnic minority groups within the UK have not always received sufficient health education concerning HIV, or health education that is culturally appropriate.

Lay health beliefs

The media also form one source of *lay beliefs* about the nature of disease in general, and of HIV in particular. It is now well recognized that people attempt to make sense of the experience of illness by actively interpreting it in terms of beliefs that are derived from a number of different sources – beliefs which on occasion may differ considerably from official medical explanations of the causes and means of transmission of disease (Fitzpatrick, 1984). An important source of lay beliefs are the traditional, 'pre-scientific' assumptions about the nature of disease that are found in all cultures, including the cultures of Western industrial nations. In the area of HIV, interesting research work by Warwick *et al.* (1988) has provided a description of a wide range of often sharply contrasting lay beliefs about HIV and its causes. They found that:

> With respect to AIDS, and in spite of recent government public information campaigns, young people continue to subscribe to miasmatic, endogenous, serendipitous and retributionist lay beliefs about its origins and modes of transmission. These may be influential in disorientating the impact of conventional approaches to health education which rely on information-giving as a strategy by which to encourage behavioural change (Aggleton and Homans, 1988, p. 6).

A recognition of the important part that lay beliefs play in mediating the interpretation that many people will make of medical and scientific information about HIV, highlights the potential difficulty of the task of communicating information about HIV in a clear, effective fashion. It also draws attention to the need for a helper to have good skills in listening and interpreting, as well as in communicating information. If information giving is to be successful, the helper may need to develop some understanding of the framework of beliefs that the client will be using to interpret any new knowledge that is being presented concerning health and disease.

To summarize some of the preceding discussion in this section of the chapter, someone giving information about HIV may encounter a number of different difficulties in communication. Problems may arise from the way in which AIDS has been represented, beliefs that people hold about disease in general, and the fact that people may have developed erroneous ideas concerning HIV and AIDS from coverage in the media. Dealing with such problems may require the helper to take some of the actions suggested in the following list. A helper needs to:

- seek information about an individual's beliefs concerning HIV and AIDS, and beliefs about how diseases in general spread, to check out for possible misconceptions;
- provide pictures, metaphors to describe HIV and AIDS which do not carry a strong, negative emotional charge;
- tailor information that is provided about HIV and AIDS very carefully to the social circumstances and world-view of individual clients; and
- use language very carefully, explain terms fully and in a concrete manner to avoid the person seeking information from developing any further misconceptions.

A number of more detailed points concerning the careful use of language will be presented later in the chapter.

Establishing the relationship, developing trust

The last few paragraphs have focused on the need to adjust the *content* of information to the world-view and personal needs of the individual client. Not only does the content have to be right, but it also requires to be communicated in a clear and appropriate fashion. Effective communication in turn is made possible by establishing a good quality of relationship with the person who has come along to seek information.

People who come along for information about HIV and AIDS are very often impelled not simply by a desire for clarification of factual matters but also by a wish to explore anxieties. They need to be put at ease and to be shown a genuine respect if they are to be able to explore these anxieties fully. To be successful in giving information about HIV, a worker will often require to have the attitudes that characterize a good counselling relationship. In particular, the attitudes of *empathy, respect for the person* and *genuineness* are called for and need to be communicated clearly to the person who has come for information or advice.

If information giving is taking place within a group where the members are expected to participate actively in learning about HIV, it is important to start off with sufficient ice-breaking activities to create a climate of trust. Even in telephone work, it is very helpful to establish some rapport before the enquirer launches into the main substance of the call.

An important action in creating a relationship of trust is establishing with the person who has come for information or advice that you will maintain confidentiality. If there are any limitations set on your ability to maintain confidentiality, these should be made explicit right away. If you are leading or facilitating a group, you need to ensure that the members respect each others' right to confidentiality.

Listening and communicating

Some general points

Interpreting the needs and motives of people who come requesting information can be a very difficult business. Attention has already been drawn to the
importance of allowing someone seeking information to express his or her
anxieties and needs fully. This is a necessary action both to allow a satisfactory
relationship to be established and as a means of giving the helper sufficient
knowledge about the person. As well as allowing a person the opportunity to
express all of his or her worries about HIV and AIDS, a helper may need to
check out the person's knowledge concerning HIV. It is advisable to start off
by discovering what people already know. They may prove to be quite
knowledgeable, or to have startling misconceptions.

As you allow people to express anxieties, seek answers to specific questions
and check out their understanding, you need at the same time to be making
and revising inferences concerning their emotional reaction to HIV and
AIDS. The understanding that you reach of the person's emotions concerning
HIV will very much determine the content, style and pacing of your
information-giving activities. As a very simple illustration of how emotional
state affects the handling of information, if people are quite upset there are
very distinct limitations on the amount of information that they can absorb on
any one occasion.

Aside from gaining a sense of the person's emotions concerning HIV, there
is also a need to be sensitive to the extent to which clients may wish to discuss
with you making decisions about testing, making changes in their life, deciding to go ahead with a particular treatment, etc. Does a particular client want
to be left to get on with things herself once you have given her enough facts to
make an informed decision, or is she indicating that some discussion which
centres on the process of decision making would be really appreciated?

Moving on to the question of the *sequencing* of the presentation of information, it makes sense to start off with less emotive, more factual information. This
allows time for a reasonably good relationship to be built up before more
difficult matters are explored. It also provides the helper with the opportunity to
gauge how the client is likely to respond to a discussion of matters which are
more likely to produce anxiety. Careful thought needs to be given to the *pacing*
of information, as well as the sequence in which information is presented. There
is a danger that a helper may try to present too many facts at once. It is sensible
to check out understanding as you proceed with giving information.

Checking out knowledge as you proceed not only allows you to pace the
giving of information, but also ensures that you continue to communicate
effectively in appropriate language. From the author's own experience of
giving information, the difficulty that some people experience in absorbing
information concerning HIV is related to the strong emotions that the subject
evokes rather than to any failure of intellect.

We all have defences against receiving unwelcome information, against really listening to information on a topic that part of us would rather avoid. There is often a need to talk through the feelings associated with HIV if information giving is to be successful, and such an exploration of feelings does take time. People may need to be given the chance to express fears safely and without feeling foolish, however irrational these fears may be, before they can come to absorb fully information about HIV. This observation applies as much to group work as it does to work with an individual client.

Moving on to look at another aspect of communicating information about HIV, helpers need to be alerted to the fact that it may be very difficult to cope with some of the messages that they receive from clients. People who wish to work in this area need to be sure that they have the personal resources and skills to deal calmly with quite hostile clients, and with clients who may express a great deal of prejudice. As well as emotional strength, mental agility is called for to deal with quite unexpected responses that may suddenly be flung at you. Helpers require the ability to be quick off the mark.

Handling uncertain information

Another area which calls for a lot of skill in the helper is that of communicating information about aspects of HIV where knowledge remains somewhat uncertain. Although helpers will wish to communicate in a clear fashion with their clients, it is important that they don't take the drive to give clear statements too far and oversimplify matters. It would be unwise to provide a very authoritative statement concerning subjects such as, say, the transmission of HIV from mother to child, on which the evidence has changed markedly in the past few years.

Where knowledge is still uncertain, helpers have to be honest about the limitations on our current information. They can say what is the most likely prediction on present evidence but indicate that we can't yet be sure about exactly how matters will turn out. There tends to be particular uncertainty around the numerical estimates that have been made of various aspects of HIV and AIDS. A lot of caution is necessary over the matter of presenting figures. A helper may need to alert a client to the way in which the values ascribed to particular quantities may change over time as the disease is studied more and understood better – to the limits of our confidence in a particular set of figures.

Helpers themselves need to keep in mind the difficulties that clients are likely to experience in trying to understand what meaning HIV statistics and numerical predictions have for their own life and actions. Linguistic qualifiers such as 'not at all likely', 'a small risk', 'a very high likelihood that', are often preferable to the use of numbers, as it is easier for people to make sense of statements of probability that are made in linguistic, rather than numerical, terms. If numbers are going to be used, a helper needs to make human sense of the statistics that he or she is presenting. The helper needs to give the client a concrete sense of what the figures mean, or do not mean, in an individual case. To achieve this, appropriate use has to be made of illustrations and anecdotes.

Using language carefully

An earlier section of this chapter discussed the problems that have arisen from the way in which HIV and AIDS have been represented in the media and throughout society. It was also noted that by using language very carefully and explaining terms fully, a helper could free clients from misconceptions and enable them to gain a more rational view of matters related to HIV and AIDS.

Aside from challenging inaccurate and negative representations of HIV and AIDS, helpers need to be alert to another important aspect of using language in a careful, sensitive fashion. A helper may unwittingly use a term to label a person or activity which a particular client may find demeaning, patronizing or somewhat offensive. For example, a fairly wide variety of terms can be used to refer to a sexual partner; but not all of these terms will be acceptable to a particular client. The helper needs to be guided by the client's own use of language as to which terms it is appropriate to use.

There is a need also to be sensitive to the fact that the same term can have different shades of meaning according to the social context in which it is used. As an example, customary linguistic usage might suggest that it is appropriate to use the terms 'victims' and 'sufferers' to refer to people who are experiencing a serious and potentially life-threatening illness. However, a number of AIDS self-help organizations and many individuals with AIDS themselves have resisted the use of the terms 'victims' and 'sufferers', seeing these terms as having connotations of passivity and hopelessness. They have preferred to use phrases with more positive connotations such as 'people living with AIDS'.

People who are being trained to give information and counsel in the area of HIV need to be made aware of the terms that people living with HIV infection themselves prefer to use to represent their condition. They also need to be aware of the meaning and emotional force that certain terms or labels may have for particular communities and groups. For example, most gay people would prefer to describe themselves by using the term 'gay', which has positive connotations, rather than the term 'homosexual' which sounds clinical and historically has referred to a lifestyle marked by humiliation and concealment.

Discussing safer sex

Another area where language has to be used in a very careful fashion is in talking about sex with people who come seeking information. Workers in the area of HIV need to feel comfortable in discussing sexual matters with clients. Helpers who feel confident about discussing sex will communicate this confidence to their clients, and make it easier for clients to ask very specific questions about what is 'safe' or 'unsafe' sex without feeling any embarrassment. Facilitating discussion about sex will also allow a helper to pick up on and to correct any misconceptions that people may have formed of what constitutes 'safer sex'.

If the language used to present safer sex is too dry and there is a focus on 'don'ts' and a lack of attention to attractive alternatives to practices which carry a risk of HIV infection, safer sex is not going to appear as a particularly desirable option. Safer sex needs to be presented as attractive and erotic, in language and images that a particular individual or group will find appealing.

Guidelines which reflect current advice on the relative risk of HIV transmission of particular sexual activities are given as an appendix to this chapter. It is important to give a sufficiently precise account of what constitutes safer sex, and the way in which this is achieved may vary considerably from client to client. Helpers need to judge sensitively what is appropriate language and images for discussing sex with different groups. The language used needs to be tailored carefully to the personal characteristics and social experience of an individual client.

Helpers are required also to be alert to the variety of ways in which clients may interpret the term 'sexual partner' and not assume that the term has a standard meaning. Clients may also have formed quite idiosyncratic definitions of what constitutes 'safe' and 'unsafe' sex, and if the helper does not use sufficiently precise, plain language to discuss sexual matters, these, possibly erroneous, personal definitions of safe sex may go unexamined.

Pursuing this theme of giving a sufficiently detailed account of what constitutes safer sex, the advice to 'use a condom' is very vague and for that reason of limited value. To be fully informed about using condoms to protect themselves, individuals may require to be advised as to which brands of condom to use, how to use them properly, how to use a spermicide together with a condom to give added protection, and how to negotiate using condoms with a sexual partner.

As the early part of this chapter established, telling individuals how to protect themselves from HIV infection without at the same time assisting them to gain the skills to negotiate safer sex with their partner may be a somewhat empty exercise. Helpers working with individuals or with groups can model and provide opportunities to practise talking about sex with a partner. Individuals can be assisted to gain skills in being assertive in negotiating safer sex with a partner. When necessary, they can also be helped to develop a greater sense of their own self-efficacy, their own ability to exercise personal control over the world around them.

Another important aspect of the language and the approach used to discuss safer sex is the need to avoid discussing safer sexual practices in too mechanistic a fashion, giving information and modelling negotiating skills without paying sufficient attention to the force of desire, love and other strong emotions which are linked with sexual expression. Clients require to be given a chance to express fully and come to terms with feelings and attitudes which may make it hard for them to practise safer sex. Staying with the example of talking about the use of condoms, using condoms may be seen by some clients as not only a way of protecting their health but also as some kind of symbolic statement about the nature and value of their current sexual relationship. They may feel that using a condom is associated with some lack of trust or love, and for such reasons find condom use with a regular partner problematic. Individuals may need to explore the meanings that surround safer sex for them before they can feel comfortable and secure about protecting themselves from the sexual transmission of HIV.

Discussion of safer sex also requires to take account of the points that have been made earlier concerning possible important inequalities between sexual partners which make the negotiation of safer sex very difficult.

Most of the published work on helping individuals to acquire the information, motivation and skills to practise safer sex has focused on the stage of starting to practise safer sex. There is a tendency to fail to consider how individuals can be assisted to maintain these changes for the foreseeable future. Previewing particular situations which might make it difficult to practise safer sex and considering ways of dealing with such situations can be useful. Similarly, it can be helpful to consider general problems that may arise for the individual in maintaining a change to safer sexual behaviour and how such problems might be resolved.

What do you need to know?

Discussion in this chapter has centred around clarifying aims in giving information about HIV and on how this information can best be communicated. Moving on now to concentrate on the information itself, helpers need to be well informed on the following areas:

- general knowledge about the natural history of the virus, its transmission, and the specific medical conditions associated with it, including knowledge concerning the way in which HIV may affect babies and children;
- general knowledge about how the body works;
- general knowledge about how to keep healthy;
- the nature of HIV tests and their possible consequences;
- knowledge of anti-viral drugs and treatments for HIV-related conditions;
- safer sex;
- how to use drugs intravenously safely;
- social and employment issues related to HIV and AIDS (these are very important issues, and shouldn't be regarded as of secondary importance in relation to the medical aspects of the disease);
- travel and employment restrictions imposed by certain countries on people who are HIV positive;

- welfare benefits, services which people with HIV-related illnesses may be able to claim; and
- support groups for people who are HIV antibody positive, or who have HIV-related illness – contact people in these groups to whom you can make a referral.

As the above checklist indicates, workers in the area of HIV require to have knowledge on a wide range of topics. They also need to ensure that their knowledge is kept up to date. One means of keeping up to date is for your organization to subscribe to the *AIDS Newsletter*, which is produced by the Bureau of Hygiene and Tropical Diseases. This newsletter provides very readable summaries of recent research work on the virus, news of the trialling of treatments, developments in various countries throughout the world, and articles on social and policy issues related to HIV. The latest issue of the *National AIDS Manual* is another very useful resource for organizations concerned with giving information about HIV. (See Chapter 16 for information on how to subscribe to the *AIDS Newletter* or the *National AIDS Manual*.)

Aside from encouraging workers to read the *AIDS Newsletter* and articles in professional journals, it is important that both voluntary and professional organizations have a programme of regular training updates for their volunteers or staff.

Another aspect of keeping up to date is to look at items concerning HIV and AIDS in a cross-section of newspapers and at current television reports. This will ensure that you keep abreast of the information that clients are receiving and allow you to make an appropriate response to their enquiries concerning a particular TV report or newspaper item.

However well you may do the job of imparting information about HIV, it is essential that clients themselves have some opportunity to look at the literature on HIV. Organizations need to keep a reference library of pamphlets, guides and, if finances permit, books on a variety of aspects of HIV.

Acknowledging our own limitations

There are certain questions which someone giving information about HIV may find it impossible to answer. In such a situation, it is important to be honest with the client that you don't know yourself. You can then either put them in contact with someone else locally who is likely to be able to answer their question, or try to find out the answer(s) to their question yourself and arrange to pass on the information you have collected on another occasion. Having a well-established network of contacts to whom people can be referred for very specific advice, information or specialized counselling is important if clients are to be provided with information and help which is tailored to their individual experience and needs. It is also important to be aware of the particular health education messages that are being given by other workers in your locality to avoid clients being presented with conflicting information.

The next chapter, *Counselling and HIV antibody testing*, looks at some other issues concerning the handling of information, and considers common reasons which people may have for seeking information about HIV antibody testing, and specific information that they require to be given if fully informed consent to testing is to be achieved.

Appendix: Safer sex

HIV may be transmistted sexually if blood, semen and vaginal secretions from an HIV-infected person comes into contact with the sensitive linings of the vagina, the rectum, or the inner lining of the penis. Transmission may also take place if HIV-infected blood, semen or vaginal secretions enter an open wound or sore. There is not a risk of transmission if these fluids make contact with intact healthy skin. Penetrative vaginal or anal intercourse without a condom are definitely high-risk sexual activities for the transmission of HIV. This risk applies to both the insertive and the receptive partner in penetrative intercourse.

Condoms act as a barrier to prevent the transmission of HIV and most other sexually transmitted diseases. It needs to be recognized that though condoms reduce the risk of transmission of HIV, they cannot be guaranteed to provide complete safety. As a form of contraception they have been found to have a failure rate estimated at upwards of 5%. Much of this failure rate is considered to be due to people using condoms incorrectly.

Condoms need to be put on carefully, making sure that no damage is done to the condom. The closed end of the condom needs to be squeezed to expel any air, and any air bubbles need to be smoothed out as they can make it easier for a condom to burst. Care also needs to be taken that the condom does not slip off during intercourse.

It is much safer when a man withdraws from his partner before coming. When a man does come inside his partner, it is necessary to withdraw before the penis becomes soft and there is a danger of semen leaking out of the condom. Holding the condom at the base as a man withdraws will stop the condom accidentally slipping off.

There is less friction or strain on a condom which is well lubricated with a water-based lubricant, such as KY. Oil-based lubricants such as vaseline, body oils and creams must be avoided as they very quickly weaken the material of which condoms are made. The use of a spermicide in addition to a condom, particularly one which contains nonoxynol-9 which has been shown to kill the HIV virus under laboratory conditions, is recommended to give additional protection. Recently, a condom for women has been developed and is marketed as Femshield. This female condom is inserted into the vagina.

Worries have been expressed about how strong and effective a barrier condoms are for the prevention of the transmission of the HIV virus in anal intercourse. For that reason, some voluntary HIV agencies have advised that the safest course is to abstain from anal intercourse. For individuals who decide that they are not going to abstain from anal intercourse, the careful use of a condom, *plenty* of water-based lubricant and a spermicide will considerably reduce the risk of transmission of HIV.

Inserting fingers deeply into the vagina or rectum, or a hand ('fisting') into the vagina or rectum can cause bleeding and consequently a risk of transmission of HIV. Fisting can also cause considerable internal injury.

Sharing sex toys which have come in contact with semen, vaginal secretions or blood could involve a risk of transmission of HIV.

There has been considerable debate about whether oral sex, where an individual may be exposed to pre-come, semen, vaginal secretions and menstrual blood, carries a risk of transmission of HIV. To what extent, oral sex carries a risk of transmission of HIV is not yet well determined. There may possibly be some risk attached to oral sex. What is clear, however, is that any risk is likely to be much smaller than in the case of penetrative vaginal and anal intercourse. Individuals who wish to continue to have oral sex can make it safer by using barriers. A condom can be used in fellatio (sucking a man's cock) and ejaculation can take place outside of the mouth. Cunnilingus, licking a woman's vagina and clitoris, can be made safer by the use of cling-film or a small latex sheet, known as a 'dental dam', placed over the vagina.

'Watersports', i.e. sex involving urine, appears not to involve any risk of the transmission of HIV, but it does involve a risk of transmitting other infections, including serious diseases.

'Rimming',i.e.tonguingtheanus,doesnotappeartoposeaparticularriskforthe transmission of HIV, although there might be some risk from blood which is sometimes contained in faeces. It does, however, carry the risk of the transmission of a large number of other infections, some of which can have serious consequences.

Any sexual activity which involves no possibility of blood, semen or vaginal secretions coming into contact with sensitive linings of the body or a wound carries no risk whatsoever of the transmission of HIV.

References

Aggleton, P. and Homans, H. (1988). 'Introduction'. In P. Aggleton and H. Homans (eds), *Social Aspects of AIDS*. London, Falmer Press, pp. 1–9.

Bandura, A. (1989). 'Perceived self-efficacy in the exercise of control over AIDS infection'. In V.M. Mays *et al.* (eds), *Primary Prevention of AIDS: Psychological Approaches*. London, Sage, pp. 128–41.

Becker, M.H. (1974). *The Health Belief Model and Personal Health Behavior*. Thorofare, N.J., Charles B. Slack.

Brandt, A.M. (1987). *No Magic Bullet: A Social History of Veneral Disease in the United States since 1880*, expanded edn. Oxford, Oxford University Press.

Douglas, M. and Wildavsky, A. (1982). *Risk and Culture*. Berkeley, Calif., University of California Press.

Fitzpatrick, R. (1984). 'Lay concepts of illness'. In R. Fitzpatrick *et al.*, *The Experience of Illness*. London. Tavistock. pp. 11–31.

Hastings, G.B. *et al.* (1990). 'Two years of AIDS publicity: A review of progress in Scotland'. *Health Education Research: Theory and Practice, 5*, 17–25.

Joseph, J.G. (1989). 'Are there psychological costs associated with changes in behavior to reduce AIDS risk?'. In V.M. Mays *et al.* (eds), *Primary Prevention of AIDS: Psychological Approaches*. London, Sage, pp. 209–24.

Nutbeam, D. and Blakey, V. (1990). 'The concept of health promotion and AIDS prevention: A comprehensive and integrated basis for action in the 1990s'. *Health Promotion International*, **5**, 233–42.

Rosenstock, I.M. (1974). 'Historical origins of the health belief model'. *Health Education Monographs*, **2**, 328–35.

Warwick, I. *et al.* (1988). 'Young people's health beliefs and AIDS'. In P. Aggleton and H. Homans (eds), *Social Aspects of AIDS*. London, Falmer Press, pp. 106–25.

SEVEN

Counselling and HIV antibody testing

CHARLES ANDERSON

Introduction

The decision to take an HIV antibody test is one that few people make lightly, and as Richard Goldstein (1989, p. 89) has remarked recently, 'for anyone in a vulnerable group, taking the test is an act of enormous courage'. Counsellors have an important role to play in assisting individuals in the decision-making process about whether or not to take the HIV antibody test. Together with medical staff, they have a duty to ensure that fully informed consent to testing has been obtained; that the person has made the decision to take the test based on a clear understanding of the nature of the test itself, and on the health and wider social implications of a positive or negative test result. Counselling that centres around HIV antibody testing also provides an opportunity for individuals to gain more information about HIV, and to empower themselves to make rational choices and take actions which will minimize their risk of becoming HIV-infected.

Much of the discussion in a pre-HIV antibody test counselling interview will centre around previewing how an individual will cope with the emotional distress, the specific practical difficulties and the problems in relationships which may follow the news of an HIV antibody positive result. This work of previewing and preparation for emotional and problem-focused coping may take quite a considerable period of time. The danger of a client becoming dependent on a counsellor to take on the decision making for him or her needs to be recognized; but at the same time counselling around decision making and the work of previewing coping with a negative or positive test result is something which cannot be rushed.

The rest of this chapter looks in detail at the range of actions that a counsellor needs to take to ensure that a client is fully informed about the nature of the HIV antibody test and its consequences, and that he or she is enabled to make rational choices about the test. It also considers the responses that a counsellor can make to assist an individual to cope with the immediate effects of receiving a positive HIV antibody test result. Chapter 8 then looks at the long-term challenges of living with the knowledge that one is HIV antibody positive, and the ways in which a helper can assist HIV antibody positive individuals to gain greater control over their lives. The present chapter also highlights the needs of people who test seronegative, problems which they may face and appropriate counselling responses.

Considering the wide range of reasons for seeking an HIV antibody test

The motives and the personal circumstances which lead people to consider the possibility of taking an HIV antibody test vary widely. Many individuals will come for pre-test counselling with a rational fear of a real risk of infection, while others will have irrational fears about an imaginary risk. Some individuals may have been advised by a doctor that certain symptoms they are experiencing might indicate the presence of HIV infection, and that they should consider having a test for the presence of HIV infection. Some people may be considering taking the HIV antibody test in connection with meeting immigration and travel requirements imposed by certain countries. A person may have had longstanding fears which have a rational basis that he or she may have been exposed to HIV infection and wish to deal with these fears in part by resolving their position on whether or not to take the HIV antibody test. Someone who has earlier not wished to take the test, may be considering taking it now that there have been some advances in the treatment of HIV-related illnesses and of HIV infection itself. People who are starting a new sexual relationship may be thinking about being tested for HIV antibodies. A woman who wishes to start a pregnancy, who is unsure about whether or not she may have been exposed to the risk of HIV infection at some point in the past, may be contemplating taking an HIV antibody test. Former or current drug users may wonder if their intravenous drug use has exposed them to HIV infection.

For some individuals, the primary motive for coming to talk about the possibility of taking an HIV antibody test may be guilt over a past sexual relationship, or deep-seated fears and concerns about their sexual identity or sexual activities. People who have a history of hypochondria may add HIV infection to the list of their fears of illnesses that may be attacking them. Irrational fears of HIV infection may feature in the system of delusions that are experienced by people who have serious pre-existing psychiatric disorders.

The illustrations that have been provided in the past two paragraphs of the varied reasons and motives that may prompt people to appear for pre-test counselling indicate the need to tailor any counselling that is provided very carefully to the needs of the individual client. However, there are certain areas which it is appropriate to explore in any pre-test counselling interview and certain counselling actions which are required in any pre-test counselling if fully informed consent is to be achieved. The following sections of this chapter examine a number of areas which will be covered in any pre-test counselling interview.

Deciding on where to go for a test

One question which a client who is receiving some pre-test counselling outside of the context of the health services may ask is where should I go to have an HIV antibody test? In responding to this question, a counsellor will need to have a clear picture of the nature of the client's existing relationship with his or her GP, and the extent to which he or she is prepared for that particular GP to know the results of an HIV antibody test.

A GP may be the appropriate person for some individuals to approach for testing. However, much of the testing which takes place at the moment is performed within Departments of Genito-Urinary Medicine, what used to be known as STD clinics. There are some advantages associated with being tested at such a site. Medical staff in such departments have expert knowledge in the area of HIV infection and the treatment of HIV-related illnesses, and can customarily be relied on to treat patients' concerns about HIV with sensitivity. There is also a measure of legal protection of confidentiality of medical information held by sexually transmitted disease clinics under the terms of the NHS (Venereal Diseases) Regulations (1974). Such clinics customarily now have associated counselling staff who will provide pre- and post-test counselling.

An important helping action for agencies concerned with HIV infection is to direct clients who are seriously considering taking an HIV antibody test to a clinic in their area which has established a good reputation for treating patients' feelings and decisions concerning the HIV antibody test with respect. The discussion of the confidentiality of the counselling relationship and of the results of any HIV antibody test may on occasion influence the decision on where to be tested.

Establishing the relationship: Allowing the expression of feelings and anxieties

An essential first step in pre-test counselling is to establish a relationship in which the client can feel secure to discuss difficult and sensitive issues. A counsellor needs to respond to a client in a way which makes it clear that he or she is being listened to very carefully, and with respect and concern. People who come for counselling concerning taking the HIV antibody test may have 'bottled up' a fear about HIV, and also have deep-seated anxieties about aspects of themselves. Before progress can be made in addressing the issues that surround the HIV antibody test, they may need to be given an opportunity to express some of their fears and anxieties and to have their experience validated by being listened to with respect. There is a lot of information about HIV and the test to be considered in the course of pre-test counselling. However, if a counsellor goes straight into the consideration of 'facts' about HIV and the test, and an assessment of the individual's risk of having contracted HIV infection, without allowing the expression of feelings and anxieties, the client may be less able to absorb this information. A client may also find counselling a somewhat disempowering experience if the counsellor concentrates too exclusively on factual matters and is not sufficiently responsive to his or her expressed needs and feelings.

A general picture of the client's situation and concerns will be gained in the earlier part of a pre-test counselling interview while the counsellor is allowing the client to state problems in his or her own terms and to express anxieties. During the early part of the interview, the counsellor can also give the client a clear statement of the nature of the counselling that is being offered, and the nature of any follow-up counselling that may be provided if the client decides to take the test, or declines to take the test but still wishes to work on problems or resolve anxieties that centre around HIV infection. The client requires to be assured that any disclosures about his or her life that are made during the course of pre-test counselling will be treated as confidential; and any limitations on the maintenance of confidentiality must be stated. The question of the confidentiality surrounding the process of testing itself and the results of testing also needs to be addressed.

An important issue that can usually be clarified in the early stages of an interview is whether the client is indeed considering testing of his or her own free will. A counsellor can explore whether particular clients have been directly or more subtly pressurized by a partner, or other person close to them, to be tested.

Providing information in a clear manner

Respecting the client's own world-view

Information that a client provides in the earlier stages of the interview will begin to give a counsellor a sense of how the client's thoughts about testing are being shaped by their general values, and their approach to coping with problems. It is important that a counsellor tries to appreciate and to respond to a client's choices in a way which stays as close as possible to the client's own values, objectives and general way of viewing the world.

Clearly, all counsellors will have some general beliefs of their own about the desirability or undesirability of testing, and some counsellors may also have opinions concerning whether particular categories of clients should be tested or not. The power that comes from the difference in knowledge and in vulnerability between the counsellor and client needs to be exercised responsibly. The counsellor's own beliefs and opinions require to be held firmly in check so that clients can make their own choices based on their own values and ideas about priorities in their lives. At the same time, the counsellor has a very important part to play in assisting clients to clarify their emotions and thoughts concerning testing. If fully informed consent is to be achieved and the individual is to have sufficient knowledge to make a rational choice about whether or not to take the test, the counsellor also often needs to impart in a very clear fashion a large amount of information about HIV and its transmission and about the test and its consequences.

Presenting information about HIV and its transmission, and assessing risk

A sensible discussion of issues surrounding the test can only be achieved if the client is in possession of basic information about HIV and its transmission. Misconceptions about HIV and its transmission also need to be corrected. Attention needs to be paid to all of the points that were made in Chapter 6, in particular to tailor information very carefully to the client's own needs and characteristics, and to be alert to the way in which lay health beliefs may be affecting the manner in which the client is interpreting information about HIV and its transmission. Information about HIV can only be fully understood if the individual receiving it has a reasonable basic understanding of the immune system and of infectious agents. Counsellors need to have the knowledge and skill to present a lucid and readily comprehensible account of how the body works.

The information that is provided about HIV and its transmission, and the correction of any misconceptions that the client has about HIV, will enable the client to make a realistic assessment of whether it is possible that there is a risk that he or she may have been exposed to HIV infection.

Presenting information about risk reduction

Pre-test counselling also provides an opportunity to provide information about safer sex, and possibly how to use drugs in a way which removes the risk of transmission of HIV. As well as being provided with information about safer sex, the client may also be helped to discuss, and perhaps find solutions to, problems that he or she has in putting safer sex into practice. It is important, however, to maintain clarity of purpose in the interview and to ensure that there is a distinct separation of the topics of risk reduction and of the decision concerning whether or not to take the test.

Explaining the HIV antibody tests

A considerable amount of time needs to be spent describing the HIV antibody tests, what they can achieve and their limitations. Misconceptions about HIV antibody tests are not uncommon, e.g. that they test for AIDS. The counsellor needs to seek out and then correct any problems in understanding of the test. Important points to include in a discussion of the HIV antibody test are the 'window period' before the development of antibodies during which the test will not detect the presence of HIV infection, and the possible need for a follow-up test if the client believes that he or she has recently been exposed to the risk of HIV infection. Understandably, people who decide to have a test and then receive a positive result often have the thought: 'Can't there have been some mistake?' In pre-test counselling, the counsellor can explain how there is a careful procedure of confirming any positive result which involves the use of another type of antibody test.

Tests which monitor the health of the immune system and the stage of HIV infection

Clients who receive a positive test result will normally be offered regular checks on their health by a medical department which specializes in the problems associated with HIV. A check-up for HIV positive patients at most clinics will involve not only a physical examination but also blood tests which provide markers of the progression of HIV disease and of immunosuppression. Tests which are commonly used to monitor the health of the immune system of an HIV positive person include a test for HIV antigen, a CD4 (T4) cell count and a test for the level of B-2 microglobulin (see Chapter 2). In a pre-test counselling interview, it may be appropriate to discuss these tests which can act as markers of progress in immunosuppression and the part that these predictive tests play in the care and treatment of HIV positive individuals.

Exploring the possible medical benefits of testing

In the first few years of testing, when there was little in the way of treatment of HIV itself and prophylactic treatment of HIV-related illnesses had not been established, the decision whether or not to test centred largely on the person's feelings and anxieties, on psychological health rather than on any benefits for physical health. However, the development of marker tests of immunosuppression which aid treatment decisions, the advances that have been made in the treatment of HIV-related illnesses over the past few years, the widespread use of zidovudine (AZT) against HIV infection and the development of new drugs which may be effective in blocking the replication of HIV, have meant that there may be distinct advantages for health in detecting the presence of HIV infection and thereby gaining access to treatment.

HIV positive individuals who may still be symptomless but whose serological tests, such as CD4 (T4) cell counts, demonstrate a progression in immunosuppression, are often now given aerosolized pentamadine as prophylaxis against PCP (*Pneumocystis carinii* pneumonia). Evidence now exists that for people who fall into the clinical definition of AIDS, early treatment with zidovudine (AZT) increases life expectancy. The existing benefits of early intervention and a belief in the potential of experimental treatments has led some clinicians to advocate that anyone who has been at significant risk of exposure to HIV infection should consider being tested for HIV antibodies.

Counsellors need to present clients who are considering being tested with a clear view of the possible health benefits of having HIV infection confirmed by a test. At the same time, however, they require to ensure that clients do not have unrealistic expectations about what medical intervention in the earlier stages of HIV infection can achieve. It is very difficult to make accurate predictions concerning whether, or at what rate, a *particular* HIV antibody positive individual who is asymptomatic will progress to a later stage of HIV infection; and there is as yet no 'magic bullet' which can prevent asympto matic but HIV-infected individuals from developing HIV-related illnesses.

Discussion of treatment options in the event of a positive result

Some people who present themselves for pre-test counselling may wish to review in detail *particular* treatment options which may be available to them should they take the test and receive a positive result. At the moment, questions about treatment options are likely to centre around the question of the possible benefits for asymptomatic individuals with HIV infection of being treated with zidovudine.

Dealing with uncertainty in current knowledge of treatment and other medical matters

Consideration of the subject of discussing treatment options in the course of pre-test counselling raises a number of important general matters concerning pre-test counselling and other types of HIV counselling. For a start, it highlights the need for a counsellor to possess a wide range of up-to-date knowledge if the client is to be given the power to make truly independent choices about testing, treatment and other aspects of care rather than being simply channelled into the treatment and care regime provided in a particular locality. A client may need to be provided with details of less commonly applied treatments and given a clear and impartial account of current evidence, and any controversy, concerning the benefits and disadvantages of a particular treatment. When current knowledge is uncertain, as it is concerning the possible benefits and risks of new or recently established treatments, it is important that in providing a somewhat simplified account of complicated matters, a counsellor does not make fuzzy knowledge appear to be clear-cut.

Clients in pre-test counselling and in other interviews concerning HIV need to be informed that the account they have been given concerning particular treatments or other areas where knowledge is incomplete is the best available at the moment, but that the knowledge is imprecise. Clients may be making very important decisions concerning the whole course of their life in pre-test counselling interviews and the limitations on the certainty of the knowledge on which they are basing their decisions require to be marked clearly and honestly.

Financial and social aspects of testing

Many of the problems associated with HIV are social rather than biological in origin. A counsellor needs to discuss not only treatment and health care issues but also the economic and social aspects of testing. Clients need to be alerted to the specific economic disadvantages that may result from discovering that one is HIV-infected. It is also useful for them to explore the ways in which HIV and people with AIDS have been represented socially and how these representations may affect their decisions concerning testing.

Insurance

An important financial matter to consider in relation to testing for HIV infection is insurance. All British insurance companies in the past few years have included questions concerning HIV and AIDS in the standard questionnaire that is filled in by applicants for life insurance. The exact wording of these questions varies, but all applicants will be asked whether they have been tested for HIV infection and the outcome of the test. Some insurance companies may also ask a more all-embracing question which probes whether the applicant has sought advice about HIV or AIDS. So far, insurance companies have not taken on individuals who are known to be HIV-infected.

Even when individuals receive a negative test result, they will be obliged to declare this in connection with any application for new life insurance. Individuals who do declare a negative test result in an application for life insurance may subsequently be asked a number of questions by the insurance company to assess their degree of risk of being exposed to HIV infection, before decisions are taken on the matter of providing them with a policy and the level of premiums.

The majority of new mortgages issued in Britain are linked to endowment insurance policies; and again the application forms for these policies will include questions concerning HIV. It is possible to take out a mortgage that is not linked to life insurance in any way; but building societies may often prefer to grant mortgages that are linked to life insurance. Private health care insurance companies also seek to investigate whether a person is infected with HIV. Questions concerning HIV in applications for insurance of any sort require to be answered honestly. If they are not answered accurately, the insurance contract may be declared void.

Employment

For some individuals who are contemplating taking an HIV antibody test, an important factor influencing their decision may be anxieties concerning the implications for employment of knowing that one has HIV infection. Sometimes, individuals present themselves for pre-test counselling because they wish to consider how they will deal with a medical for a new job in which they believe, possibly with good reason, that the question of testing for HIV may arise. Some individuals may also wish to use a pre-test counselling interview to explore how to cope with medicals that may be required in connection with membership of a private health insurance scheme provided by their company.

Restrictions on travel and work permits

A number of countries, particularly in the Middle East, are at present requiring proof that applicants for a visa or work permit have been tested recently for HIV infection and are denying entry to individuals who have a positive test result. Some individuals who feel that they may have been at risk of contracting HIV infection will wish to discuss the test in relation to the prospect of a job in a country which places restrictions on people with HIV infection.

Exploring the effects of negative representations of HIV and of people with HIV infection

The anxieties that some people seeking pre-test counselling experience in connection with HIV are fuelled not only by a rational, or irrational, belief that they may have been exposed to a potentially life-threatening disease. They also derive from the negative social representations of HIV and of people with AIDS; from the ways in which HIV infection has been portrayed as an evil disease and one that does not afflict 'normal people'. Powerful destructive emotions of fear, anger and rejection have been associated with HIV. People who think that they may have been at risk from HIV infection and who present themselves for pre-test counselling are not immune from the effects of these negative social representations of the disease. It may be important to explore with some clients the extent to which they have been influenced by certain of the representations of HIV and AIDS – whether they themselves see HIV as a shameful disease which sets people who have it apart from the rest of society. They can then be provided with a very different view of the disease which emphasizes that it is only one serious infectious disease among others. A counsellor can help a client to strip the disease of the negative metaphors, images and moralistic overtones which have surrounded it (see Chapter 8).

Dealing with the reactions of others, exploring how the test decision is influenced by others

A counsellor may be able to assist some clients to develop a more 'objective' view of HIV, and to appreciate that there is nothing inherently shameful about the infection itself. However, there is no escaping the facts that AIDS has been a heavily stigmatized condition and that individuals with HIV infection have met with real hurts, even from people close to them. Clients need to consider how they might deal with the reactions of partners, family and friends to a positive test result. They also need to make a realistic assessment of the social support that they may require, and are likely to receive, if they get a positive test result. Breaking the news of an HIV antibody positive test result to some family members may also often require individuals to make an additional revelation concerning their sexual preferences and sexual activities, or concerning their illicit use of drugs. Some clients who are insecure in their own feelings about being gay may find the prospect of making disclosures both about being HIV antibody positive and being gay distressing and possibly even quite threatening to their personal identity. This topic may need to be treated with considerable care and sensitivity in a pre-test counselling interview.

With some individuals, it may be appropriate for a counsellor to look in detail at the support services provided by various voluntary services to people who are HIV positive as well as exploring the sources and extent of support in the person's own social network.

In addition to looking forward and anticipating the possible reactions of significant people in the client's life to a positive, or indeed a negative, result, some of the session is likely to focus on the question of how the client's present decision to contemplate taking an HIV test is being influenced by the actions of other people and by the quality of his or her personal relationships. Although an aim of pre-test counselling may be to enable clients to make decisions in an autonomous manner, clients are not isolated, asocial individuals. A counsellor can help clients to examine carefully the way in which thoughts and feelings about testing are being shaped by their personal and social circumstances.

Looking carefully at testing and behaviour change

For some clients, the decision to take an HIV antibody test is motivated principally by the belief that knowledge of their HIV antibody status will enable them to make changes in their behaviour. They believe that taking the test will be a turning point in their life and that after this point a change in sexual behaviour, in their pattern of drug use, or towards a more generally 'healthy' lifestyle, will be achieved. Knowledge of a test result may indeed, in some instances, prove to be an important incentive to make major life changes. However, it is also possible that some clients may have somewhat unrealistic expectations about the extent to which a positive or negative test result will assist them to move to new ways of living. A counsellor can assist such clients to explore *in detail* how they believe the test will enable them to change aspects of their life; and to consider what skills they may need to acquire and what support they will need to bring about changes in behaviour, irrespective of the decision that they finally come to concerning testing.

It is important also that counsellors themselves (a) do not have unrealistic expectations about the extent to which testing can bring about changes to more 'rational' behaviours, and (b) do not subtly guide a client towards testing in the belief that this will aid a change in behaviour. Anthony Pinching, a leading British physician in the area of HIV, has commented recently that: 'Many proponents of testing seem to imagine some very direct linkage between a test result and a behavioural change, which is at variance with much clinical experience' (Pinching, 1990, p. 33). Decisions concerning the extent to which testing may assist behaviour change need to remain firmly with the client.

Exploring anxieties and ways of coping

So far in this chapter, the possible treatment advantages of testing, the economic and social aspects of testing, and the issue of testing and expectations of behavioural change have been explored. For many clients, however, the principal focus of attention in a pre-test counselling interview will not be on any particular tangible advantage or disadvantage, or aspect of their relationship with other people, but on how they will achieve greater peace of mind. In the earlier part of a pre-test counselling interview, clients will normally have had an opportunity to express in general terms the anxieties that they feel about HIV and the test itself. Later in the interview, a counsellor can provide them with the opportunity to explore in a more focused way particular anxieties that they are experiencing concerning HIV. Clients can be helped to consider for themselves whether realistically the knowledge of a positive or negative test result will reduce or exacerbate their anxieties. For some clients, the reduction of uncertainty may be of prime importance. Other clients may decide that they would prefer to live with some degree of uncertainty rather than risk being given a positive test result which they would find very distressing and threatening.

There are a number of ways in which counsellors can assist clients in the process of reviewing how the test will affect their emotional well-being. Counsellors can help clients to look in considerable detail at exactly how they might react to a positive or negative test result, to identify how they customarily react to and cope with uncertainty or emotionally distressing situations, to consider other ways of coping that might be available to them, and the sources of support on which they might draw. The counsellor can also provide clients with an account of the 'normal' feelings that are experienced on receiving a positive test result.

Making a decision about testing

Gaining clarity about one's feelings and thoughts concerning testing, deciding how best to deal with anxieties concerning HIV and the test itself, and carefully weighing particular advantages and disadvantages of the test can be a very emotionally taxing set of tasks. It may also require quite a considerable period of time before some people are ready to make a definite decision to take, or not to take, the HIV antibody test. For some clients, the issues surrounding testing are relatively straightforward and they are prepared to proceed immediately to a decision about testing. For other clients, however, the decision about the test may be much more problematic; and it is important that such clients do not feel pressurized and are not hurried to make an immediate decision.

Counsellors can make clear at a first pre-test counselling interview that another appointment will be available in a few weeks when the client can return and explore further his or her thoughts concerning the test. It may often be appropriate for a counsellor to discuss with a client whether he or she intends to talk through the decision about testing with a partner, friend or associate in this intervening period, and to explore whether this would be a desirable course of action. Clients can also be provided with literature on HIV, and on HIV antibody tests, which may be helpful to them in coming to a decison about the test.

Counsellors can also suggest to clients methods which may be useful in structuring the process of deciding whether or not to take an antibody test. Marks and Goldblum (1989) suggest the use of what they term as a 'Benefit–Risk' analysis. They describe this procedure in the following terms:

> The client lists the potential benefits and risks of being tested. Each benefit is scrutinized to determine whether it can be accomplished using a method other than antibody testing that does not have a concomitant risk . . . If a greater overall benefit has been established to proceed with the test, a careful review of risks must be undertaken . . . After a careful examination of the benefits and risks, the final choice – an educated decision – is the client's alone to make (Marks and Goldblum, 1989, p. 56).

A decision-making framework, such as that suggested by Marks and Goldblum, may be a useful aid to some clients in clarifying their thoughts and feelings about testing. It must be recognized, however, that where powerful emotions and important life choices are involved, it may be very difficult to perform a clear-cut balancing of risks against benefits. Some clients may find it difficult to come to a definite decision about testing because they are faced with a very real conflict of reasons for and against taking the test. It may take them some time to establish which aspects are crucial in the decision concerning testing and to accept that where there are two conflicting sets of purposes both cannot be satisfied. They need to accept that whatever decision is finally reached, it may well have disadvantages as well as advantages associated with it.

Coping with the period of waiting for test results

Clients who decide to take an HIV antibody test should nowadays have to wait for only a few days or at most a week before they receive test results. (Delays in delivering results admittedly do occur, but such delays are difficult to justify.) These few days may seem like an eternity, however, to the person who is waiting. A counsellor can assist clients to plan how they are going to cope with this period of waiting. Particular leisure activities can be planned which will go some way to help to occupy the person's time, and consideration given to how the person can best find emotional support. A counsellor can instruct clients who are very anxious about the result in ways of coping with panic and of minimizing the distress caused by intrusive thoughts.

Further work in realistic preview

In some texts on counselling in HIV and AIDS, a fairly tight division is made between pre-test counselling which centres around decision making concerning the test and post-test counselling where attention is focused on the task of coping with a positive test result. In the present author's opinion at least, however, the tasks of pre- and post-test counselling do not separate out in quite as clear-cut a fashion. Someone who does receive a positive test result normally feels shocked by the news and is not in a state where he or she can readily take in information or make plans to deal with immediate difficulties and challenges. For that reason, it is useful in pre-test counselling to look in some detail at immediate practical problems which the client might be faced with if he or she receives a positive result and to consider how best to meet these problems.

Previewing the emotion that may be experienced on receiving a positive test result cannot take away the pain and distress that are likely to result from receiving a positive test result. However, work done in previewing emotional reactions may enable a person who receives a positive test result to feel in somewhat greater control of these powerful emotions and to appreciate that his or her feelings are in no way 'abnormal'.

The questions of who to tell about a possible positive test result and when, can be addressed more profitably in pre-test counselling than in a counselling interview in which the individual is actually given a positive test result. On some occasions, it may be useful for the counsellor and client to role-play telling someone close about a positive test result. This role-playing exercise can be used to consider how the client may cope with a range of different possible reactions from the person who is being given the news of the test result.

It is appropriate that the counsellor who is providing pre-test counselling gives a clear indication of the extent to which he or she will be able to provide counselling in the event that the client receives a positive result. Other sources of counselling and support, statutory and voluntary, which may be available to an HIV positive person in that locality can also be mentioned.

Giving a positive test result

The exact procedure for giving a test result will vary from clinic to clinic. In many clinics, it is common for a doctor to check out whether a patient still wishes to receive a test result and, if requested, to proceed to give the test result. Someone who receives a positive test result would then be given the opportunity to see a counsellor immediately afterwards. The most useful actions a counsellor can perform at this time are to allow the person to have the opportunity to express his or her feelings in an unrestrained manner and to have the space to absorb some of the shock of receiving a positive test result. Once the person has had a chance to express some of his or her feelings, and may be a bit more composed, it may be appropriate to help them to plan how they are going to cope emotionally and in practical terms with the week ahead. A counsellor can indicate to a client that the more extreme emotions that are often experienced on receiving a positive test result are time-limited and are a normal reaction. The client can be assured that control over thoughts and feelings will be re-established. It is important that the client is offered another appointment a week or so ahead where there can be a further opportunity to work on absorbing the impact of the news. The counselling actions which are appropriate at this follow-up meeting and subsequent meetings with an HIV positive person are detailed in Chapter 8.

Being alert to the needs of people who receive a negative test result

Most people who receive a negative test result feel relief and a reduction in anxiety. However, this is not a universal reaction. Some people who receive a negative test result may still experience considerable anxiety concerning HIV. They may be very fearful of sexual activity and attempt to reject all sexual behaviour to remain seronegative, feeling isolated as a consequence of this decision and guilty should they break their resolution to be celibate. In areas of the USA where the incidence of HIV infection has been high among the gay community, it is common for gay men to have seen a partner or close friends live with and die from AIDS. It has been found that in such communities, gay men who receive negative test results can be burdened by feelings of 'survivor guilt'. It is important that people who receive a negative result but who appear not to be reassured by this result, or who still have considerable problems which centre around HIV, are given the opportunity of further counselling in which they can explore and attempt to resolve troubling thoughts and feelings. Voluntary agencies may also consider setting up support groups for gay men who are seronegative, but who may be experiencing some difficulty in coming to terms with a negative test result.

The worried well

In the area of HIV, the term 'worried well' is customarily used to refer to individuals who (a) experience high levels of anxiety about the possibility that they may have been infected with HIV and (b) have little rational cause to believe that they are infected with HIV. Such individuals will either have received negative test results, or have a life-history in which it is very unlikely that they have been at risk of contracting HIV infection.

Some individuals who have been presented with clear information concerning HIV and its transmission and appear to have had no problems in understanding the information may remain very worried that they may be infected with HIV after they have received a negative test result. In this situation, a counsellor can review with clients relevant areas of their life-history and emphasize that the negative test result is providing an accurate reflection of the fact that they have not been at any significant risk of being infected with HIV.

Exploring why the client remains worried

There is a need, then, to explore with the client exactly why he or she remains so worried about HIV. Aside from providing information which can guide helping actions, this process of exploring fears in a detailed manner can in itself have a therapeutic value. The level of anxiety of some clients will be reduced when fears that they have experienced as all-encompassing, are given a much more limited and definite shape. Being able to look directly at fears in the presence of an understanding, supportive person may also serve to rob these fears of some of their power. A counsellor can also often perform a useful function in helping clients to appreciate that symptoms which they have interpreted as related to HIV are in fact symptoms associated with feeling very anxious.

As well as exploring the precise nature of clients' fears surrounding HIV, it may be necessary to look carefully at the particular set of meanings, metaphors and visual images that make up their conception of HIV and AIDS. A counsellor can then work with the client at constructing an alternative, more 'rational' picture of HIV and AIDS.

Concerns about some unsatisfactory aspect of their life or relationships is sometimes chanelled into and given expression in severe worries concerning HIV. For example, guilt concerning infidelity or about inconsiderate behaviour within a sexual relationship may lead a person to develop serious worries which centre around HIV infection. In such a case, looking carefully at the origins of the worries concerning HIV and pointing out in a sensitive manner the self-defeating nature of this guilt may enable the person to gain greater control over his or her fears about HIV infection and to experience much less anxiety.

A full exploration of why a person is very worried about HIV infection, even although he or she has not experienced any significant risk of contracting HIV, is likely to involve the counsellor in taking a very careful history. The person's worries often need to be understood not only within their present life situation, but also in relation to any emotional difficulties that they have experienced in the past. A counsellor can question 'worried well' clients in a sensitive manner to establish whether they have a history of hypochondria, have experienced episodes of severe depression, states of severe anxiety, obsessional states, or psychiatric illnesses which featured delusional thoughts.

In cases where concerns about HIV seem to be linked in some way or other to a pre-existing psychiatric illness, it is important that counsellors attempt to ensure that clients are referred on to receive appropriate psychiatric treatment. Part of the process of taking a careful history with the worried well will involve exploring whether their anxiety about HIV has led them to have had some thoughts of suicide or even made plans concerning suicide; and also establishing whether they have thought about or attempted suicide in the past. It is important that clients who have persistent thoughts of suicide receive prompt and appropriate psychiatric help.

There may also be occasions where a client has no history of psychiatric illness, and his or her worries about HIV do not fit clearly into any established psychiatric diagnostic category; but it is appropriate because their fears are so disabling or overwhelming that they receive psychiatric help. Referral on to a psychiatrist or clinical psychologist needs to be made in such a way that the client does not feel that his or her concerns about HIV are not being taken seriously. Counsellors can indicate that they will still be available to assist such clients to deal with their worries concerning HIV, but that additional help is also in their best interest.

Helping actions with the 'worried well'

These 'worried well' clients whom the counsellor is confident can be effectively helped to deal with their concerns without receiving psychiatric help may be assisted in a number of ways. The beneficial effect of allowing clients to give expression to specific concerns about HIV and more general problems in their lives was described earlier in this section, as was the effect of giving a more definite and limited shape to their worries about HIV. This process of delimiting worries can be taken a stage further by actively assisting clients to redefine the worries that they may have concerning HIV. Techniques for 'restructuring' irrational, troublesome thoughts can be used by a counsellor working with a 'worried well' client (some of these techniques are discussed in Chapter 8). The counsellor can also teach the client skills of relaxation and of coping with panic attacks, which can be very helpful in reducing anxiety. It may also be appropriate to do some work with clients on how they can solve problems and reduce stress that they are experiencing in their life at the moment.

Clients may have found their thoughts, feelings and actions have become very centred around worries and anxieties. A counsellor can present them with an alternative perspective on their life in which their attention is not focused exclusively on worrying and painful matters. Clients can be encouraged to consider the possibility of relaxation and pleasure. Counsellors can help clients to identify and pursue pleasurable activities which will help them to banish worrying thoughts for a time at least and to reduce their level of anxiety.

Working with clients using the methods that have been suggested in the last few paragraphs can be effective; but in instances where people are experiencing considerable anxiety and are very much 'caught up in' a web of troubling thoughts, progress may be slow. A counsellor will need to display patience and to possess considerable skill. It is important also that counsellors respect their own limitations and recognize that some of their 'worried well' clients may have serious problems which will require psychiatric treatment.

References

Goldstein, R. (1989). 'AIDS and the social contract'. In E. Carter and S. Watney (eds), *Taking Liberties: AIDS and Cultural Politics*. London, Serpents Tail, pp. 81–94.

Marks, R. and Goldblum, P.B. (1989). 'The decision to test: a personal choice'. In J.W. Dilley *et al.* (eds), *Face to Face: A Guide to AIDS Counselling*. San Francisco, AIDS Health Project, pp. 49–58.

Pinching, A. (1990). 'AIDS: Clinical and scientific background'. In B. Almond (ed.), *AIDS – A Moral Issue: The Ethical, Legal and Social Aspects*. London, Macmillan, pp. 25–33.

Suggested reading

On the 'worried-well': Green, J. (1989). 'The worried well'. In J. Green and A. McCreaner (eds), *Counselling in HIV Infection and AIDS*. Oxford, Blackwell Scientific, pp. 167–73.

EIGHT

Living with HIV

CHARLES ANDERSON

Introduction

This chapter looks at the situation of individuals who have recently received an HIV antibody positive diagnosis, and suggests a number of helping actions which may assist them to cope effectively with such a diagnosis. The chapter also looks at the longer-term challenges faced by someone who is living with HIV infection. The need for helpers to have a wide focus of attention and to be able to respond appropriately to any of the wide range of problems that may be experienced by an HIV antibody positive client is emphasized. Attention is directed to the way in which clients may be constructing a new set of meanings for their life after an HIV antibody positive diagnosis, and the actions that a helper can take in assisting clients to question unnecessarily bleak interpretations of their situation. Throughout the chapter, the accent is on looking at how helpers can provide people who are living with HIV infection with information and skills which will assist them to cope with present anxieties, uncertainty about the future and the stigma which has been attached to HIV infection. The first topic that is considered is defining with the person who is living with HIV infection the nature of the helping relationship that will be established with him or her.

Negotiating the nature of a helping relationship

An individual who has recently received an HIV antibody positive diagnosis is likely to be feeling vulnerable, and ready to accept help and support without questioning too deeply the nature of the help that is being provided. If helpers are to respect the vulnerability of their clients and to act responsibly, it is important though that the type of helping which is on offer is described clearly and that consent is obtained (see Chapter 1). This applies as much to a voluntary, informal helping relationship as it does to the help offered by a professional counsellor.

An individual who is coping with the shock of receiving an HIV antibody positive diagnosis may be in need of warm, non-judgemental emotional support from a helper. Care needs to be exercised, however, in the way that emotional support is provided. The client's own longer-term interests will not be served by giving support in a way which encourages a very heavy reliance on the helper and a corresponding devaluing of the client's own strengths and abilities to cope.

It is common for people who have just received an HIV antibody positive test result to wish to receive counselling on a regular basis for the first few months after diagnosis. However, after that period, many individuals may wish only occasional help from either professional counsellors or volunteers. Once an individual has begun to cope with the initial impact of an HIV antibody positive diagnosis, it can be useful for a helper to negotiate with him or her the exact nature of the help that they see themselves requiring in the future. The question of how often they want to meet can be discussed at the same time. Any arrangements that are made concerning the nature of the counselling that is on offer and when meetings with a helper should take place need to be flexible. It is important that helpers respond appropriately to the marked variation over time that there may be in the needs of someone living with HIV for both emotional support and assistance with practical matters.

Coping with the news of an HIV antibody positive test result

Variations in the response to a positive HIV antibody test result

The period immediately following an HIV antibody positive result is often one of considerable confusion and emotional distress. Individual reactions to an HIV antibody positive result vary greatly, however, and not everyone experiences an immediate, or somewhat delayed, large increase in anxiety (Perry *et al.*, 1990).

It was argued in Chapter 2 that it is important that general descriptions of how people react to loss and to stressful situations are not used by helpers in a *prescriptive* way. Although many people will feel great distress on receiving a positive HIV antibody test result, this does not mean that *all* individuals will or should experience and express distress. Some clients may even experience a certain amount of relief from the strain that uncertainty about their HIV antibody status was causing them. Helpers need to base their responses on a sensitive and accurate assessment of the ways in which a client is in fact responding to the news of an HIV positive antibody test, rather than being driven by a set of assumptions concerning how an individual *ought* to react to such a situation.

Common responses to receiving a positive HIV antibody test result

Even with careful pre-test counselling and a lot of personal work to prepare for the possibility of a positive result, many individuals do experience a profound sense of shock when they are given the news that they have tested positive for HIV antibodies. This sense of shock will affect feelings, thoughts and behaviour, and may manifest itself in a number of different ways. Some individuals will respond by feeling 'numb'. In addition, they may become withdrawn, finding it very difficult to communicate with anyone. Others will experience very great emotional pain and express it by crying, or possibly by being aggressive and abusive. Often individuals will respond by feeling emotionally 'numb' on some occasions, and quite overwhelmed by powerful emotions at other times.

It is common in the aftermath of receiving distressing news of any kind to experience sudden intrusive troubling thoughts which it does not seem possible to control. Competing worries and uncertainties about the future, and frightening images of the future, may fill the mind in quick succession to each other. People may also be seized by sudden strong feelings of anger, which are both frightening and difficult to control.

The feelings and thoughts experienced by an individual who has received a very disturbing piece of news are particularly hard to bear, because in addition to being more intense than normal they also tend to be unpredictable. Disturbing images of the future may appear suddenly, and strong feelings of sadness or anger may also occur without any warning. Consequently, some people may feel that they have 'lost control' of their thoughts and feelings. Shock also affects an individual's thinking abilities, and some impairment in the normal powers of concentration, memory and communication may in itself be a further source of worry.

At a time when the world may seem very uncertain and troubling, it is important that an individual who has received a positive HIV antibody test result, or a diagnosis of HIV-related illness, is provided with a caring, helping relationship where he or she can feel secure and fully accepted. Within such a relationship, an individual can express the strong emotions which he or she is experiencing and have their feelings of grief and loss validated.

While listening to a client's expression of distressing feelings, a helper needs to emphasize that although these feelings are intense, they are not 'abnormal' in any way. Clients may need to be told very clearly that the distress that they are experiencing does not mean that they have 'become mad' or that they are coping badly. It is a natural reaction to a difficult situation. Clients may feel less troubled by a lack of customary control over thoughts and feelings, when they are reassured that what they are experiencing is a normal response to very distressing news.

The need to gain information

Having questions about HIV answered in a clear, calm and honest fashion may also be an important need for many individuals who have received a positive test result, and are seeking to gain greater control over the new situation that they find themselves in. Some worries may also be eased by the provision of information. Explaining the biology of HIV and clarifying medical terms can help to 'demystify' HIV, to make it seem less alien and threatening. While it is important that clients are provided with the opportunity to explore any worries about HIV and to have all their questions about HIV answered, a helper also needs to avoid overwhelming a client with information. There are very distinct limits to the amount of information that anyone who is feeling somewhat confused by shock can absorb. The helper very much needs to take the lead from the client as to what information is required and the pace at which information is presented.

Clients may also be helped towards a greater sense of control over their lives, if a helper presents a clear picture of the ways in which shock and grief affect thoughts, feelings and behaviour. It is particularly useful to explain the connections between thoughts and feelings of anxiety and the physical manifestations of anxiety. Clients who have been suffering from panic attacks, or who fear that they may suffer from panic attacks, can be instructed in a number of techniques, such as re-establishing a normal pattern of breathing, to manage such attacks. Various means of controlling anxiety, for example by distraction, by using relaxation techniques, by 'defusing' the power of anxiety-provoking thoughts, can also be suggested. Exploring with some clients how they have coped with difficult situations in the past and reminding them of strengths that they possess for coping with adversity can be a very useful helping action.

Some clients may react to an HIV antibody test result by feeling that all aspects of their life are now totally changed. Helpers can acknowledge these feelings. At the same time, they can point out to clients that, although they may be viewing their life in very different terms at the moment, an HIV antibody positive diagnosis does not necessarily mean that large changes are required in everyday living or a reduction in the quality of life.

Occasionally, clients may feel that they wish to cope with the news of a positive HIV antibody test result by making immediate large changes in their life, or by broadcasting the news widely among their circle of friends and acquaintances. While respecting the client's right to cope with the news in his or her own fashion, helpers can advise some caution over making any sudden, large changes. Helpers can work with clients to explore carefully the costs and benefits that may be associated with specific changes, and with giving the news of the test result to particular people. They can also present a different perspective on the time over which changes can be made and the ordering of priorities for change. Often, it can be pointed out that there is no urgency to take decisions or make changes, and that for the moment priority can be given to allowing personal adjustment to the test result to take place. Clients can be reminded that they will be in a stronger position to make changes once their feelings have quietened a bit, they have learned more about HIV and its effects and they have had time to understand what the diagnosis means for them personally.

Helpers can assist clients who have recently received the news of a positive HIV antibody test to give their life a bit more structure and enhance their sense of control by previewing in very concrete terms how they plan to cope in the next few days, or weeks. There is a need to identify both ways of coping with emotional difficulties and with practical problems. They can consider what activities will be most useful in filling up leisure time and in giving some sense of reassurance, and how stresses at work and at home can be managed. Helper and client can discuss carefully the extent to which a partner or close friends can be relied on for support, and how best to call on and make use of the support that may be available to them.

If appropriate, clients may also be referred to local self-help groups for HIV antibody positive people where their concerns will be readily understood and they will come to appreciate that they need not be isolated or view being HIV positive as stigmatizing. 'Buddies', volunteers trained by agencies such as Scottish AIDS Monitor, can also be a very valuable source of support for an individual who is experiencing considerable shock as a result of receiving the news of a positive HIV antibody test. Buddies often make a time commitment to an HIV positive individual which professional helpers would not be able to match, and can provide solid emotional support and friendship.

In conversation with a helper, a person who has recently received the news of a positive test result is also likely to make some exploratory moves to give meaning to the diagnosis. The next section looks at some of the varying ways in which individuals make some sense out of the news of a positive HIV antibody test result, or the diagnosis of an HIV-related illness.

Looking for meaning in an HIV antibody positive diagnosis

It is difficult for anyone who is given a definite diagnosis of illness, or the prospect of an uncertain future inherent in an HIV antibody positive diagnosis, to regard this situation as coming about by 'chance'. We seem to need to construct an explanation, to give meaning, to the experience of illness or the possibility that we may be faced with a serious illness in the future. The meanings that we do create to make sense of illness, or difficult situations of uncertainty, are likely to be linked to any religious beliefs that we may have and to our general beliefs about the nature and purpose of life. For example, in describing her experience of working with cancer patients and their families, Simonton (1984, p. 31) observes that: 'In asking, "Why me?" patients are also asking a theological question. It may be stated as, "Why is there evil in the world?" or "Is this really God's will?" or "What did I do to deserve this?".'

An individual's general world-view and customary ways of responding to difficulties will influence how he or she attributes the causes of becoming infected with HIV. Some individuals may attribute becoming infected with HIV to factors within themselves, such as 'lack of self-control', while others attribute infection to factors outside of themselves, such as the social environment in which they were living. These different styles of attribution, of accounting for infection with HIV, may lead to corresponding differences in adjustment to an HIV antibody positive diagnosis or a diagnosis of AIDS. A study conducted in California by Jeffrey Moulton, as reported by Mandel (1986), found that among men with AIDS attributing illness to external factors, such as bad luck, appeared to give some emotional protection. A different set of outcomes was found for individuals who attributed infection to factors within themselves. In Mandel's (1986, p. 78) words: 'Attributing responsibility to oneself for a life-threatening condition can be devastating. If experienced as a "death warrant", a diagnosis of AIDS may involve blaming one's character or behavior for a condition for which no redress may be available.'

The possibility of reacting to an HIV antibody positive diagnosis by blaming oneself for becoming infected with HIV is increased by the social stigma that has been attached to HIV infection. Some of the discussion of AIDS within the media, and throughout society, has tended to blame the 'victims' of HIV infection for the situation in which they find themselves. Under the shock and strain of an HIV antibody positive diagnosis, some individuals may be led to internalize these social perceptions of blame and to wonder whether they have in fact done something in the past which was wrong. They may come to reinterpret their past and to feel guilty about actions which previously caused small, or no, concern. Internalizing blame for becoming infected with HIV is likely to lead to feelings of inadequacy and lack of self-worth, which in turn make it difficult to cope effectively with the challenges of HIV.

The search for meaning may thus lead individuals to 'reconstruct' their past and to have a new, darker vision of their life history. Some individuals may also come to construct their future in very negative terms and in a way which fills their present experience with despair. Dorothy Rowe (1983, p. 46), writing about the world-view of people suffering from depression, notes how: 'If you have written a scenario for yourself which includes much pain and suffering, or circumstances which produce a terrible death scene, then this scene can take on a strange reality and haunt all your waking and sleeping moments.'

Assisting a client to construct a different set of meanings

When clients are expressing a view of the future which is similar to the scenario that Rowe describes, it can be tempting for helpers to react with reassurance and an attempt to provide a positive, optimistic account of the future. However, such a surface imposition of a more positive view of the future on a client is not likely to be particularly effective in addition to being ethically somewhat suspect. Clients may need to be helped to explore very carefully the particular view of their present and future world which they have created in response to an HIV antibody positive diagnosis before any real change in outlook is possible.

Part of this careful exploration of their view of the world is likely to involve considering *exactly* how their general view of the future and particular trouble-some thoughts are causing them emotional pain and limiting their freedom of action. As this process of exploring their thoughts about the present and the future proceeds, clients are likely to find themselves more able to replace global, 'catastrophic' worries about the present and the future with a more clearly defined set of concerns. All-encompassing fears that have a vague threatening shape may be transformed into a more sharply focused set of difficult, but manageable, worries.

One important way in which a helper can assist HIV antibody positive individuals to create a more hopeful view of their present and future is by exploring with them in some depth how they think about HIV and AIDS. One aspect of this joint work of looking at beliefs and knowledge about HIV and AIDS involves giving information which may correct unnecessarily nega-tive views that the person has about matters such as the amount of life that may be left for him or her.

A sense of hope can also be found by some clients in looking in detail at the possibilities for antiviral treatment and prophylactic treatment for HIV-related illnesses that may be available to them. Much of the discussion of AIDS in the media has presented the picture that little can be achieved in the way of treatment. It is understandable, therefore, that some people with HIV infec-tion take a fatalistic and hopeless attitude to their future. While acknowledg-ing both the potentially life-threatening nature of HIV infection and the reality of a client's feelings of hopelessness, a helper can also point out what can be achieved in the way of treatment and in maintaining the quality of life of individuals with HIV-related illness.

Chapter 1 pointed out the damaging effect on HIV antibody positive individuals of the ways in which AIDS has been socially represented, and people with HIV infection have been stigmatized. As that chapter identified, a very important helping action may be to identify with HIV antibody positive clients whether they are thinking about HIV and AIDS in terms of the frightening and stigmatizing images that have been used in the media. If a client is thinking about HIV and AIDS in such images, a helper can work to strip these images of AIDS of their destructive power and to negotiate with the client new, less emotive meanings for HIV.

An earlier part of this chapter described how some HIV antibody positive individuals may come to 'internalize' the social stigma and the attitudes of blame that have been attached to people with HIV infection. Helpers may often find it appropriate to consider with an HIV antibody positive client the way in which people with HIV have been stigmatized, and the harmful and hurtful effects of this process of stigmatization. More positive, caring and hopeful ways of seeing their situation can then be discussed. Such discussion of social stigma and of the way it can be internalized into feelings of self-blame and 'uncleanness' can be very helpful to a person with HIV infection. However, a more powerful influence may be meeting and talking with other HIV antibody positive individuals who have managed to develop a fairly positive outlook and an assertive attitude towards the world. Some people with HIV infection have also said that they found it very encouraging to read accounts of how other people had experienced living with the knowledge that they had HIV. An excellent book of this type is *Living With HIV In Self and Others*, by Richie McMullen, in which he reveals his 'own vulnerabilities as a man with HIV disease', and at the same time celebrates 'being fully human and fully alive' (McMullen, 1988, p. 5).

Living with uncertainty

Whatever sets of beliefs individuals use to make sense of the experience of discovering that they are HIV antibody positive, they are faced with the task of living continuously with a large degree of uncertainty about how the future will turn out. This uncertainty is a source of stress, and often makes a large qualitative difference to an individual's experience of the world. If they are to respond appropriately to HIV antibody positive clients, helpers need to attempt to view the world from their clients' perspective, and try to gain at least some sense of how such a degree of uncertainty may change one's felt experience and view of the world. It was indicated at the beginning of this chapter that the amount of support and counselling help required by people living with HIV may fluctuate considerably over time. Uncertainties and anxieties about the future may remain at a low level for long periods and then become acute again, possibly as a result of a minor, or more serious, illness or of stresses experienced in relationships or at work. Helpers need to make themselves readily available when uncertainty and anxiety are acute; and they can take care not to be too intrusive at times when an individual is feeling more secure and experiencing little anxiety.

Coping with HIV

Different coping styles

There is quite marked variation in the way that individuals cope with the uncertainty about the future, and stress, of an HIV antibody positive diagnosis. An individual's general style of coping with HIV may be determined by quite a large number of factors. One critical determinant of how they cope with living with HIV is the way in which they view their present and future situation. Earlier sections of the chapter have looked in some detail at the effects of differing sets of meanings that an individual may attach to HIV, and of different ways of viewing the future. HIV may be regarded as a challenge to be combated vigorously, or as a 'fate' that limits the person's powers of action. The ability to see HIV as a challenge to be met vigorously will also be influenced by the beliefs that individuals have about their general *self-efficacy*, their ability to control and influence events.

Other important influences on the way in which an individual copes with living with HIV will include their manner of coping with difficult situations in the past, the social support which they have available to them, their past experience of illness, and the ways in which they think about health and illness. The style of coping with HIV which an individual adopts may also be heavily influenced by cultural norms of how to respond to difficult situations and to illness. As Chapter 1 described, individuals in some cultures may not share the Western preoccupation with establishing 'control' over external events, and may be more concerned to control their thoughts and emotions.

A number of studies have indicated that the use of an 'active' or 'positive' coping style by people living with HIV and AIDS has beneficial consequences. For example, in discussing the results of a study of the coping strategies of people with AIDS, Namir (1986, pp. 91–2) writes that: 'participants in our study who were better psychologically were using an active form of coping called positive involvement. This includes taking vitamins, maintaining a healthful diet, developing themselves as people, being involved in political activities related to AIDS, and enjoying everyday things more than previously.' Namir's list thus identifies as a successful style of coping one which involves the elements of actively maintaining health, dealing with emotional issues and enjoyable social involvement.

Given that this active style of coping which deals with both practical and emotional challenges has very positive outcomes, there is a danger that some helpers in HIV might give it the status of an ideal type of coping which clients *ought* to use. As the preceding paragraphs have described, there are many factors which influence an individual to use, this or other, styles of coping. It is important that clients are presented with the possibility of dealing with the challenges of HIV in this active manner and encouraged to see themselves as having the ability to control aspects of their lives and to live fully. At the same time, though, helpers need to avoid *imposing* this or any other style of coping on a client, either in a direct or more subtle fashion.

For some individuals, a more stoical, somewhat less active, style of coping with HIV may represent an effective and appropriate strategy viewed from within the context of their personal history, cultural background and present experience. A helper will encounter individuals living with HIV who are having difficulty in constructing any general way of coping, or who have adopted a style of coping, such as attempting to totally avoid recognizing the challenges posed by HIV and avoiding social contact, which is causing them considerable difficulties. In such cases, the challenge for the helper is to work with clients to try to identify particular, more constructive ways of coping, which will meet their own goals in life and be tailored to their own personality and the resources that they have for managing stress.

Managing stress

Helping clients to cope in a positive manner with the challenges of HIV may involve working with them to identify sources of stress in their life and working out ways in which they can reduce or eliminate these sources of stress. Clients may, for example, consider how they can relieve themselves of some tasks which are causing them a lot of stress. They can learn techniques of relaxation and work to introduce, or re-introduce, more pleasurable activities into their lives. They can also learn to view social or work situations which cause them stress in a way which makes them appear less threatening, and how to be assertive in stressful situations. Dealing with relationship difficulties often may help an individual to feel much less stressed.

Active work to reduce levels of stress may give back to some individuals living with HIV the sense of control over their present and future that had been threatened by anxieties and uncertainty about the future. Reducing stress leads to a greater sense of well-being and an ability to cope with challenge. Aside from the beneficial effects on emotional health and social life of reducing stress, there may be benefits for physical health. The results from some studies suggest that stressful experiences may somewhat reduce the ability of the body to combat infection (Endler, 1988). It needs to be noted, however, that the exact relationship between stress and immunological functioning is not clearly understood and is likely to be complex. The effects of stress on immune functioning seem to depend in part on the individual's ability to cope with stress (Endler, 1988). Individual's beliefs about their capabilities to cope and exert control over themselves and over their social world, their sense of self-efficacy, may also influence the effects that stress has on the immune system. Bandura (1989, p. 129) notes that 'perceived coping inefficacy increases vulnerability to stress and depression and activates biochemical changes that can affect various facets of immune function'.

Although reducing stress may have a number of positive effects in the life of a person who is HIV antibody positive, care needs to be taken by people living with HIV in the way that they go about reducing stress. In particular, sudden large changes in behaviour, even if they have the purpose of creating a less stressed life, may themselves be a source of disruption and stress for at least a short period of time. Sometimes, individuals may force themselves to make changes towards 'healthier living' but lack any intrinsic motivation to alter their lives. They may be making changes towards a less 'stressed' life, simply because this seems to be a good idea or because they're being pressured by friends or helpers. Individuals who are forcing themselves to make changes against the grain of their real inclinations, who don't have their heart in the efforts that they are making, may often create tension for themselves rather than reduce stress.

Some simple ways to reduce stress were presented in the first paragraph of this section. However, implementing these individual ways of reducing stress needs to be tailored very carefully to the situation of each individual who is living with HIV. Helpers need to avoid the belief that there can be a standard treatment for reducing stress. Much recent work by psychologists on understanding stress and its effects has emphasized that the way in which people respond to stress is very heavily influenced by the manner in which they view potentially stressful experiences (Lazarus and Folkman, 1984). The same event may seem very threatening and stressful to one person, but be regarded as a challenge by another person. The way in which people respond to stress is also very much affected by the way in which they judge both their own options for coping with stress and how effective they may be in putting these options into practice (Lazarus and Folkman, 1984). Aside from these important differences in the perception of potentially stressful experiences, people vary considerably in their vulnerability to stress.

Taking these important individual differences into account requires that helpers assist people living with HIV to identify what aspects of their situation *they* find most stressful. Some ways of reducing these sources of stress can then be discussed which fit well with the person's own aims in life.

There is a danger that stress can be thought about in too 'individualistic' a fashion, and all the responsibility for dealing with stress placed on the individual who is living with HIV him- or herself. Studies on stress have found that social support is very important in buffering individuals from stress and in enabling them to cope with stressful experiences. Having strong support from partners, friends and helpers can enable individuals to experience stressful events, such as learning that you are HIV antibody positive, as less devastating and enhance their abilities to cope with everyday life. Not everyone living with HIV, however, can rely on concerned friends to provide support in an appropriate, sensitive fashion. Even in cases where friends are initially very supportive, they may find it difficult, or not see the need, to sustain this support over a long period of time. The social network of some people living with HIV may be a source of stress, discord and rejection rather than a resource which supports them in times of stress. Helpers need to be very aware of the resources that individuals living with HIV have for managing stress, and the constraints that their social situation may impose on reducing stress.

Many people living with HIV have very stressful living conditions, such as very poor housing and being desperately short of money. Attempts to encourage HIV antibody positive individuals who have difficult living conditions to 'reduce stress', aside from being insensitive, are not likely to be particularly effective until their living conditions are improved. Helpers who wish to assist such individuals to 'reduce their stress' may as a first step need to fight hard with them to get better housing, or benefits to which they are entitled.

Locating helping efforts firmly within a social context

As the preceding paragraphs on managing stress have argued, helpers may risk responding inappropriately to a client if they do not take his or her social situation fully into account. Chapter 1 argued very vigorously for the need to set helping efforts firmly within a social context and to consider carefully how a person's response to living with HIV is shaped by the relationships within their social world. The effects on people living with HIV of social stigma, and the fact that many of the hurts which they suffer come from others, and are not simply a problem of 'internal adjustment' to a difficult situation were also highlighted.

Much of the discussion in the present chapter has focused on how helpers can work with clients to allow them to meet the challenges of HIV and to exercise greater control over their lives. There are times, though, when the reactions of other people in the life of an HIV antibody positive person make it very difficult for him or her to exercise greater control over his or her life. HIV may deeply affect not only the emotions of the person infected by HIV, but also his or her partner, family and friends. The way in which significant people in the life of a person living with HIV respond to the news of the diagnosis may limit his or her possibilities for positive emotional coping and action. If a partner reacts very angrily and disruptively to the news of the HIV antibody positive diagnosis, or reacts by totally denying the reality of the diagnosis, it can make life very difficult indeed for the person who is living with HIV. Effective helping in HIV often requires a careful exploration of the way in which significant people in the client's life are reacting to the HIV antibody diagnosis, and how these reactions are affecting and possibly limiting the emotional response and daily life of the person who is living with HIV. In some cases, it may be necessary to attempt to provide support and counselling for a partner, family member or friend in order to reduce stress on the person living with HIV and to increase his or her freedom of action (see Chapter 14).

Helpers also need to be sensitive to the ways in which the social roles that women play will affect their perception of living with HIV and their styles of coping with HIV. The worries of HIV antibody positive women with dependent children are often likely to focus largely on their children rather than on themselves. For them, coping with HIV cannot be focused solely on their own needs.

Sexual difficulties and pleasures

One possible source of stress for a person living with HIV is sexual difficulties, which may arise after the news of an HIV antibody positive test result. Loss of sexual desire is a common response to highly stressful events. Individuals who have recently received the news that they are HIV antibody positive can often be assured that in time they will regain their normal level of sexual desire. A loss, or a considerable reduction, in sexual desire often accompanies depression. Such a loss of desire can itself be an additional worry and source of strain and create difficulties in a stable sexual relationship. Illness, whether or not it is HIV-related, also commonly leads to a reduction in sexual desire.

Some individuals living with HIV may feel a sense of grief at what they see as the loss of their past sex life. A helper can assist them to acknowledge and deal with this sense of loss. Some women may feel a great sense of loss if they decide that they now cannot have children. This decision in turn may affect their self-image and their sexuality. Some clients may also wish to discuss, and discover ways of dealing with, emotional or practical difficulties that they are having in practising safe sex.

A smaller number of clients may have continuing difficulties with sexual expression which are related to their understandable fears about HIV. It may be necessary to explore with such clients exactly how they see their own sexuality, how they see HIV, and how they are linking together HIV and sexual expression in their minds. Different ways of thinking about HIV and about their own sexuality can be considered. They can also work to re-establish the association between sex and pleasure, and to challenge any recent associations that they have established between sex and distress and danger. Clients who continue to have problems with sexual desire, or sexual expression, may benefit from receiving help from a psychologist or psychiatrist who specializes in the treatment of sexual problems.

Aside from wishing to talk about and resolve any problems they are experiencing in sexual desire and expression, people living with HIV may simply want detailed information from helpers on how to practise safer sex (see Chapter 6). One important point to bear in mind here is that current safer sex guidelines advise that even when both individuals in a relationship are HIV antibody positive, they should consider practising safer sex. This is because of the variability in the HIV virus, i.e. the fact that there are slightly different strains of the virus. Talking about and negotiating safer sex with a partner can be particularly problematic for a less sexually experienced, younger person, and also for women (see Chapter 10).

Maintaining and making relationships

The problems that some individuals find in sexual desire and expression may not be caused by shock, depression or the way that they view the links between HIV and sex. Some individuals living with HIV have found that their partners have been unable to cope well with the news of their HIV antibody positive test result and that their relationship has become troubled. A very important aspect of helping in HIV involves assisting people living with HIV to express problems that they are having with a partner, and to identify how they are going to deal with these problems. Sometimes, these problems may be directly related to HIV, and sometimes they may result from existing stresses in the relationship.

Often, an individual living with HIV will be firmly committed to a stable sexual relationship and wishes to resolve whatever difficulties exist. At other times, however, the question of whether the person living with HIV wants his or her present sexual relationship to continue may be much more open. They may find it very useful to talk through with someone else their feelings and situation, and identify more clearly the advantages and disadvantages associated with the relationship. In such circumstances, it will often be important for the individual to identify whether he or she wants to take the risk of leaving the present relationship. For women with dependent children, this process of deciding whether or not to stay in a relationship may be particularly difficult. Their assessment of what they should do is often likely to centre around the needs of the children. They also may need to cope with social pressures to 'keep the family together'.

Helpers need to appreciate the difficulties and isolation which may be experienced by someone living with HIV who does not have a sexual relationship, and may also have few, if any, close friendships. Some individuals living with HIV have described how they have been reluctant to take the risk of starting a new close relationship, which they are aware may bring with it not only advantages but also the possibility of experiencing more hurt and loss. On occasion, it may be important for helpers to encourage or 'to back' individuals to take the risk of starting a new relationship.

Starting a new relationship can be very difficult for someone who has been feeling isolated and emotionally somewhat vulnerable. John MacLachlan (1991) expresses these difficulties very clearly in the account that he has written of living with AIDS: 'I wanted desperately for someone to hold me, comfort me, to take away the pain, the fear and the loneliness. . . . I sought salvation from the first person available. Inevitably, it didn't work.' Helpers may need to give a great deal of support and work carefully on problem solving with someone who is trying to establish a new relationship under difficult circumstances.

Telling partners and friends the news of a positive test result

Often, someone living with HIV may wish to explore with a helper how best to give the news to a prospective, or indeed an established, sexual partner that he or she is HIV antibody positive. They can look at the difficult feelings that may be involved for both parties, consider how best to give the news, and preview how the individual will cope and respond to a number of different reactions.

For many individuals living with HIV, the support of friends, and possibly also of family, who are aware of their HIV antibody positive diagnosis can be of very great value. However, the reaction of significant people in an HIV antibody positive person's life to the news of their HIV status is not always as favourable, and sometimes can be the source of great pain and feelings of loss. Even on occasions when an individual is very sure that they will meet with support and acceptance, the actual act of telling someone the news of the diagnosis may be a fairly stressful experience. It is particularly likely to be stressful when disclosure of the news of an HIV antibody positive diagnosis to a family member also involves disclosing for the first time being gay or having been involved in intravenous drug use. Individuals who are living with HIV will often wish to work with a helper to decide who they should tell about their diagnosis and when, exploring disadvantages and advantages of giving the news. If they decide that they do want to go ahead and break the news to some friends or members of the family, they may also wish to look at how best to go about giving the news.

Helping others living with HIV

Many individuals have found a source of new friendships and a sense of real purpose in becoming actively involved in the politics of HIV and AIDS or in a helping, befriending role with other people who are living with HIV. Coping effectively with HIV and the stresses it brings does not need to be centred largely on self. It may involve an active commitment and a very positive contribution to other people who are living with HIV infection.

Providing information on practical matters and gaining access to services

An earlier section of the chapter emphasized that enabling some people living with HIV to reduce stress will involve dealing with pressing practical problems and improving living conditions. Chapter 6 gave a checklist of topic areas on which helpers need to possess up-to-date information if they are to provide an effective service to individuals who are affected in some way or other by HIV infection. Chapter 6 also emphasized the importance of helpers establishing a good local network of contacts which would give a client access to more specialized information and services. This is particularly important for dealing with practical problems which are faced by a client. For example, it is important to know where a client can receive sound and sympathetic advice on legal matters related to HIV or on other legal problems. Legal advice may often be required around employment issues. Individuals with HIV infection need good advice on how best to protect their position, and what rights they have, within their particular place of work. Legal advice may also be urgently required should an employer, or prospective employer, make any demand for HIV antibody testing. Good advice is also required when the question of HIV antibody testing arises in relation to private health insurance schemes which are linked to employment.

One area of practical concern faced by many people is how to deal with different sorts of insurance problems (see Chapter 7). These problems might relate to life insurance, mortgage-related insurance or private health insurance. Helpers need to be well informed on the general aspects of insurance and HIV. Clients can also be given information about other financial options – how they may borrow money and meet financial obligations without facing the demands associated with taking out an insurance policy. However, clients may often have enquiries about insurance which are not altogether straightforward and would benefit from more detailed advice from a lawyer or insurance broker. Such advice can be obtained from the legal centre of the Terrence Higgins Trust, or from the legal service provided by Scottish AIDS Monitor. It can also be useful to attempt to establish contacts with local lawyers or sympathetic insurance brokers who are knowledgeable about the problems faced by individuals affected by HIV in obtaining insurance and the options which may be available to them.

Chapter 9 looks at the question of the housing needs of people living with HIV and HIV-related illness. The quantity and quality of the provision of housing services to people who are living with HIV varies considerably over the UK as a whole. Good local knowledge and contacts are again important.

It is useful if all helpers have a fair knowledge of the welfare benefits and various types of financial help to which people living with HIV may be entitled. The booklet *HIV and AIDS Welfare Rights Guide* (Hillier, 1990) provides a good introduction to the subject. However, detailed knowledge of benefits and a working knowledge of how best to ensure that clients receive payments to which they are entitled is required in many cases. Some agencies, such as Scottish AIDS Monitor, employ welfare rights officers to advise and press the case of individuals who are living with HIV and HIV-related illness. Citizens Advice Bureaux, and Citizens Rights Offices in Scotland, can also be a useful source of advice. A successfully-functioning local network of advice on welfare rights and financial matters can be a very valuable resource for people living with HIV.

Life is for living

Much of the discussion in this chapter has centred on the actions that a helper can take to enable a person living with HIV to gain a sense of emotional well-being and an ability to cope effectively with the challenges of HIV. Even when helpers have established a fairly democratic relationship where the emphasis is on the transfer of knowledge and skills, there is a danger that the way in which these skills are handed over may limit the client's possibilities for action.

Careful attention needs to be given to the *spirit* in which helpers work with clients to meet the challenges of HIV. Much work may need to be done on dealing with particular troublesome thoughts, identifying assets, clarifying the nature of problems and looking for appropriate solutions to these problems, and helping clients to learn new skills which will enhance the quality of their life. As they look at ways of dealing with particular challenges, however, there can be a tendency on the part both of helpers and people who are HIV antibody positive themselves to see living with HIV solely as a 'set of tasks' which has to be managed successfully. If some individuals living with HIV are to avoid being dominated by a 'task-centred' view of the world, helpers may need to emphasize their freedom of action, to remind them that HIV has not robbed them of the ability to act spontaneously and to feel joy. The necessary concentration on careful planning to meet the challenges of HIV and to increase control over life may need to be balanced by a willingness to back clients to take risks and to encourage them to act and feel without fear. Life is for living, not just about coping successfully with a series of tasks and challenges.

Ensuring that some clients receive appropriate specialist help

As Chapter 1 emphasized, it is important that helpers acknowledge their own limitations, and ensure that clients who are experiencing particularly severe psychological problems receive appropriate expert treatment. Among individuals who are coping with HIV-related illness, it can also be very difficult to diagnose whether or not severe disturbances in thoughts and feelings are directly related to some organic cause (see Chapter 4). Careful assessment may be required to make sure that clients receive the appropriate treatment.

To facilitate a client's access to psychiatric intervention, both voluntary and professional helping agencies need to maintain good links with psychiatrists and clinical psychologists in their area. Any referral of a client on to psychiatric help needs to be done in a very sensitive fashion. A helper may also need to deal with any fears or stigmatizing attitudes that the client may attach to seeing a psychiatrist. It is important that clients are not left with the perception that they are being rejected by the helper or being 'passed on' because they are too difficult for the helper to handle. The ways in which the helper can continue to provide a client with caring support, while he or she is at the same time receiving more expert psychiatric care, may need to be emphasized. It is particularly necessary to ensure that a client receives appropriate expert care when he or she is suffering from *suicidal* thoughts and feelings, severe *depression* and persisting *obsessional* thoughts or behaviour.

Suicidal thoughts and feelings, and dealing with feelings of 'hopelessness'

Looking first at suicidal thoughts and feelings, it is not uncommon for people who are experiencing grief and loss, or any large traumatic change in their life, to think about the possibility of suicide. It is important that helpers take care to provide clients with an opportunity to express any suicidal thoughts and feelings which they may have experienced. Even in cases where there may be very little risk of the person committing suicide, it may be a great relief to be able to talk about such feelings. Discussion of suicidal thoughts may also make it easier for the person to express feelings of anger or hopelessness which may be associated with such thoughts. Similarly, feelings of grief which may be accompanying thoughts of suicide may be validated. Where appropriate, clients can be assured that having some thoughts about suicide is a fairly common experience for people who are suddenly faced with distressing news and uncertainties concerning the future.

Thoughts of suicide and suicide attempts are most likely to occur when an individual feels a sense of hopelessness about the future and a lack of power to change this bleak future for the better (Beck *et al.*, 1985). When clients are overwhelmed by a sense of hopelessness, helpers can assist them to explore the ways in which their feelings are linked to the particular vision that they have created of what the future holds. An earlier section of this chapter suggested some ways in which clients can be helped to rethink some of their current beliefs and to construct a less troubling view of the present and the future. When a client is exploring the effects of a general bleak vision of the future, or the effects of particular troubling thoughts, it is important that a helper allows any painful feelings associated with these thoughts to be expressed fully. Once these feelings have been expressed, a helper can assist a client to rekindle a sense of hope.

Hopelessness, whether or not it is accompanied by suicidal thoughts, can also be decreased by reminding individuals of the strengths that they possess to cope with difficulties, and the ways in which they can *act* on the world. In addition to reminding people of their strengths, a helper can also assist individuals to enhance their abilities to act confidently. When people who have been beset by feelings of hopelessness manage to set and achieve goals which matter to them, the belief that they are 'victims' and cannot control their future is likely to be weakened.

In studies in the general population of factors which may place people at risk of committing suicide, social isolation, i.e. a lack of any strong social support in times of difficulties, emerges clearly as a risk factor. It may be very necessary to ensure that some clients who possess little in the way of social support are provided with a befriending relationship with a voluntary worker who can provide commitment and care.

Some clients may have considerable sources of support available to them in their ordinary social network, but feel alienated from everyone and perceive themselves as being very much alone. Helpers can work with such clients to examine and possibly resolve these feelings of alienation. Feelings of alienation may have been created in some clients by the very real hurts that they have recently received from friends or other significant people in their lives. In such cases, helpers can work with the individuals to acknowledge and begin to heal the hurts that they have received, and to encourage them not to 'give up' on trusting other people, to risk looking for warmth, acceptance and joy in new social or sexual relationships. A helper can also work with a client to resolve feelings of alienation that have arisen from difficulties that a client is experiencing with his or her partner.

Whenever clients discuss suicidal thoughts or plans for suicide, a helper needs to assess very carefully how serious they may be in their intentions to commit suicide. There is also a need to consider the degree of hopelessness which the person is feeling, and a number of other factors which may increase the likelihood of a person putting an intention to commit suicide into practice. These factors include earlier suicide attempts or episodes of suicidal thinking, a history of psychiatric problems, lack of social support, problems related to drug or alcohol use, and coping with severe pain or discomfort.

Where clients have expressed an active intention to commit suicide, or appear to be at considerable risk of making a suicide attempt, psychiatric help needs to be arranged immediately. Even when suicidal thoughts do not appear to be accompanied by any active planning to put them into practice, it may still be appropriate to suggest psychiatric assessment and care. Continuing powerful thoughts concerning suicide can in themselves be a source of great distress and also be associated with other problems, such as severe depression, which may require psychiatric help.

Responding appropriately to depression

Depression is a common reaction to discovering that one is HIV antibody positive or to receiving a diagnosis of HIV-related illness. In addition to the distress caused by the lowering of mood, lack of enjoyment in life and loss of a sense of purpose, depression has disabling effects on thought and action. People suffering from depression often lose their appetite and experience disturbances in their pattern of sleeping. It is also more difficult to control feelings, such as irritability with others. Some individuals may have frequent episodes of crying. Feelings of tiredness and a loss, or at least a reduction, in sexual desire are common. An individual's powers of concentration are also reduced by depression, and it may be difficult to order one's thoughts clearly.

For many individuals, depression disappears or declines to less troubling proportions, once they have time to adjust to an HIV antibody positive diagnosis without any skilled intervention from a helper. When individuals are continuing to suffer depression some time after receiving an HIV antibody positive diagnosis, there are a number of actions that a helper can take to assist them to deal with depression and its effects.

A simple but useful action is to inform clients about what is known concerning depression, its effects and its treatment. This action gives more power to clients to understand and decide on treatment options. It also gives them a somewhat different perspective on depression, as a condition that they can study and gain control over rather than just a force which is imprisoning their lives. There are also a number of good, clearly written books such as *Coping with Depression* by Ivy Blackburn (1987), and those written by Dorothy Rowe, in particular *Depression: The Way Out of Your Prison* (1983), which a person with depression may find very helpful. These books present the experience of individuals with depression, discuss the nature of depression and suggest ways of coping with it.

An important set of actions for a helper working with individuals with depression is to assist them to examine and challenge the set of beliefs that is leading them to see the future as hopeless. Earlier sections of this chapter have looked at ways in which helpers can work with clients to explore the effects of a bleak vision of the future or the way in which particular thoughts can lead to feelings of hopelessness. It is also important to help depressed individuals to develop a greater sense of their ability to act and take control of their life. They need to feel that they are in charge, not HIV. Exercises in creative visualization, where a depressed individual concentrates his or her attention on the healing power of particular calming or energizing images, may also be helpful in dispelling negative thoughts and images.

People who are considerably depressed commonly find routine tasks and even social activities, which they used to consider no effort, fatiguing and difficult to manage. Individuals who find themselves in this situation can be helped to structure their everyday activities in a way which enables them to build up motivation to work and enjoy life. For example, they may set out gradually to increase their level of daily activity in very small steps which they feel they can manage. More pleasurable activities can be built into their daily routines and used consciously as 'rewards' for getting through everyday tasks which are perceived as tiring or somewhat threatening. It is also valuable for depressed individuals who are in reasonable health to incorporate some, fairly vigorous, physical exercise into their daily routine.

A depressed person can feel very alone, imprisoned in a despair which cuts them off from the social world. Being provided with very warm, caring support from loved ones and from professional and voluntary helpers, can be very important in helping to break down these feelings of isolation and imprisonment.

Although helpers can assist individuals who are depressed in the ways that have been listed above, it is important that they also respect the limitations on their own helping capacities. People who remain very depressed for a period of time may require both medication and specialized counselling before they begin to improve. In terms of more formal counselling interventions, cognitive therapies have been shown to have the most success in the treatment of depression. Any helper in HIV should try to ensure that individuals who have been seriously depressed for some period of time receive the skilled intervention that they have a right to receive, and arrange for a referral to be made to a psychiatrist or clinical psychologist who has a good track record in the treatment of depression.

Obsessive thoughts and disabling anxieties

The same advice concerning the need to make appropriate referrals applies when helpers find that their clients are very troubled by obsessional thoughts or disabling anxieties. Being troubled by particular persisting worries concerning the present or the future is a normal response to being suddenly faced with uncertainties about the future. The 'automatic' nature of these thoughts, the fact that the individual is unable to exercise much control to prevent these thoughts from occurring, makes them particularly distressing. Some individuals may also experience a compulsive need to check physically that they have not developed any illness and that their appearance is unaltered.

Use of the method of 'restructuring' these obsessional thoughts, exploring them and trying to alter their character may often be helpful to a client. As with other problems that have been discussed earlier in the chapter, providing information about HIV may be useful together with an explanation of the nature of obsessive thoughts and their effects. It may also be important to work with a client to identify what are effective methods of distraction from these thoughts for him or her personally. The general methods of enabling people to reduce the anxiety that they are experiencing which were discussed earlier may also be helpful. In some cases, individuals may find it very difficult to regain control over obsessive thoughts or patterns of behaviour and, as Chapter 4 indicates, more specific psychiatric assessment and treatment may be necessary.

Maintaining health

The importance of monitoring health regularly

Hospital units which specialize in the treatment of HIV infection and HIV-related illnesses now usually provide regular monitoring of the general health and the immune function of all HIV antibody positive individuals. This monitoring is required to ensure that an HIV antibody positive individual will be able to benefit from early treatment intervention. It allows an individual to receive appropriate antiviral drugs and prophylactic treatment against HIV-related illnesses whenever there are signs of a potentially damaging decline in the functioning of the immune system. Some of the principal tests used as 'markers' of immune functioning and progression of HIV disease are described in Chapter 2.

A helper has an important role to play in providing an HIV antibody positive individual with information concerning this monitoring of general health and immune function and its benefits. HIV positive individuals may sometimes feel somewhat ill at ease and find difficulty in knowing exactly how to formulate questions and express worries that they have about their health during an interview with a doctor who is monitoring their health. Helpers can assist clients to communicate with doctors and possibly even role-play, practise communicating with a doctor. Helpers also have a role to play in ensuring that some clients do not make unnecessarily pessimistic interpretations of a particular set of test results which they have been given by a doctor.

Although hospital units which specialize in the treatment of HIV infection will customarily offer regular health monitoring as a routine part of the care of their patients, there may be hospitals which have less experience in the treatment of HIV infection where sophisticated monitoring of health is not offered on a routine basis. In such cases, a helper may require not only to explain to a client the type of monitoring which he or she has a right to receive, but also to pursue the matter with medical staff. Effective helping in HIV infection may on occasion involve the helper fighting on behalf of a client or a group of clients.

Contact with GPs and dentists

Many people with HIV infection obtain most of their health care from a hospital clinic. GPs, however, also often play a very important part in the overall health care of an individual living with HIV. They are able to provide a rapid response to any symptoms which may suddenly emerge, and having the services of a good GP may enable some individuals with more severe HIV-related illnesses to receive much of their care at home rather than in hospital. GPs often form a good point of contact for access to a wide range of social services. Developing a good relationship with a sympathetic GP can also provide someone who is HIV antibody positive and asymptomatic with the security that they will be able to receive appropriate care at home should they become ill at some point in the future.

Understandably, many people who learn that they are HIV antibody positive worry that their present GP may not treat them in a sympathetic manner, or may worry about the reactions of a new GP to whom they give the news that they are HIV antibody positive. A sympathetic attitude and a good working knowledge of HIV-related illnesses and their treatment cannot be guaranteed. It is very useful when individual helpers and voluntary agencies in an area attempt to gather information which allows them to advise clients on which local GPs have a reputation for providing a good quality, sympathetic service to people with HIV infection. Chapter 3 emphasized the importance of good dental care for individuals with HIV infection. As in the case of GPs, clients may be fearful of how dentists will respond to someone with HIV infection. Helpers and agencies need to be able to direct clients to dentists who will react sympathetically and provide an appropriate standard of care.

Giving information on how to maintain health

Chapter 3 highlighted the importance of good nutrition, physical exercise and sufficient rest for maintaining health, and various alternative therapies that an individual may use to increase well-being and health. Helpers can provide people living with HIV with detailed information about how to maintain health. Such information can be a vital asset for achieving a good quality of life as well as physical health. It is important, though, that this information is not presented in a prescriptive way. The benefits of following sensible guidelines for maintaining health are obvious; but at the same time, it needs to be recognized that a change to 'healthier living' can involve costs as well as benefits. Changes in health-related behaviour can affect a person's whole manner of living. Helpers might consider how they would feel and react to suddenly changing to a regime where they have little alcohol, eat sensibly and go to bed earlier.

It is necessary that individuals living with HIV are presented with the knowledge and enabled to acquire the skills which will allow them to meet the challenges posed by HIV. However, it is up to them to decide what changes in actions and in thinking are appropriate and realistic for them to make. If respect for individual choice and freedom are to be maintained, helpers need to avoid imposing any ways of adjusting to the challenges of long-term uncertainty on an individual who is living with HIV.

References

Bandura, A. (1989). 'Perceived self-efficacy in the exercise of control over AIDS infection'. In V.M. Mays *et al.* (eds), *Primary Prevention of AIDS: Psychological Approaches*. Newbury Park, Calif., Sage, pp. 128–41.

Beck, A.T. *et al.* (1985). 'Hopelessness and eventual suicide: A 10 year prospective study of patients hospitalized with suicidal ideation'. *American Journal of Psychiatry,* **145**, 559–63.

Blackburn, I.M. (1987). *Coping with Depression*. Edinburgh, Chambers.

Endler, N.S. (1988). 'Hassles, health, and happiness'. In M.P. Janisse (ed.), *Individual Differences, Stress, and Health Psychology*, New York, Springer-Verlag, pp. 24–56.

Hillier, I. (1990). *The Benefits Research Unit's HIV and AIDS Welfare Rights Guide, 1990–1992 edition*. Nottingham, Benefits Research Unit, University of Nottingham.

Lazarus, R.S. and Folkman, S. (1984). *Stress, Appraisal, and Coping*. New York, Springer-Verlag.

MacLachlan, J. (1991). 'When you ache for life it's worth taking risks'. *The Observer,* 13 January 1991.

McMullen, R. (1988). *Living with HIV in Self and Others*. London, GMP.

Mandel, J.S. (1986). 'Psychosocial challenges of AIDS and ARC: Clinical and research observations'. In L. McKusick (ed.), *What to do about AIDS: Physicians and Mental Health Professionals Discuss the Issues*. Berkeley, Calif., University of California Press, pp. 75–86.

Namir, S. (1986). 'Treatment issues concerning persons with AIDS'. In L. McKusick (ed.), *What to do about AIDS: Physicians and Mental Health Professionals Discuss the Issues*. Berkeley, Calif., University of California Press, pp. 87–94.

Perry, S.W. *et al.* (1990). 'Psychological responses to serological testing for HIV'. *AIDS*, **4**, 145–52.

Rowe, D. (1983). *Depression: The Way Out of Your Prison*. London, Routledge and Kegan Paul.

Simonton, S.M. (1984). *The Healing Family*. London, Bantam.

NINE

Coping with illness

CHARLES ANDERSON

Introduction

Individuals who experience HIV-related illness have to meet a considerable number of challenges. During a period of fairly acute illness, there is a need to cope with what some writers have described as 'the grind of being ill', to deal with pain, fatigue and a restriction on activity over a period of time. An individual who is ill with an HIV-related infection may also have to deal with new treatment procedures and to adjust to the experience of being in hospital. There is a need to cope with the emotions which are evoked by illness, and with an increase in anxiety and uncertainty about the future. Relationships with partners, friends and family require to be maintained under the stress of illness. Individuals may sometimes need to redefine their goals in life to meet the difficulties imposed by illness and a less certain future. The variability in the course of illness in very many individuals with HIV infection, the fact that they may have acute episodes of illness interspersed with long periods of well-being, or of comparative well-being, can also cause stress. For people with advanced HIV disease, there are all the changes and difficulties that face anyone who is coping with a terminal illness.

People living with HIV-related illness face not only the challenges and difficulties that accompany any serious medical condition, but also the additional problems of stigma and discrimination. Self-help groups, and many individuals with HIV-related illness, have reacted vigorously against the stigmatization of people with AIDS, and against the doom-laden images that have been used to represent AIDS. They have preferred to talk about 'living with AIDS' rather than 'dying from AIDS' and have emphasized the possibilities of coping positively with a diagnosis of HIV-related illness. This chapter looks in some detail at the challenges which have been identified in the preceding paragraph, and considers how helpers can best aid individuals living with HIV-related illness to meet these challenges.

Giving information, communicating with medical staff

Any type of serious illness can be very frightening. A particularly frightening aspect of illness is the feeling that one is no longer in control of events. For some individuals, finding out more about the nature of the particular illness that they are experiencing, its likely course and the nature of the treatment that they are receiving, is important not only in allaying anxiety but also in helping them to re-establish a sense of control over events. As well as passing on information which they possess themselves, helpers may have an important role to play in assisting clients to ask medical staff questions. Not everyone, however, will wish to cope with illness by becoming as well informed as possible about its nature and treatment. Members of medical staff and other carers need to take their cue from individual clients as to how much information they wish and when they wish to receive it.

It is much easier for individuals experiencing a fairly serious HIV-related illness to have a sense of being in control of events when the medical team which is treating them very much involves them in decisions about their care. It is also easier for individuals to cope with aspects of their illness, if they are given the opportunity to express fully any fears about the illness to medical staff. Being treated with respect and having one's concerns taken seriously enables individuals who are ill to maintain a sense of dignity and of control over their lives.

Individuals may experience difficulties in communicating to doctors which symptoms they find most troublesome or are causing them most anxiety. Doctors necessarily are going to focus their attention on the aspects of an illness which are most critical for health, and they may sometimes give less attention to symptoms such as an irritation or a skin rash which are causing a patient considerable distress. Individuals with an HIV-related illness can be encouraged to communicate clearly with medical staff about the symptoms which they are finding most troublesome so that they can obtain appropriate relief of these symptoms. Some people may even find it useful to write down a list of things that they want to say before they meet with their doctor.

New types of medical examination and treatment procedures can sometimes appear quite frightening. This fear may often be reduced, and individuals given a sense of greater control over what is happening, if information is given in a clear fashion about the nature of the procedure itself and how the procedure may affect them, i.e. if they will feel no discomfort or some pain. Again, though, it is important to take the cue from the individual who is living with HIV-related illness as to how much information he or she wishes to gain.

On occasions when an individual is asked by medical staff to consider taking a treatment for HIV disease itself, or for an HIV-related illness, which is still being trialled, he or she will need a considerable amount of information from medical staff about both the treatment and the purposes of the clinical trial if informed consent is to be obtained. An individual with HIV-related illness may often find it useful to talk through with a helper any decision about whether or not to take part in the clinical trial of a new treatment, carefully evaluating the possible advantages and disadvantages.

Pain control

Sometimes, an individual with an HIV-related illness may be experiencing a considerable amount of pain, but not wish to complain about the pain. He or she may even have the belief that it is 'natural' for someone with a serious illness to experience considerable pain. In such a situation, a helper can encourage the person to seek from medical staff medication which will provide him or her with appropriate pain relief. It is important also that drug users are provided with sufficient analgesic drugs to relieve any pain and discomfort which they may be experiencing.

Aside from ensuring that people with HIV-related illnesses receive appropriate pain-killing medication, helpers can assist by providing information about pain and its effects, and by instructing an individual in a number of different techniques for controlling pain. Pain can be easier to bear if its cause is clearly explained.

It is now recognized that pain is a complex phenomenon, and that the perception of pain is influenced by a large number of factors. One important determinant of the perception of pain is the psychological state of the individual who is experiencing pain. Pain is likely to be experienced as more severe by individuals who are feeling very anxious. An important part of pain relief may involve helping people in a variety of ways to reduce the anxiety that they are experiencing. It may also be important for pain reduction to help people to express feelings of sadness, anger and hopelessness and to deal with these feelings. The relief of emotional suffering can help individuals to cope more readily with physical pain.

The muscle tension that is associated with feelings of anxiety can in itself increase the intensity of pain which an individual experiences. Teaching people muscle relaxation techniques can, therefore, be valuable in the relief of pain as well as contributing to a greater general sense of well-being. Individuals can also be helped to find ways to distract themselves from the pain and discomfort that they are experiencing, to find pleasurable activities which will take their attention away from the pain.

For some individuals, the use of imagery, i.e. creative visualization exercises, may be a very effective way of gaining control over and reducing pain and discomfort. Using imagery to deal with pain and discomfort is likely to be more successful if the individual first practises a relaxation technique to get rid of tension in the muscles. Then the individual can concentrate on an image, or set of images, which he or she finds particularly healing and calming. One commonly used image for pain relief is simply to picture pain flowing out of the body as you breathe out, and healing and calm flowing into the body each time that you breathe in. Individuals can also imagine in great detail, and using all their senses, a very relaxing scene, such as lying on a warm beach by a calm sea. They can then concentrate on the deep feelings of relaxation that come from being in this scene.

Aside from a wide range of medication, relaxation techniques and the use of imagery, there are a large number of techniques which may bring relaxation, comfort and the relief of pain. They include massage, acupressure and hypnosis. It is not possible to predict accurately which technique will bring most benefit to a particular individual. It is important that people are presented with choices, and given a sense of control over how they can deal with any pain or discomfort which they are experiencing.

Looking for meaning in the diagnosis of an HIV-related illness

A section of Chapter 8 looked in some detail at how people create meaning out of an HIV antibody positive diagnosis, and at appropriate helping actions in cases where individuals are constructing an unnecessarily bleak view of the present and the future. Similarly, it may often be necessary to explore with clients how they are giving meaning to a diagnosis of HIV-related illness, and to assist them to construct a different, more positive set of meanings.

Individuals who have been given an AIDS diagnosis may on occasion see this diagnosis as meaning that they will have only a very short time to live. A considerable number of specific infections and cancers are regarded as 'indicators' of a case of AIDS. These infections and cancers, which are regarded as indicators of AIDS, vary considerably in their effects and in their prognosis. Episodes of most of these infections can be treated with success. Gaining more information about HIV-related illnesses and their treatment, and meeting others who have coped successfully for a long period of time with HIV-related illnesses, may enable some individuals to form a less negative view of the amount of life that they can expect and the quality of that life.

Expressing feelings and dealing with loss

It is important that individuals with HIV-related illness are presented with information which may allow them to construct a more positive picture of the future and enhance their will to live and to enjoy life. At the same time, however, it is essential that they are given the opportunity to express fully fears that they have concerning the future. It is also likely to be much easier to construct a more positive view of life once such fears have been expressed and have been acknowledged by another person.

Aside from the loss of certainty about future health, individuals with HIV-related illness will often experience a number of serious losses. As an earlier section of the chapter described, serious illness can cause people to have less control over the daily circumstances of their lives and to feel that they are no longer in control of events. When people who have been used to leading a full, active life find their activities considerably restricted by illness, they are likely to experience a considerable sense of loss. Illness may bring with it an inability to work full-time and financial difficulties. Individuals with serious HIV-related illness may fear the loss of independence and find it difficult to have to rely on others for practical care and emotional support. Relationships may not survive the strain of coping with illness. Serious illness may also cause individuals to realize that they will have to relinquish important goals and plans for the future, for example, to start a family.

For very many people, being healthy, vigorous and physically attractive are central parts of their self-image, and of their sense of self-worth. Becoming unwell, and believing that one is no longer physically attractive, can often be quite threatening to an individual's sense of self. Individuals may also believe that they are no longer sexually attractive to other people and may suffer a loss of sexual desire which can accompany serious illness.

Chapter 1 emphasized the dangers of helpers imposing their own conceptions of what constitutes 'good adjustment' to situations of loss and uncertainty on people who are living with HIV-related illness. Individuals will have their own unique ways of expressing grief at the losses which they have experienced and their own ways of making practical adjustments in their everyday lives to deal with loss. Helpers can try to create the type of relationship where individuals will feel safe to express their sense of grief at the losses which they have experienced, or which they anticipate. Helpers can also assure people living with HIV-related illness that intense emotions, such as sudden bursts of deeply felt anger, are normal reactions to loss. In cases where individuals react to the experience of suffering multiple losses by becoming severely depressed, helpers need to ensure that they receive appropriate skilled counselling and medication to deal with this depression.

Helpers can play a useful role in assisting individuals with HIV-related illness to make plans to deal with the practical difficulties, and the adjustments that are required in everyday living, as a result of the restrictions imposed by ill health. They can also aid a person living with HIV-related illness to focus on what is still possible to achieve, to set realistic and self-enhancing goals. Some individuals who are living with HIV-related illness may come to see themselves in negative terms, and they can be helped by being reminded of the positive aspects of themselves and of their own potential for living.

People with HIV-related illness may sometimes be unsure about carrying out some action or starting a project which is dear to them, because it carries a certain element of risk. This might be risking to start a new relationship, achieving an important project at work, taking a particular holiday which they have always dreamed about. Talking through the decision about pursuing a goal which involves some risk in a careful manner with someone else may be very helpful. On occasion, it may be important for a helper to demonstrate clearly that he or she is backing the individual living with HIV-related illness to take the risks involved in pursuing some important goal.

Living positively

Having goals which give a sense of purpose to living not only improves the quality of life of a person who has an HIV-related illness, but can also enhance the will to live and to fight back against illness. These goals can include working to maintain health. As Chapter 8 described, an 'active' coping style where an individual is positively involved in maintaining physical and emotional health and enjoyable social activities has beneficial results. Individuals can be encouraged to take active control over aspects of their life in the face of illness, and to live as fully as they can within the restrictions that illness may impose. However, Chapter 8 also emphasized that there is quite marked variation in the way that individuals cope with stress and uncertainty about the future. It is necessary to avoid *imposing* this active style of coping, or any other style of coping with HIV-related illness, on a client. People living with HIV-related illness can be assisted to find a style of coping which fits well with their individual circumstances, personality, values and social background.

A number of writers (e.g. Tatchell, 1990) have stressed that 'a positive mental attitude' is of great importance for people living with HIV-related illness. People can affirm to themselves their will to live, can enhance their self-image, and find love for themselves and others. They can also use imagery exercises to visualize the HIV virus being destroyed, and their immune system being strengthened (see Tatchell, 1990, pp. 124–6).

Trying to impose such a set of positive attitudes on a person with HIV-related illness from outside, though, is not likely to be particularly effective, as well as being an insensitive action. People can be encouraged, and given the support from loved ones and helpers which can assist them, to adopt a positive mental attitude; but such a mental attitude cannot be forced.

Actively promoting a positive mental attitude is likely to bring hope and purpose into the life of someone with an HIV-related illness, but 'positive thinking' can also on occasion contain dangers for some individuals. Occasionally, individuals who are following a programme of responding positively to the challenge of HIV-related illness may feel too much responsibility for the course of the illness and even self-blame should they experience another episode of illness. People also need to recognize that it is very difficult to find the energy to feel and think positively at times when illness is acute. This point is made very clearly by David Miller (1987, p. 27), writing about the situation where other people are exhorting a seriously ill person to fight and react positively to illness: 'The good intentions of others may cause *guilt* to pile up on top of sickness. One of my patients called it "the tyranny of positive thinking". He felt guilty because his illness was so overwhelming at the time he was diagnosed that he simply couldn't find the energy for "positive" thinking.'

The actions and needs of partners, family and friends

Chapters 1 and 8 drew attention to the need to set helping efforts firmly within a social context, and to be aware of the ways in which the actions of other people may limit or enhance an individual's ability to cope with the challenges of HIV infection. How individuals cope with HIV-related illness will be influenced to a fairly large degree by the amount and the type of support that they receive from others. In many cases, people with HIV-related illness have gained strong, loving support and appropriate practical care from partners, family and friends. Sadly, however, this has not always happened and some individuals have had to cope with rejection in private life, as well as with the social stigma that has been attached to HIV infection and AIDS. Sometimes, also, troubled relationships and rivalries among the significant people in their life have created great distress for individuals living with HIV-related illness. It can be particularly difficult if the family of a person living with HIV-related illness try to exclude his or her partner or friends in the later stages of illness. When people are isolated and have few sources of emotional support and practical help, voluntary helpers, buddies, can be of very great value.

Friends and family may find it difficult to sustain their initial level of support throughout a long period of illness, and the individual who is ill may then feel 'let down'. It is also recognized from the study of other serious diseases that partners, family and friends may sometimes find it particularly difficult to sustain the quality and quantity of their support in the terminal stages of an illness. They may directly avoid the person who is dying, or more subtly communicate their own feelings of pain and social awkwardness.

Helpers can aid some individuals to plan when and how they are going to tell partners, family or friends about the diagnosis of an HIV-related illness. They may also be able to assist some individuals to deal with emotional and sexual difficulties that are occurring within a relationship as the result of the strain of coping with illness. Women with HIV-related illness who have children are likely to be very concerned that appropriate arrangements are made for their children's care, and may need both emotional support and practical help with the task of safeguarding their children's interests.

Partners themselves may need considerable support if they are to respond effectively to the needs of an individual who is living with HIV-related illness (see Chapter 14). In addition, they may need to gain a lot of information about HIV-related illnesses and their treatment. This information will allow them not only to understand more clearly the situation of the person who is ill, but also possibly to gain a greater sense of control over events. Often partners or flat-mates of a person with HIV-related illness will need to learn a good deal about the practical aspects of looking after someone who is very ill at home. Instructing partners and other carers in how best to respond to the practical needs of an individual who has a serious HIV-related illness should be seen as an important part of his or her care. The manner in which partners and others provide nursing care and deal with other household tasks is also crucial. Care needs to be provided in a way which respects the dignity and autonomy of the person who is ill. When an individual with HIV-related illness is in hospital, it is usually helpful if a partner is made to feel that he or she is still actively involved in the person's care and that his or her contribution to the person's well-being is recognized.

The diagnosis of an HIV-related illness is likely to cause considerable anxiety to the people close to a person who is living with HIV. A partner, close friend or family member may be feeling so upset that he or she is unable to respond appropriately to the needs of the person who is ill. Strong feelings of anxiety or anger felt by a carer may also be conveyed directly to the person who is ill, increasing his or her anxiety and decreasing his or her ability to cope. In such cases, it is very important that the carers of people with HIV-related illness are given support and careful counselling to assist them to deal with their own feelings.

Difficulties may arise when an individual who is ill and his or her partner wish to cope with illness or with the prospect of death in very different ways. For example, an individual who is terminally ill may wish to talk about the imminence of death and how he wishes to be remembered in the future, whereas the partner may still wish to cope by avoiding the topic of death. Skilful and sensitive helping work may be required with both partners in a relationship when there are marked differences in their ways of coping; but it also needs to be recognized that difficulties which arise from divergence in ways of coping may not always be easy to resolve.

Dealing with practical matters

Coping with illness can be a very difficult business indeed for people who have pressing financial problems, who are ill-housed or are suffering problems of discrimination. Chapter 8 highlighted the need to provide people living with HIV with a successfully-functioning local network of advice on welfare rights and financial matters. There are quite a number of different benefits which a person living with HIV-related illness may be able to claim. It is important that people with HIV-related illness are made aware of these benefits and any other sources of financial support, and are assisted to claim them. The welfare rights officers employed by HIV agencies in the voluntary sector will also be able to advise on matters concerning confidentiality and the claiming of benefits.

In addition to helping people living with HIV-related illness to receive expert welfare rights advice, there may be a need to assist them to obtain appropriate legal advice if they are suffering problems of discrimination in housing or in employment. People living with HIV-related illness may also require the services of a lawyer to draw up a will and to help them to settle financial matters at present and in the event of their death in the way that they wish.

People who are worried that they may at some point not be able to manage their own affairs can, with the assistance of a lawyer, give someone else a 'power of attorney'. In other words, a legal document is drawn up which permits an individual whom they choose to act on their behalf and deal with their affairs.

People who are living with HIV-related illness may sometimes be unsure as to whether or when they should give up permanent employment. Talking through this decision with a helper can sometimes be very useful. The benefits and disadvantages both of staying at work and of leaving work can be looked at in detail and weighed up.

Individuals living with HIV-related illness may have to face a number of housing problems including discrimination, homelessness, difficulties in keeping up with rent or mortgage payments as a result of illness, and living in accommodation which is not well suited for home nursing care. To maintain health, people with HIV-related illness require good quality, well-heated accommodation where they can feel secure from any threat of discrimination or attack. National and local voluntary HIV agencies can often provide advice on housing and referrals on to appropriate housing associations. The provision of housing services by local authorities for people living with HIV-related illness varies considerably throughout the UK. Some authorities have implemented very good policy guidelines and have responded well in providing housing and support services. It is possible, though, that in some areas workers in the area of HIV may need to help people with HIV-related illness be assertive about having their housing needs met.

People in the later stages of HIV disease are likely to wish to spend as much of their time at home as is possible. However, a measure of choice about whether to be treated at home for most of the time, as opposed to a hospital or hospice, is usually only possible when there is good provision of services for home care within an area. There also needs to be good co-ordination between different services in the community, and between hospital and community services.

When people are very ill and their movement is restricted, simple adaptations to the home, such as the provision of strategically placed handrails, can allow greater independence and comfort. Occupational therapists and social workers who specialize in the housing needs of people who are ill or disabled can assess what adaptations and aids are required, and arrange for their provision. When someone is housebound, a telephone is not only essential to summon aid but is very important for maintaining social contact with friends and family. Finding financial assistance to meet the telephone bills of individuals who are seriously ill with HIV-related illnesses can be a very valuable piece of practical help.

Talking about death

Individuals who know that they are dying, or who are experiencing serious HIV-related illness, may find it very valuable to talk about their thoughts and feelings concerning death. At the same time, helpers need to take their lead from the person who is experiencing HIV-related illness, and not force a discussion about death on someone who is dying.

Helpers may sometimes find it difficult to respond appropriately to someone who is dying and wish to avoid the topic of death as a result of their own anxieties or past experiences of bereavement. The training of helpers in the area of HIV needs to provide individuals with an opportunity to explore their own thoughts and feelings about death and dying, and how their interactions with a person who is facing death may be influenced by their own experiences of loss and death. Worries that helpers have about talking to people who are dying also need to be addressed directly. Even when carers do not feel any social awkwardness in talking about death and in listening to people who are dying, they may still communicate more subtle changes in their perception of someone who is now terminally ill. There is a danger that they will focus attention primarily on the fact that they are talking to a 'dying person' and, as a result, change their behaviour towards him or her in ways which may be hurtful. Someone who is dying expects and needs to be accepted, and responded to, as the person that he or she has always been.

There is very considerable variation in the way that individuals who are terminally ill respond to death and the process of dying. Some individuals accept death calmly and do not show distress, anger or fear. When individuals who are terminally ill are very fearful or depressed, helpers can assist them to express the specific fears which they possess about death and dying and to explore the causes of their depression. Depression may on occasion be related to regrets about aspects of the past, feelings that important goals have not been achieved or that difficulties in relationships have not been resolved. Worries may also centre around other people. There may be concern about the present difficulties being experienced by partners, friends or children, and worries about the future of loved ones. There may also be concern and guilt about being a burden to other people.

Fears about the process of dying commonly include concerns about a loss of dignity and independence, changes in physical appearance, physical pain and the possibility of being abandoned by others when death is near. Helpers can often provide reassurance that some fears about the process of dying are unnecessary. They can also take practical steps to ensure that the individual who is terminally ill is treated with dignity, receives appropriate pain relief and has the companionship and support of other people.

Individuals can sometimes be helped to accomplish projects which really matter to them. The accent in helping efforts with people who are terminally ill does not need to be solely on matters of death and dying. People can be assisted to live as fully as they can within the considerable limitations imposed upon them by serious illness, and to achieve goals which are important to them.

An individual who is facing death is likely to need to make quite a number of practical arrangements. Dealing with practical matters such as making a will or organizing funeral arrangements can also give someone a greater sense of control over the process of dying. Individuals can ensure that their property, including personal belongings, is passed on in the way that they wish, that people whom they would like to know of their death are notified and that their funeral takes place according to their wishes. The process of dying is also likely to appear less uncertain and frightening when individuals are actively involved in matters such as their own pain control and consulted on treatment decisions. This active involvement in their own care, is very important in giving individuals a sense of power and of control over the process of dying.

A large number of people interpret the experience of dying in terms of the religious beliefs which they hold, and also wish to deal with religious and spiritual aspects of dying. A useful guide to providing sensitive pastoral care to people with HIV-related illness who are facing death is provided in Bill Kirkpatrick's (1988) book, *AIDS Sharing the Pain: Pastoral Guidelines*.

For many individuals, whether or not they hold religious beliefs, the prospect of dying in the near future causes them to reflect on the meaning of their own life and possibly to question more widely the purpose of human existence. In conversation with someone who listens with care and interest, individuals who are facing death can construct a narrative of their life which gives meaning to the past, the present and the future.

References

Kirkpatrick, B. (1988). *AIDS Sharing the Pain: Pastoral Guidelines*. London, Darton, Longman and Todd.
Miller, D. (1987). *Living with AIDS and HIV*. London, Macmillan.
Tatchell, P. (1990). *AIDS: A Guide to Survival*, 3rd updated edn. London, GMP.

Looking at particular needs

TEN

Women and HIV

PATRICIA WILKIE

Introduction

Women have contracted HIV. Women have developed AIDS. Women have died of AIDS. Women have transmitted HIV to their new born infant. HIV can affect sexually active women. Women have lost daughters, sons and partners who have died of AIDS. HIV has created very specific difficulties for women because of the many roles women play as mothers, carers and sexual partners, and as a result of the expectations of how women should behave. Women are particularly at risk of contracting HIV from unprotected inter-course with an infected man and from needle sharing in intravenous drug use. Furthermore, HIV can be transmitted by an infected mother to her baby during pregnancy, labour or delivery.

Background

In the UK, where the number of women affected by HIV and AIDS is still relatively small, women themselves have not in general appeared particularly concerned about their risk of contracting HIV. Until 1990, government and health education HIV prevention policies have tended to focus on groups at high risk of contracting HIV, in particular homosexuals and intravenous drug users. This concentration of health education programmes about HIV on specific risk groups makes it easier for sexually active women who may be involved in risk behaviour, to disassociate from or forget their risk and their need to take preventive action. In addition, the geographical concentration of HIV infection can mean that women living outside of these areas of high incidence may never have known or met a person with HIV.

In order to prevent the further spread of HIV, women have to learn about and accept that they are at risk of contracting HIV. Women have to learn how to protect themselves from contracting HIV sexually. The use of a condom is necessary to prevent the spread of infection and is recommended for women setting out on a new sexual relationship. For women accustomed to controlling their own fertility by oral contraception, the use of dual protection, i.e. the woman using some method of contraception as well as her partner using a condom, may seem problematic and particularly so when their partner is uncooperative. To suggest that their partner use a condom is likely to be very difficult for younger, less sexually experienced women because of lack of familiarity in the use of condoms and because of the woman's fear of being considered 'cheap' by the male. In addition, the use of alcohol reducing inhibitions and caution is often associated with early sexual encounters making it more difficult for the woman to be assertive.

Women have also to consider the possibility of transmitting HIV to their unborn child and then be faced with the choices of whether to continue with the pregnancy or whether to terminate. This area raises some of the most difficult and delicate issues for helpers, including the dilemma facing a mother who knows that the baby she is carrying may not be born healthy; the guilt surrounding a decision to have a child when the mother herself is HIV positive; the problems surrounding termination of pregnancy on the one hand and the need to be fulfilled as a mother on the other.

Traditionally, women are carers in their roles as a mother, as a partner and as a daughter. The implications for women should a partner, an offspring or another relative be affected by HIV are clearly very great. What particular problems arise when caring for a child who is HIV antibody positive or has AIDS? How much information needs to be given to other sibs and relatives, neighbours, other parents and school? How does a woman cope with her own grief when a partner is affected and she is not? What particular psychological and emotional support do women in these situations need and what is available?

Being diagnosed as HIV positive is for some women the first indication that their sexual partner or previous partner is or was infected with HIV. This information can cause a very profound sense of betrayal as well as distrust of their partner, adding to the emotional crisis caused by the diagnosis of HIV.

A further consideration concerns services for women living with HIV and HIV-related illness, as well as for those women seeking information and advice about HIV. Because the great majority of those with HIV and HIV-related illness are male, services, counselling agencies and health education have all tended to focus on and reflect their needs.

In the UK to date, the majority of men affected by HIV have either come from, or moved into, larger conurbations or cities. In these areas, large hospitals have departments of genitourinary medicine, formerly often known as STD clinics, which many gay men have attended before the appearance of HIV. These departments offer confidential counselling concerning HIV and medical care, but it is not known whether many women will initially seek counselling and advice about HIV from departments of genitourinary medicine. Moreover, such clinics tend to be attached to large hospitals in major cities. Should HIV spread more widely through the female population, it will be necessary to develop appropriate advice and counselling services that will be acceptable to women.

Women with HIV will often have children, and when these women become ill and require in-patient treatment, arrangements for the care of their children will be needed. In some cases, the children may be able to remain at home; in others, it will be preferable for the family to remain together, but be taken into care. In some cases, the mother and her child may both be ill. In these last two situations, the development of special facilities for mothers and their children are needed.

The gay community has taken the initiative and lobbied most effectively on behalf of those with HIV, as well as pioneering the dissemination of educational material. As a result, health education material has come to focus on all sexually active people warning them of the risks of contracting HIV. Although the emphasis in most health education material about HIV and AIDS is now on all sexually active people, there is a concern among some health educators that there is insufficient material which is tailored to the needs of women and which is likely to engage women's interest. These health educators are worried that much of the health education material supposedly designed for *all* sexually active people is more geared in terms of content, style and language used to appeal to men than to women. More effort needs to go into identifying and producing literature which will focus on women's needs and will have greater appeal to women.

Difficulties faced by women in negotiating safer sex

Safer sex guidelines recommend the careful use of a condom when partners wish to have intercourse, and if these guidelines are followed it is not considered necessary to know the HIV status of one's partner. To follow safer sex guidelines does require cooperation between the partners. There is also an underlying assumption that there is an equality between the partners. This is certainly not the case in all heterosexual relationships where often the woman feels vulnerable and is physically weaker. Women not only have to protect themselves from becoming infected with HIV, but also have the additional responsibility of protecting an unborn child. In order to protect themselves from infection, women are dependent upon their partner to use a condom. Safer sex guidelines do recommend other methods of sexual satisfaction without having intercourse. However, these alternatives may be far from easy for women to implement, particularly for young people in new relationships. In the young male heterosexual culture, the common assumption is that sex equals intercourse, and it can be difficult for women to counter this assumption.

Given the inequality in power that often exists between men and women, some writers such as Kaplan (1987) have argued that women should be recommended to be assertive about knowing the HIV status of their partners before getting into bed with them. Some caution needs to be exercised over this recommendation, however, given that a partner's claims about his sexual history and HIV antibody negative status may need to be treated with a degree of scepticism; and the inability of HIV antibody tests to identify recent infections.

The difficulties that women may face in negotiating safer sex, and their inability to trust their sexual partner to be honest with them, has led some women to view the confidentiality of medical information as being a relative rather than an absolute right. Members of the gay community, conscious of their vulnerability as a group and of the discrimination to which they may be subjected, have justifiably and vigorously argued for the absolute right to confidentiality of medical information for all HIV positive people. However, when one considers the position of a woman who may have little power in the relationship that she is having with an HIV positive partner who has chosen not to disclose his seropositive status to her, the moral issues concerning the confidentiality of medical information become less clear-cut. Bringing women's needs into sharper focus is likely to complicate the debate over the aspects of the politics of HIV which concern the question of civil liberties and individual rights.

Helpers also need to consider the way in which HIV positive women are portrayed in the media and the implications of this for prevention. Many of these issues which are peculiar to women and which have begun to arise as women have become affected by HIV have not been adequately addressed. They are examined in more detail in this chapter.

HIV and women: Some special considerations

Any woman who learns that she is HIV positive is likely to feel a variety of emotions including disbelief, hurt, anger, fear, sadness, panic and concern for loved ones. Indeed, these emotions are similar for anyone, male or female, when learning of this diagnosis. However, there are specific issues surrounding the diagnosis of HIV which are peculiar to women and which require special consideration in counselling.

Mothers will be concerned about what will happen to their children should they become ill. Will children be taken away into care? Some women may be pregnant when they learn that they are HIV positive, and others may be considering pregnancy.

To date, the media image of people with AIDS is that if they are male they are either gay, in which case 'they have only themselves to blame', or they are haemophiliacs and hence 'innocent victims'. The image of a woman who has HIV or AIDS remains also uncompromisingly harsh. She must either be a prostitute or a drug user and if she is neither of these she must be 'promiscuous'. These attitudes to women with HIV increase their isolation not only from friends and family but also from statutory services, e.g. maternity services, which the woman may need. Financially, HIV positive women may have specific problems. Some of these women will have a partner who is also HIV positive, and some will have dependent children.

Women are traditionally the carers; and mothers in middle years have once more found themselves looking after HIV positive offspring at a period in their life when they have had the first opportunity to have more time to themselves.

There has been considerable discussion about whether or not to screen all pregnant women for HIV. The main aim of such screening is for epidemiological purposes, to assess the prevalence of HIV in the female population. Normal obstetric care in pregnancy involves testing the mother for different conditions including hepatitis and syphilis. Those investigations involve taking a sample of blood and it has been argued that to test for HIV would not inconvenience the mother. There have been objections to such general screening for HIV among pregnant women. Midwives and the National Childbirth Trust both stated that the mere use of women for purposes not aimed at their own personal good is offensive.

Two methods have been suggested for testing pregnant women. The first is voluntary testing, where women would be informed that testing for HIV would be offered to them and they could decide whether or not they wished to accept testing. Statisticians have criticized this proposal on the grounds that even a few refusals from women who may be HIV antibody positive would invalidate the findings. The other suggestion is to test all pregnant women anonymously, that is, to remove any identification of the patient before the sample is sent to the laboratory. The disadvantage of this method is that should a patient be found to be HIV antibody positive, there is no method of identifying her to inform her.

In anonymized voluntary testing, all women would be told that HIV testing will be included in the range of screening tests that are normally carried out on pregnant women in the early stages of pregnancy. This form of testing pregnant women for HIV has already been introduced into some maternity units. It is important that when such anonymized voluntary testing is carried out, a comprehensive HIV pre-test counselling service is available (Boyd, 1990).

Women and the transmission of HIV

It is now well documented, and is referred to in Chapter 2, that the most common routes of transmission of HIV are through vaginal and anal intercourse, through transfusion of infected blood or blood products and through the sharing of contaminated needles in intravenous drug use. Women, therefore, have become infected with HIV by having intercourse with an already infected man, by sharing needles in intravenous drug use and by having recieved a transfusion of contaminated blood.

A woman who is already HIV positive can transmit the virus by sharing needles in intravenous drug use, or through vaginal secretions during intercourse to her sexual partner. HIV and HIV-infected cells can enter the body when they come into contact with the mucous membranes of the genital organs, the anus, the rectum and possibly of the mouth. The female sexual organs are covered by moist mucous membranes that allow infected cells an easy point of entry. (The dry skin that covers the outside of the body is very different from the moist mucous membranes that line the openings of the body. Dry skin has a layer of cornified material which acts as a barrier to many germs as well as protecting the body from injury.) During vaginal intercourse when the man is infected, his pre-ejaculatory secretions, pre-cum, the little drops of clear fluid that precede ejaculation, and the seminal fluid are passed into the vagina and can infect the woman. When the woman is HIV positive, her infected vaginal secretions cover the moist open entrance of the urethra at the tip of the penis and can infect her partner. If the skin of the vagina or penis has tiny cuts or abrasions, the chance of becoming infected with HIV is higher because the infected fluids have direct access to the bloodstream. It is also possible that there could be an accidental exchange of secretions after intercourse and the removal of a condom when a couple cuddle and embrace.

Anal intercourse is also very risky, especially for the receptive partner. In contrast to the vagina, the anus is tighter and more likely to be damaged during intercourse allowing infected secretions direct access to the bloodstream.

It is also possible that there may be a risk of transmission of the virus in oral sex. During oral sex, when a woman stimulates the penis of an infected man, she is exposed to pre-ejaculatory fluid and semen. The man, on the other hand, may also be at risk if he kisses, sucks or licks the genital area of an infected woman.

Women who are HIV positive can also transmit the virus to their child. The possible routes of transmission from mother to child are across the placenta (transplacentally) before the baby is born, through the birth canal during delivery of the baby and post-natally through breast milk. Mok (1988) suggests that it is most likely that the infection is transmitted transplacentally before the child is born.

What is not known is the exact risk of the virus being transmitted from an HIV positive mother to her child. It is now known that all babies born to HIV positive mothers will themselves be HIV antibody positive at birth. This is because there is transmission of maternal HIV antibody *in utero* to the infant, and infants do not produce IgM antibody to HIV.

The European Collaborative Study reported in 1988 that it had followed a sample of 271 children born to HIV positive mothers from birth for varying periods of time. By June 1988, 45% of these children had been followed for over 1 year. They found that most of the infants in the study had cleared the

HIV antibody acquired from their mother, with a median age of antibody loss of 10.3 months. Of the children in the study, 234 were immunologically normal and clinically well. Ten infants had developed AIDS, of whom five had died. A further 22 children had symptoms or signs suggestive of HIV infection. However, some of the HIV antibody negative infants have also been shown to be positive for HIV, i.e. virus can be detected in their blood (Mok *et al.*, 1987). It is clear that establishing a diagnosis of HIV infection in infants is difficult.

It is not known whether the infants found to be virus positive, but HIV antibody negative, will develop symptoms of HIV infection, nor whether they will be able to pass on the infection while remaining symptom-free themselves. It is therefore essential that all babies born to HIV positive mothers are followed up for some years.

Further considerations in mother-child transmission of HIV are the state of health of the mother at conception, the effect of HIV on pregnancy and the effect of pregnancy on the progress of HIV infection in the mother. There is still conflicting evidence about the degree of infectivity of the mother and her ability to transmit infection to her unborn child. Some workers (e.g. Minkoff, 1987) suggest that women with more advanced immunocompromise transmit the virus more effectively. Current evidence would appear to suggest that HIV infection has no deleterious effect on the pregnancy of the expectant mother who is asymptomatic for HIV infection (Johnstone *et al.*, 1989). In this study mothers tended to book late, deliver prematurely and have babies with intrauterine growth retardation. Small for date babies and prematurity occurred three times more commonly than in a population of non-HIV mothers. But it should be pointed out that the majority of the sample studied were intravenous drug users, and that there were factors over and above HIV which may well have been affecting the pregnancy.

Early work suggested that pregnancy had an adverse effect on the course of HIV infection (Scott *et al.*, 1985). This conclusion was not confirmed by a prospective study by MacCallum (1987), which found no difference in the rate of development of AIDS in HIV positive mothers compared with the rate of development of AIDS in non-pregnant women. However, this is an area where there is still insufficient information. The study by Rutherford *et al.* (1990) shows that the proportion of people who develop symptoms of HIV in any period depends considerably on the duration since first infection. But information about the date of first infection is often not known. Unless this date is known for all the subjects in a study, any conclusion from such a study may be unreliable.

Prevention of HIV: Women and sexual relationships

For the last 20 years in the Western world, women have been able to take the responsibility for the control of their own fertility through the widespread availability of oral contraception. This, combined with a freer attitude to sexual relations, has meant that women can be involved in a sexual relationship and enjoy that relationship without the fear of becoming pregnant. In this respect, women using oral contraception are independent of their partner in their ability to prevent pregnancy and also, should they wish it, to become pregnant. HIV is sexually transmitted and oral contraception does not protect women from becoming infected. In order to safeguard themselves from contracting HIV, it is essential that women learn how to protect themselves. This discussion does not concern women who are in a longstanding relationship with the same partner and where neither partner is involved in intravenous drug use nor has had a sexual relationship with another partner in recent years.

Women may be at very great risk of acquiring HIV when they have vaginal or anal sex without the use of a condom with a partner whose sexual history is unknown, or with a partner with a known high risk or with a partner who is known to be HIV positive. Sex in any of these circumstances would be described as high-risk sexual activity and women can risk becoming infected from even a single exposure. Following current safer sex guidelines, oral sex is seen as involving a much smaller, and not well determined, risk of becoming infected with HIV.

'Safe sex' describes sex where there is no mingling of 'body fluids', i.e. blood, vaginal and seminal fluids, which may be infected with HIV. This safe sex could include stimulation of each other's genital organs to orgasm without the mingling of body fluids. It would be absolutely safe to masturbate in each other's presence without touching each other, to caress each other's bodies omitting the genital areas, to talk about sex and to talk about each other's sexual fantasies. Counsellors can help women to increase the discussion of pleasurable activities, and as Patton (1985) suggests to 'eroticize measures that reduce transmission of all sexually transmitted diseases'.

When the riskiness of different sexual practices is examined, it seems essential for a woman in order to protect herself from sexually transmitted disease, to avoid unprotected intercourse with a partner whose sexual history is unknown and until she is sure that the partner is free from infection. It follows that it is important when a woman is getting involved in a new sexual relationship that she discusses with her partner what they are going to do to protect each other from HIV. Many women, in particular those who are more sexually experienced, may not find it difficult to have such a discussion before they get into bed. But this is not always the case. Studies of contraceptive use and young women indicate that despite the easy availability of effective contraception, many young women do not regularly use contraception. One possible explanation for this behaviour suggested by Gebhard (1980) is that women in deference to established social expectations are frequently 'emotional' rather than 'logical' in their attitude to sexual behaviour, not wishing to acknowledge to themselves or to their partners that they are anticipating intercourse. Some women seem to believe that the premediated use of contraception spoils what they like to think of as romantic spontaneity. In addition, there is always the thought that 'just this once could not possibly make me pregnant'.

A recent survey of sexual practices of female university students at a US university showed that sexual practices seemed to have changed little in the past 15 years (De Buono *et al.*, 1990). Comparisons of behaviour in 1975, 1986 and 1989 cohorts of students showed no difference in the number of male sex partners reported nor in the types of sexual activity. Fewer women used the pill in 1989 than in 1975, and still less than half the women used a condom. Most of the women in the study seemed to think that they knew enough about their partner for 'it to be all right'; and both male and female students were prepared to lie about the number of previous partners that they had had, about the existence of another partner and about episodes of infidelity in order to have sex (op. cit.).

How women perceive the risk of contracting HIV may affect their attitude to protecting themselves. The number of women with HIV and women with AIDS in the UK is still small. It is, therefore, not surprising that women, particularly if they have no association with drug use, do not perceive a risk to themselves of contracting HIV. The attitude of women to protecting themselves from contracting HIV and to taking a positive approach to safer sex can also be affected by a fear of being perceived by their partner as inferior, a fear of being rejected by their partner, and a fear of being humiliated by their partner.

If a woman wishes to protect herself from infection and have intercourse with a partner whose sexual history is unknown to her, then she needs to ensure that her partner uses a condom. The use of a condom can be combined with the use of a barrier spermicide cream such as nonoxynol-9 to provide an additional safeguard. Nonoxynol-9 is known to kill HIV in laboratory settings (Hicks *et al.*, 1985). This does not necessarily guarantee that it will kill the virus in other settings, but its use should lower the risk of transmission of the virus. The female condom is a new contraceptive method that has been undergoing clinical and laboratory studies. It has been shown to prevent the passage of HIV *in vitro*. Female condoms are marketed as Femshield and may offer a useful barrier method of protection for women.

The actual use of a condom can, however, present problems for both partners. Women accustomed to controlling their own fertility with a non-barrier method of contraception do not readily welcome the idea of using additional barrier methods. Some women have reported that they no longer feel 'in control of the situation', as they are dependent on their partner to protect them from infection. The use of a condom and a spermicide is not always readily welcomed by women who have been sterilized, often on completion of their family. Often such women say that it is only with the fear of pregnancy permanently removed that they have really enjoyed their sex life.

In addition, some women who are in a stable long-term relationship and whose partner is HIV positive have found the wearing of a condom creates an emotional barrier with their partner, reminding them of the seriousness of their situation, the risks to themselves and the illness of their partner.

Many men, however willing they are to cooperate in the use of a condom, are frequently unaccustomed to them as so many sexually active women use oral contraception. Furthermore, there is a commonly held belief that the use of a condom during intercourse interferes with the man's pleasure. According to Rainwater (1960), in his now classic study of contraception and family planning, it is possible that 'the man's dislike of condoms (like taking a bath with your shoes on) is as much based on the psychological meaning of lack of contact as on actual diminished physical sensation'. It is suspected that this belief is still held among men in widely different socioeconomic groups and ethnic backgrounds, making it difficult for women, however assertive, to gain their cooperation in the use of a condom. A recent survey by the Family Planning Research Network reported a negative attitude towards condom use by the partners of women studied, with 86% considering that men dislike using condoms. The same study found that 46% of women stated that they also disliked using them with only 7% stating that they enjoyed using them. The most common reason given by women for using condoms was the safeguard they provided against infection (UK Family Planning Research Network, 1988).

For many women, having sex is not just about having intercourse but about having a sexual relationship which includes love and affection. In their study of the sexual experiences of British women, Chester and Walker (1980) report on the importance of the physical expressions of affection such as kissing, cuddling and hugging which women felt should be part of everyday living and not solely associated with a preamble to love making. The Hite Report (1981) also had similar findings with US women who stressed the importance of close physical contact and touching. In the UK study, women frequently complained about what they called the 'wham bang' approach to love making, with very little consideration being given to the feelings and wants of the women. It is important to remember that the desire and need for affection remains relatively constant while the desire for love making may fluctuate, and that is particularly true when people are ill, in pain or undergoing considerable stress.

HIV, women and pregnancy

Some women may be pregnant when they learn that they are HIV positive. Some of these women will be helped in their coping with the diagnosis of HIV by the fact that they are pregnant. While others will experience feelings of panic, fear, despair and indecision. What are they to do; what are the choices available to them? Some women will wish to continue with the pregnancy, while others will have no choice but to continue with their pregnancy because it is too far advanced for termination to be carried out.

Other women may not wish to continue with the pregnancy. Whatever decision is reached, women should be given all the information available to enable them to reach an informed choice.

There are some HIV-related issues which should be considered when counselling this group of women. This is a very difficult area for counsellors, and it is not helped by the still imperfect knowledge with which counsellors must work. It is therefore important that counsellors keep abreast of information on women, pregnancy and HIV and are able to say to women that this is the most accurate information that is known to date.

An important consideration in counselling this group of women is to consider the implications of having a child who may be HIV positive. We have already referred to the current evidence that the majority of babies born to HIV positive mothers will be HIV negative after some months. However, a minority of these children will remain HIV positive and go on to develop AIDS. It may be helpful in counselling for prospective parents to consider the implications for them of having a child who may be HIV positive and go on to develop AIDS, who may have a very short life and who may predecease the mother.

These topics constitute part of what genetic counsellors would refer to as the burden of the disease (Sorenson *et al.*, 1981). Counselling this group of clients requires considerable skill and it is most likely to be done by members of staff in an obstetric or other specialist unit. However, this is not always the case, and counsellors particularly concerned with HIV may be involved. It is important to remember that clients or patients do not share the same, or even a similar, frame of reference as the counsellor and the burden of HIV and AIDS may not be perceived to be important by the prospective parents.

It is usual for pregnant women to ask whether their baby will be healthy. HIV positive mothers often ask if it is possible to know whether their baby will be one of the babies to remain HIV antibody positive and to develop AIDS. It is not possible to tell what will happen in individual cases. In these situations, it is only possible to say to the woman that some babies will be HIV positive and go on to develop AIDS, but at the moment we understand that will not happen in the majority of cases. This uncertainty and lack of knowledge is difficult for people who wish to make a decision and feel that medical science should have the answers.

It is emerging that pregnancy may mask the symptoms of HIV-related illness. Minkoff *et al.* (1988) suggest that non-specific symptoms of infection such as fatigue may be dismissed as 'normal' in pregnancy, thus delaying the onset of treatment. However, it may not be possible to give some treatments for HIV-related illnesses during pregnancy because of the possible deleterious effect on the foetus. For example, it may not be possible to start treatment with zidovudine (AZT) due to the unknown effect on the foetus.

Some prospective mothers and fathers ask about the health of the mother during her pregnancy. Some ask about dying and whether pregnancy will aggravate HIV-related illnesses and cause the premature death of the mother. Once again, it is not possible to say what will happen in individual cases; and, as has already been stated, there is still a lack of knowledge about the effect of pregnancy on the mother's health with respect to HIV-related illnesses.

One of the very great concerns expressed by HIV positive mothers is what will happen to their children should the mother die. While this is not an easy subject to talk about, particularly when the mother is in good health, it is often a relief for them to have discussed what sort of plans could be made for their child or children in the event of their death. Women who have had such a discussion have also said that it has helped them to feel that they have some control. However, many people live in the hope that the inevitable will never happen and HIV positive pregnant women are no different. There is always the hope that a cure for HIV will be found soon. Pregnant women are often younger women who normally would not be considering their own mortality. When they do not know others who have become ill with HIV or who have died from HIV-related illnesses, it may not occur to them to raise the subject themselves.

Some women will have planned their pregnancy. Other women will not have planned their pregnancy and may feel ambivalent about being pregnant. Some workers have suggested that women who feel that they have not achieved much in their lives and who believe that the future does not have much to offer them either, often perceive pregnancy as a desirable option. Authors such as Bury (1984) suggest that such women have little incentive to prevent pregnancy. Being pregnant in the first instance and then being a mother gives these women a status and a role in life which they feel they have not had. Some of these, often younger, women say that they get respect (which they have never previously experienced), they have someone to love and at least one person who now needs them. And at a practical level having a child in some instances enables the mother to live independently and to be rehoused.

When a woman is ambivalent about her pregnancy and unsure about what to do, it is helpful for her to consider the support she has: whether she has the support of the father of the child or her partner; the proximity of family or close friends who could give practical help; and how she will manage financially.

Medical care during pregnancy and delivery

Most pregnancies are relatively uncomplicated as are the majority of births. The presence of HIV in the mother may cause some complications and give rise for concern to the obstetrician who is concerned for the health of both the mother and the child. For many years, women have been complaining about the over-medicalization of pregnancy and labour. When the mother is HIV positive, it is likely that her pregnancy and birth will be very closely monitored. The medical care of many non-HIV pregnancies involves shared care, i.e. the care of the mother during pregnancy is shared between a GP and hospital with most of the routine check-ups of early pregnancy being carried out by the GP. This arrangement offers the mother the expertise of the hospital and the convenience of her GP for the majority of the visits. At the moment, it is likely that the majority of HIV positive mothers will be cared for entirely by the hospital for the duration of their pregnancy. If a mother wishes to have some other antenatal care carried out by her GP, she should ask whether this is possible. It is likely that there are variations around the country as different obstetric units and GPs gain experience in the care of HIV positive expectant mothers.

A concern about the delivery of the baby is the possibility of transmission of infection. In some labour units, obstetricians prefer to deliver HIV positive women by caesarian section. While in individual cases there may be a medical reason for this form of delivery, there is no evidence to suggest that this route of delivery prevents mother–child transmission of HIV. It is important that staff take appropriate precautions to protect themselves from infection from contaminated blood during delivery. This will mean wearing protective clothing throughout delivery. Mothers will understand that this is necessary provided that the wearing of protective clothing and any procedures considered necessary for the safe delivery of the baby are explained to the mother. Much distress can be caused to expectant mothers during delivery through lack of explanation by thoughtless or inexperienced staff. Mothers should be encouraged to ask questions about what will be, or what is, happening to them (see Nursing Guidelines, 1986).

Classes for the preparation for childbirth that pregnant mothers are encouraged to take should also be available for those who have HIV. Information about pregnancy, birth and the process and procedures of delivery can help reduce fear and tension. The concern to maintain confidentiality has possibly meant that HIV positive women do not attend antenatal classes, thus isolating them from their peers. Similarly, recently delivered HIV positive mothers should be encouraged to do some post-natal exercises to help regain their figure and to give them a feeling of well-being.

Injecting drug use, HIV and pregnancy

Female intravenous drug users are particularly vulnerable to HIV. First of all, the majority of these women are the sexual partners of male intravenous drug users (Brown and Primm, 1988). Furthermore, a considerable proportion of HIV positive pregnant women will have contracted HIV through intravenous drug use. It is important to try to attract pregnant HIV positive women into the maternity services as early in pregnancy as possible. However, the lifestyle that often accompanies intravenous drug use is such that drug-using women are often poor attenders at clinics. Moreover, these women frequently perceive that society views them negatively, is critical of them and author-itarian. Many of these women often feel very guilty about their lifestyle and are fearful that if they admit to drug use they may be considered unsuitable as a parent.

As a result of a combination of these factors, many drug-using pregnant women often book late into antenatal clinics. One result of late booking is that some women lose the choice of whether or not to continue with the preg-nancy. Some women may also book late for fear that they may be pressurized into having a termination and there is some supporting evidence for this fear from both workers and women themselves.

Any drug-taking pregnant woman will be regarded as having a high-risk pregnancy, but the antenatal care for intravenous drug-using pregnant women is no different from the antenatal care of any non-intravenous drug-taking pregnant woman who is considered to be at high risk obstetrically because of her previous obstetric history, or because of other medical problems.

Once a woman has come to the attention of the maternity services, it is clearly desirable to encourage her to attend clinics on a regular basis. Many drug-using women either fail to attend clinics or express a reluctance to do so because of a fear of the attitudes of the staff to their problems and to their lifestyle, and also because of a concern that their baby may be taken into care. It is important that staff acknowledge these fears and stress that the mother's drug use and her ability to be a parent are issues that will be assessed separately and will not affect her antenatal care (Gerada, 1990). There is a need for a flexible and non-judgemental approach, and the provision of this approach has been pioneered by doctors such as Dr Mary Hepburn and her colleagues at the Royal Maternity Hospital, Rottenrow, Glasgow.

While pregnant intravenous drug-using women should try to stop taking drugs during their pregnancy, many find it difficult or impossible to do so. One major aim in the management of drug-dependent pregnant women is to reduce the risk to the foetus of withdrawal. Women who cannot stop taking drugs can be helped to control their use better. Oral methadone can be substituted for opiates, although the organization DAWN has suggested that pure, i.e. non-street, heroin may be less dangerous to the foetus than meth-adone. It is also important that women have access to sterile needles and syringes.

For intravenous drug-using pregnant women, the management of labour and the incidence of caesarian section are no different from the situation of women in a non-drug-using population. Intravenous drug-using women can be given analgesia during labour and delivery as there is little evidence that opiates are harmful to a foetus already sensitized to opiates during pregnancy. Furthermore, studies by Fraser (1976) suggest that respiratory depression at birth is not an important problem for these babies. It is important that women can be reassured that, when they are in labour, pain will be controlled, and that a sufficiently large amount of analgesia to give relief will be prescribed.

Because intravenous drug-using mothers generally have not attended ante-natal classes, and as a result may not be familiar with routine procedures, it is very important that explanations are always given about procedures that need to be carried out. This is particularly crucial post-natally, when actions involving removing the baby from the mother are necessary, e.g. taking the baby to the neonatal baby unit. When unfamiliar procedures are explained, tension is re-duced and the patient may feel that she is being treated appropriately. Anxieties may, therefore, be alleviated; and the chances of the mother discharging herself early, and thus disappearing from the helping services, are reduced.

The HIV positive pregnant drug user is a woman who needs care for the safe delivery of her baby, and in this respect is no different from any other pregnant woman. However, she may also have some medical, obstetric and social problems which require the resources of a multidisciplinary team. Preg-nancy can present an excellent opportunity to develop good relationships with these women by helping them to feel that as people they are worth bothering about and by increasing the awareness of the importance of the maternity services. Drug dependence is a condition where there may be periods of heavy drug use, which alternate with periods of minimal or no use. It is possible that by developing a good relationship with the mothers during their pregnancy, that in the future they may be helped to control their drug use.

Termination of pregnancy

When some HIV positive women learn that they are pregnant, they would prefer not to carry on with the pregnancy. However sure and steadfast a woman is in her reasons for this decision, counsellors should work through her reasons with her and discuss some of the implications of termination. For example, even though a woman is quite sure that termination was the right decision, she may continue some time after termination to feel weepy, de-pressed and even doubtful that she did the right thing. That is a normal response to abortion. A failure to offer women an opportunity to work through the decision process prior to termination can result in greater psycho-logical morbidity afterwards. It may also help such women to consider that they can enjoy life without the additional responsibility of a child or another child and without the guilt or anxiety of bringing into the world a child who may be HIV positive.

There are many reasons why HIV positive women may decide to terminate the pregnancy. Some may be concerned about their own health and feel that they will not live to see the child grow up. Others may already have symptoms of HIV-related disease and this may be considered a strong medical contra-indication for continuing with the pregnancy. Some women will also be intravenous drug-dependent, which may cause medical problems for both the mother and the baby during pregnancy. There is a danger that HIV positive women, particularly drug-using women, will be pressurized either explicitly or implicitly into agreeing to termination. The time for good pre-termination counselling is often short, as it depends upon what stage in her pregnancy the woman appears for counselling. Whatever decision the mother reaches about termination, it is important that it is supported and accepted by counsellors and other professional staff.

The father of the baby

In working with a woman towards a decision whether or not to continue with the pregnancy, it is important to establish her relationship with the father of the baby. In some cases, there may be no contact with the father. In others, the woman may feel particularly bitter towards the father whom she believes infected her with HIV. Some women may be carrying the child of a deceased partner. Some fathers may be very much involved and supportive and some of these fathers may themselves be HIV positive, making the total family situation very complex. In other cases, the father will be HIV negative. If the parents wish to, and the father is able to look after the baby should the mother's health deteriorate, this can be a very great reassurance to the mother and can help in her decision about the future of the pregnancy.

Post-natal care

Mothers with HIV require supportive post-natal care for the successful social, emotional and psychological development of the new family unit. Feelings of not being able to cope, irritability, weepiness, loneliness and lack of self-esteem are often experienced by recently delivered mothers. Because of their situation, HIV mothers may experience these emotions acutely. They may be very tired, partly because of HIV-related health problems and partly because they have just had a baby. Some mothers may be very lonely. Some will be single parents and the new baby temporarily restricts their ability to get about, thus increasing their isolation. It is important that mothers are helped to maintain a balanced perspective and not to attribute all their problems to HIV. Some HIV mothers may become depressed and clinical post-natal depression has been identified as a problem in some cases. All recently delivered mothers need good nutrition, exercise and as much rest and relaxation as possible.

It has already been said that the progress of children born to HIV positive mothers should be monitored carefully and that clinical examination, laboratory evaluation and developmental studies be carried out. Children who are then found to have clinical evidence or laboratory evidence of HIV disease can be treated appropriately.

Breastfeeding

All new mothers have to decide how to feed their baby. There is some evidence that HIV can be transmitted in breast milk and until more is known about this possible route of infection there is a tendency to discourage HIV positive mothers from breastfeeding (see Chapter 2). The government has also introduced rules for the screening of mothers for HIV who donate milk to milk banks and for the heat treatment, i.e. pasteurization, of the donated milk. However, in view of the lack of conclusive evidence about infectivity, medical and nursing staff who are advising the mother may need to consider each case on its own merits. Breastfeeding is cheap and convenient as well as emotionally satisfying for the mother and the baby. Being unable, or 'not allowed', to breastfeed because of HIV can be very problematic for some women. Cows' milk is not advised for very young babies and proprietary baby milk is expensive and therefore difficult for those on low incomes to afford. Furthermore, some mothers, because of their lifestyle, may find it difficult to prepare the feed and clean the bottle in a hygienic way.

Women who wish to breastfeed and who are unable to do so for whatever reason are likely to be very disappointed. Some feel a failure and feel that they have not been able to do the best for the baby. HIV positive mothers have similar emotions, often exacerbated by any guilt they have about HIV. There is still very little known about the feelings and attitudes of HIV positive women who have become mothers. Women who have given birth to a child suffering from a genetically transmitted disease which has been passed onto the child by the mother are known to express strong feelings of guilt. Mothers who wish to breastfeed but who are unable or discouraged from doing so should be told that many babies are never breastfed and these babies thrive and develop normally. At a practical level, mothers can be encouraged to bottle feed their baby snuggled against their body without the barrier of clothes. Feeding this way makes the mother and baby feel good.

The possible risk of transmission of HIV through breast milk also means that a woman with HIV should not donate milk to the breast-milk bank nor should she breastfeed another person's baby (wet nursing). It is known that wet nursing is becoming popular among certain groups of women and is common in certain developing countries. The Department of Health has issued a circular to all doctors and regional nursing officers recommending that wet nursing be avoided.

Foster care and adoption

It is the ideal that the natural mother looks after her own child and it is generally assumed that this will happen with HIV positive mothers. However, the mother's ill health or problems associated with drug use on the part of some mothers has resulted in alternative care having to be sought for the child. Sometimes care can be maintained within the family. The father of the child may be able to look after his child with help from other extended family members. When this is not possible and when no other appropriate close relative is able to help, it may be necessary for children to be placed with foster families. Black and Skinner (1987) have looked at ways of developing foster care services, taking into consideration the needs of the child and the whole foster family. These authors emphasize that this is an evolving area of care requiring very close cooperation between the foster parents, the medical profession and the social workers. Foster care raises many questions in relation to HIV, including confidentiality. When the child is HIV positive, the question of who should know about the child's HIV status outside the foster family is raised. It is of course necessary to protect the privacy of the child. It is also necessary that the foster family can live normally with the support that they may need from friends and neighbours. It is hoped that this problem will become easier to deal with as the public gain more knowledge and understanding about the nature of HIV.

Black and Skinner discuss the placing of an HIV positive child in foster care. There may, however, be other older and HIV negative children in the family. Some mothers are very concerned to keep the whole family together. It is important that the mother is involved from the beginning in any plans for the placing of the baby in foster care. It may be difficult for social workers to find families who are willing to take an entire family including an HIV positive child. This is a new and challenging task for social work and social service departments. Some HIV babies will go on to be adopted and there is now a moderate amount of experience in the adoption of HIV positive children.

Mothers sometimes ask what will happen should both the mother and her child become ill at the same time. At the moment there are few facilities where mother and child can be nursed and receive medical care together or in close proximity, and there are regional variations in what can be offered. Often, the best that can be offered is to assure the mother that every effort will be made for her to see her baby, but this will depend on her own state of health and that of the child and how easily they can be moved.

Women living with HIV

A very common response among women who have learned that they are HIV positive is an enormous feeling of isolation. Many of these women do not have a partner and some are estranged from their family. Women who have HIV do not form a homogeneous group. Some have contracted HIV through heterosexual contact, others through intravenous drug use and some from infected blood transfusion. Some are quite young and others are older. Some are childless and others have dependent children. This lack of homogeneity and of a common unifying sense of identity has meant that the establishment of self-help and advocacy groups for HIV positive women has followed a slower course than that of other groups who have been affected by HIV.

Since the advent of AIDS, the gay community has developed an articulate and powerful lobby of self-help groups; and the haemophilia community has an established organization to speak on their behalf. In the past few years, however, organizations such as Positively Women have been established and it is hoped that they will provide a focus for the special needs of women with HIV as well as establishing a network of self-help groups around the country.

A further consideration is that while there is now a relatively open attitude among women towards sex and sexuality, society is not particularly accepting or understanding of women who have contracted a sexually transmitted disease. As Patton (1985) has pointed out, good girls do not enjoy sex. There is a fear among women with HIV of criticism and therefore a reluctance to say what the problem is, thus increasing their isolation. This is also true for those women who have been involved in intravenous drug use. Many of these women say that they find it very difficult to know who to talk to and which friends to trust. Often they do not tell anyone that they have HIV. When such women do find their way to counselling, a very common request is to meet other women in similar circumstances to themselves. As more women are identified with HIV, there is an increasing need for the establishment of group support for HIV positive women. Helpers need to work to reduce the isolation experienced by HIV positive women, and to liaise with other workers in the statutory and voluntary sectors.

People with HIV-related illness tend to have periods when they are well and without symptoms and then periods of infection. When women suffer from HIV-related illness, they often complain about feeling unattractive. In Western societies, there is very great emphasis and pressure on women to be attractive. Advertising in magazines, on television and in the high street emphasizes how women should look and what they should be wearing to make themselves sexually attractive. Women with HIV-related illness who feel unattractive also say how much they dislike their own bodies. Counsellors can help these women to like themselves (see Kirkpatrick, 1988) and look for the positives in themselves and in their lives.

Feeling attractive is closely linked with being and feeling loved. It is also associated with status and a feeling of confidence. Some HIV positive women may be in a stable and supportive relationship, and some may have the support of family and friends. Those are the more fortunate ones. Some women will have a job with the status and financial security that that brings. However, many HIV positive women are unemployed and dependent on social security where the involvement of a welfare rights officer would be helpful. Some women will have dependent children, while others have none. The counselling response to women must reflect their social circumstances.

Everyone who is HIV positive is concerned and frightened about developing illness and those who have serious HIV-related illnesses are concerned about death. These are some of the major uncertainties that both the affected person and the helper are facing and are addressed in Chapters 8 and 9. There is, however, an additional problem for counsellors working with HIV positive mothers, which concerns who is the client. A mother with HIV receives counselling and the counsellor then becomes concerned about the child.

Social work counsellors may be obliged to take action in a statutory capacity making the mother feel that her best interests are not being met. For example, in certain circumstances, social workers may have to take a child into care. It is essential that helpers clarify in their own mind and with the woman what precisely is the situation. This is particularly a problem for helpers from the statutory agencies.

A similar situation faces probation officers who have female clients with HIV in prison. One solution is to have a counsellor for HIV-related matters who will also continue to see the woman once she is discharged. This allows the probation officer to focus on statutory matters.

Prostitution, women and HIV

A varied sexual exposure to large numbers of sexual partners and thus to sexually transmitted diseases means that prostitutes can be at risk of HIV infection. Early in the AIDS epidemic, there was considerable media coverage about the possibility of prostitutes being the source of the spread of HIV to heterosexual men (Shilts, 1987). This blaming, or scapegoating, of others was not based on scientific evidence available at the time and seems similar to the double standard attitude to prostitution in which women are punished and men are not (Brandt, 1987).

Studies by Rabkin *et al.* (1987) and Chaisson *et al.* (1988) found no associa-tion between HIV infection and prostitute contact among non–intravenous drug-using men attending a New York STD clinic. On the other hand, Wallace *et al.* (1988) reported an HIV infection rate of 1.1% in a similar group of men, all of whom reported having had contact with a prostitute. Studies such as these of the customers of prostitutes are rare in Europe and the USA and are complicated by the fact that seropositive men are likely to attribute their infection to contact with a prostitute because of the stigmatization of homosexuality, bisexuality and intravenous drug use.

In the West, it is very difficult to determine precisely the role that pros-titutes play in the spread of HIV. It is known that prostitutes can and do become infected with HIV through the sharing of contaminated needles in intravenous drug use. There is also evidence that women turn to prostitution in order to finance their need for drugs (Richardson, 1989; Perkins and Bennet, 1985). Prostitutes also become infected with HIV through sexual contact with infected partners.

There are, however, many social, geographical and cultural variables associ-ated with prostitution. These variables can include which groups of people are involved in prostitution as well as the attitudes of society, the customer and the women to prostitution. In the West, the boundary between sex for money and sex for love is often separated by disassociating the two by geography and by culture. For example, studies of clients of prostitutes have shown the extent of interest in buying sex abroad (Day, 1988). By buying sex abroad the client has greater anonymity. Furthermore, it makes it easier for Western clients to maintain this very important boundary between sex for money and sex for love. This pattern of behaviour is supported by data from prostitute women in countries known for their sex industry which shows that the majority of prostitutes see foreign clients (McGrath, 1984). The economics of prostitution, therefore, would appear to suggest potential routes of HIV transmission between tourists and local women, and between those who buy and sell sex.

Research with prostitute women has focused on their working lives on the assumption that these women are at risk from HIV infection from their clients as well as from intravenous drug use. However, as Day (1988) and other workers have discovered, the private sexual relationships of prostitutes may be very important in the transmission of HIV to the women and particularly when the male partners are at risk of infection.

In her study of London prostitutes, Day (1988) found that a distinction between home and work was made by the women in their use of condoms. These women used condoms with their clients protecting themselves, but also emotionally distancing themselves from their clients. However, they did not necessarily use condoms with their regular partner. According to Day, this distinction between 'work' sex and private sex has important implications for health education, as it may be easy to persuade prostitutes to use condoms all the time. In some areas, prostitutes have been advocated as 'safer sex educators' (*World Wide Whores News*, 1986).

It is important that the labelling of prostitute women as a high-risk group is discouraged as this separates them from other women who are lulled into a false sense of security that they are not at risk of HIV.

Women, HIV and rape

The reporting of rape and the incidence of rape appear to be on the increase. Women who are raped suffer great emotional distress with a common fear being that they may have conceived. Termination of pregnancy can be offered to any woman who conceives following rape. Workers in rape crisis centres have reported that women are being told by the rapist that he is HIV positive or has AIDS. This sadistic twist, whether the information about the HIV status of the rapist is true or not, merely adds to the torment of the woman and makes her rehabilitation even more difficult.

Lesbians and HIV

Lesbians have experienced the adverse consequences of the increase in the stigmatization of homosexuality which has occurred since the advent of AIDS, and some lesbians have been insulted or threatened in connection with HIV and AIDS (Richardson, 1989). Lesbians have felt that they have been marginalized in the discussion of HIV and AIDS within the media, and that their needs for appropriate information about safer sex have not been met. Lesbians have also expressed concern about attitudes of hospital staff to lesbian women who have HIV infection.

Reports of female-to-female transmission of HIV have been rare, and there is conflicting evidence about the cases that have been discussed. This lack of many clearly documented cases of female-to-female transmission of HIV should not, however, be taken to mean that lesbians can set aside any worries which they may have about the possibility of contracting HIV infection. The fact that identified HIV infections have been far fewer in number among lesbians than in other identified 'risk groups', does not mean that lesbian sex is safe *per se*.

Lesbian women may become infected with HIV as a result of having 'unsafe' sexual relationships with men, or from 'unsafe' sex with other women. Women who are concerned that they or their partner might be HIV antibody positive should practise 'safe sex', i.e. avoid contact between bodily fluids, such as vaginal secretions or blood, and the sensitive mucous membranes of the body. This can be achieved by using latex barriers during oral sex, by avoiding sharing sex toys, and by ensuring that vaginal secretions do not come into contact with any cuts or sores.

There is then a need for greater attention to be focused on the possibility of woman-to-woman transmission of HIV and for appropriate safer sex education for lesbians. Due recognition also needs to be given to the needs of lesbians as carers for people with HIV-related diseases. As health care workers, lesbian women have been involved in the care of people with AIDS. Lesbian women have also cared for, and grieved for the loss of, gay friends through AIDS.[1]

HIV and AIDS and women as carers

Women are daughters, mothers and partners; and in all these roles they are also carers. While the focus of this chapter has been about women who themselves are living with HIV or HIV-related illness, counsellors may also be involved with women who are caring for someone with HIV-related illness or who have cared for someone who has died of AIDS. There are a variety of possible situations when this occurs and some are more common than others, e.g. the partner of a man with AIDS, the mother of haemophiliac sons who may or may not be her only children, a widowed mother caring for her son who is dying of AIDS, and a mother caring for her daughter with AIDS.

Each of these situations will present different social, emotional and psychological problems for the carer and may depend upon her relationship with the affected person, her feelings about how the affected person contracted HIV and the degree of support that she may have. Tension can occur because the carer is torn at times between looking after the person with HIV and finding time for herself. This is critical when the carer is also HIV positive; but it is also an important factor for all carers. Women often tend to feel very guilty when they spend time on themselves. An additional factor concerns care in the community. In theory, this is an excellent concept, but its success depends upon sufficient support for the principal carers from the statutory and voluntary sectors. Resources are scarce and counsellors may find themselves in the position of an advocate for the patient or client in helping the family find support.

Women also play a major part as professional carers and particularly in the nursing profession, where there is considerable awareness and concern about burnout among staff. Burnout is described as the situation where a person is so emotionally and physically depleted by their work situation that they are no longer able to work efficiently. Staff support groups are helpful (see Chapter 15), but these do not exist in all situations where staff are looking after someone with HIV-related illness.

A counsellor can assist by looking with the member of staff at her total work and domestic situation. In some cases, work may have filled the whole of the person's life and in these circumstances they need to be encouraged to find some leisure pursuit or hobby. In other cases, the person may need to be helped to speak to a senior member of staff about the situation and perhaps be moved to a different working environment. This could be on a temporary or permanent basis.

Conclusion

This chapter has focused on HIV-related problems that have particular relevance for women. There is still very little known about the effect of HIV and HIV-related illnesses on the female population and the wider implications for society. Any advances in drug therapy for HIV-related illnesses will benefit women. Women must learn to assert themselves and to ensure that they and their unborn child are protected from infection. Working with women who have HIV or HIV-related illnesses, or who are caring for someone with these illnesses, is both a privilege and a challenge for helpers.

Note

1   Readers who wish to look at a more detailed treatment of the way in which HIV has affected lesbians, are recommended to read the relevant chapters in Richardson (1989) and Patton (1985).

References

Black, A. and Skinner, K. (1987). 'Placement of children at risk of HIV infection'. In D. Batty (ed.), *The Implications of AIDS for Children in Care*. London, British Agencies for Adoption and Fostering, pp. 36–47.

Boyd, K.M. (1990). 'Institute of Medical Ethics: Working party report. HIV infection: the ethics of anonymised testing and of testing pregnant women'. *Journal of Medical Ethics*, **16**, 173–8.

Brandt, A.M. (1987). *No Magic Bullet: A Social History of Venereal Disease in the United States since 1880*, expanded edn. Oxford, Oxford University Press.

Brown, L. and Primm, B. (1988). 'Sexual contacts of IVDU: Implications for the next epidemic of AIDS'. *Journal of the American Medical Association*, **80**, 65–6.

Bury, J. (1984). *Teenage Pregnancy in Britain*. London, Birth Control Trust.

Chaisson, N.A. *et al.* (1988). 'No association between HIV-1 seropositivity and prostitution contact in New York city'. *Fourth International Conference on AIDS*, Stockholm, June (abstract 4053).

Chester, R. and Walker, C. (1980). 'Sexual experience and attitudes of British women'. In W.H.G. Armytage *et al.* (eds), *Changing Patterns of Sexual Behaviour*. London, Academic Press, pp. 71–92.

Day, S. (1988). 'Prostitute women and AIDS: Anthropology. Editorial review'. *AIDS*, **2**, 421–8.

De Buono, B. *et al.* (1990). 'Sexual behaviour of college women in 1975, 1986, and 1989'. *New England Journal of Medicine*, **322**, 821–5.

European Collaborative Study (1988). 'Mother to child transmission of HIV infection'. *Lancet*, **ii**, 1039–43.

Fraser, A.C. (1976). 'Drug addiction in pregnancy'. *Lancet*, **ii**, 896–9.

Gebhard, P. (1980). 'Sexuality in the post-Kinsey era'. In W.H.G. Armytage *et al.* (eds), *Changing Patterns of Sexual Behaviour*. London, Academic Press, pp. 45–57.

Gerada, C. (1990). 'Management of the pregnant opiate user'. *British Journal of Hospital Medicine*, **43**, 138–41.

Hicks, D.R. *et al.* (1985). 'Inactivation of HTLV111/LAV infected cultures of normal human lymphocytes by nonxynol-9 *in vitro*'. *Lancet*, **ii**, 1422–3.

Hite, S. (1981). *The Hite Report: A Nationwide Study of Female Sexuality*. New rev. ed. New York, Dell.

Johnstone, F.D. *et al.* (1989). 'HIV infection and pregnancy outcome'. In *Proceedings of Silver Jubilee of British Congress of Obstetrics and Gynaecology*, July, p. 48.

Kaplan, H.S. (1987). *The Real Truth about Women and AIDS: How to Eliminate the Risks without Giving up Love and Sex*. London, Simon and Schuster.

Kirkpatrick, B. (1988). *AIDS: Sharing the Pain*. London, Darton, Longman and Todd.

MacCallum, I.I. (1987). 'Presentation at International Hospital Infection Society Conference'. *AIDS Alert*, **2**, 162.

McGrath, A. (1984). '"Black Velvet" Aboriginal women and their relations with white men in the northern territory, 1910–1940'. In K. Daniels (ed.), *So Much Hard Work: Women and Prostitution in Australian History*. Sydney, Fontana/Collins.

Minkoff, H.L. (1987). 'Care of pregnant women infected with human immunodeficiency virus'. *Journal of the American Medical Association*, **258**, 2714–17.

Minkoff, H.L. *et al.* (1988). 'Routinely offered prenatal HIV testing'. *New England Journal of Medicine*, **319**, 1018.

Mok, J. (1988). 'Children born to women with HIV infection'. *The AIDS Letter*, no. 7, Royal Society of Medicine.

Mok, J.Q. *et al.* (1987). 'Infants born to mothers seropositive for human immunodeficiency virus: Preliminary findings from a multi centre European Study'. *Lancet*, **i**, 1164–8.

Nursing Guidelines on the Management of Patients in Hospital and in the Community Suffering from AIDS (1986). *Second Report of the Royal College of Nursing AIDS Working Party*. London, RCN.

Patton, C. (1985). *Sex and Germs: The Politics of AIDS*. Boston, South End Press.

Perkins, R. and Bennet, G. (1985). *Being a Prostitute*. Sydney, George Allen and Unwin.

Rabkin, C.S. *et al.* (1987). 'Prevalence of antibody to HTLV-11/LAV in a population attending a sexually transmitted diseases clinic'. *Sex Transmitted Diseases,* **14**, 48–51.

Rainwater, L. (1960). *And the Poor get Children: Sex, Contraception and Family Planning in the Working Class*. Chicago, Quadrangle Books.

Richardson, D. (1989). *Women and the AIDS Crisis*. London, Pandora.

Rutherford, G.W. *et al.* (1990). 'Course of HIV-1 infection in a cohort of homosexual and bisexual men: An 11-year follow-up study'. *British Medical Journal*, **301**, 1183–8

Scott, G.B. *et al.* (1985). 'Mothers of infants with AIDS: Evidence for both symptomatic and asymptomatic carriers'. *Journal of the American Medical Association*, **253**, 363–6.

Shilts, R. (1987). *And the Band Played On*. London, Penguin.

Sorenson, J.R. *et al.* (1981). 'Reproductive pasts, reproductive futures: Genetic counselling and its effectiveness'. *Birth Defects: Original Article Series*, vol. XVII, no. 4. New York, Alan R. Liss.

UK Family Planning Research Network (1988). 'Patterns of sexual behaviour among sexually experienced women attending family planning clinics in England, Scotland and Wales'. *British Journal of Family Planning,* **14**, 74–82.

Wallace, J. *et al.* (1988). 'HIV-1 exposure among clients of prostitutes'. *Fourth International Conference on AIDS*, Stockholm, June (abstract 4055).

World Wide Whore's News (1986). No. 2, Winter. Amsterdam International Committee for Prostitutes' Rights.

ELEVEN

Gay men and HIV

CHARLES ANDERSON

Introduction

In the first few years following the appearance of HIV infection, there were many gay people in the UK who, although concerned about its progress, did not perceive it as a problem which would have any direct impact on them. It was a real threat, but a threat to people remote from them geographically and socially.

Now, in 1991, there can be very few gay people whose lives have not been deeply touched by HIV. An increasing number of gay men each year develop HIV-related symptoms. Very many others, although in good health, live with the fear that a past sexual encounter may have put them at constant risk. There are few gay people who have not experienced the pain of seeing a friend die from AIDS, or felt anxiety when a friend or lover has been diagnosed as HIV antibody positive.

Lesbians are in a position of relative safety from HIV infection in com-parison with all other sexually active groups in the population. However, the lives of many lesbians have none the less been powerfully affected by the advent of HIV. The recent increase in the stigmatization of homosexuality which has come about as a result of the way in which AIDS has been represented hits gay men hardest, but also has effects on gay women. In addition, lesbians have felt that their needs for appropriate information on safer sex have been overlooked by health educators, and that they have been marginalized in public discussion of issues concerning HIV. Women's role as carers, and the anxiety and stress that they may feel as a result of the illness of male friends, also needs to be acknowledged.

In the second part of this chapter, there is an attempt to alert readers to the particular problems that HIV infection has created for gay people, and to suggest appropriate responses to these problems. The positive responses that the gay community itself has already made to the challenges posed by HIV and AIDS will also be highlighted.

There is a tendency in writing on counselling and helping to see problems in a very individualistic fashion, to look at how an individual can be aided to cope with personal difficulties, and with immediate social circumstances; and to neglect to consider the social determinants of these personal diffi- culties. Many of the problems faced by gay people centre around the need to cope with prejudice and to forge for themselves a worthwhile identity in the face of the stigmatization of homosexuality. The first section of the chapter therefore attempts to give a brief sketch of the social context within which gay people come to define their sexuality and to make choices about how to express it.

Orientation and identity

Attempts to explain homosexuality

There is no shortage of lay, or scientific, theories that aim to explain the aetiology of homosexuality. Scientific accounts of the causes of homosexuality can be divided into three main classes of explanation.

First, there are those accounts which have explained the emergence of a homosexual orientation in terms of social experience during childhood and early adolescence. Homosexuality is seen as the product of a particular pattern of child–adult relationships. The claim has been made that very intimate relationships with mothers or distant, poor-quality relationships with fathers may predispose children to grow up to be homosexuals. A number of writers have also put forward the hypothesis that specific experiences in childhood may cause some children to develop a fear of heterosexual relationships, and that this fear leads these children to make an adaptive switch to homosexual relationships. Research studies have found that adult homosexuals are some- what more likely than heterosexuals to report that their mothers were strong individuals and are more likely to describe their fathers as rejecting or cold (Fisher and Greenberg, 1977; Bell *et al.*, 1981). However, there is little evi- dence to suggest that parents may cause their children to become homosexual, and very little support whatsoever for the idea that adult homosexuality is linked to particular traumatic incidents in childhood. Given the prevalence of the belief that dominant mothers may 'make' their sons homosexual, and the guilt that parents sometimes experience when they discover that their children are gay, it may be important for a helper to point out that we do not have sufficient evidence at the moment to support the idea that the origins of a person's homosexual orientation can be traced back to a particular pattern of adult–child relationships.

Another class of explanations has centred around the search to show that homosexuals differ from heterosexuals in physical characteristics, or in their body chemistry. The attempt to differentiate homosexuals from heterosexuals in terms of physical appearance and body build has not met with success. The claim that adult homosexuals differ from heterosexuals in their level of hormones has also been difficult to establish in practice.

Another class of explanations has attempted to explain homosexuality in terms of genetic influences and of the possible role that homosexuality may play within the process of evolution. Many of the explanations that so far have been produced within this class have been made in rather general theoretical terms and *much* more evidence would need to be gathered to support them.

In summary, we do not have definite knowledge at the moment as to the causes of differences in sexual orientation. It seems that any successful explanation will need to take a large number of factors into account, rather than looking for a single, root cause. West (1977), a leading researcher on homosexuality, points out that: 'No single causal explanation will ever suffice. Moreover, the key influences need not be the same in every case; different people may reach a similar sexual orientation by very different routes. Generalisations for many cases will not apply at all'.

Leaving aside the crucial question of whether one can ever justify the attempt to change someone's sexual orientation, there is a consensus nowadays that interventions which aim to change someone from a homosexual to a heterosexual orientation are not likely to meet with success. Contemporary psychotherapy and counselling has the aim of assisting people to accept their sexual orientation, and regards the idea of change as impractical as well as rejecting the assumption that homosexuality is in any way a less 'adequate' or valuable form of sexual expression.

Evidence from a number of research studies indicates that it would be wrong to think of homosexuality as necessarily being a fixed characteristic, or to claim that there is a very sharp divide between being heterosexual and homosexual. For example, the Kinsey Report in 1948, the first large-scale study of sexual behaviour undertaken in the USA, found that at least 37% of the male population had had at least some homosexual experience during the course of their life, 13% had had more homosexual than heterosexual experience for at least 3 years of their life, and 4% had always been exclusively homosexual (Kinsey et al., 1948).

Later surveys of sexual behaviour have also found that a large proportion of men, and a somewhat smaller, but still considerable, number of women, have had homosexual experiences at some point in their lives. Rather than thinking of people as being necessarily either 'homosexual', 'bisexual' or 'heterosexual', it probably makes more sense to think of sexual orientation in terms of a continuum. Kinsey et al. (1948) were forced to distinguish seven categories on what they described as a 'heterosexual–homosexual rating scale'. Sexual orientation can be seen as a varying, and somewhat fluid, potential for sexual response.

Sexual expression and sexual identity

The discussion so far in this chapter has centred around the notion of sexual orientation – the desire or inclination to have sexual relations with someone of your own, or of the opposite sex. Turning to behaviour, it is important to emphasize the diversity of ways in which gay men express their sexuality. Some have sought out many pleasurable, short-lived encounters – a lifestyle which has been so pilloried in the popular press in recent years. Others have sought out anonymous sex and avoided longer-term commitments through fear of being identified as gay. Some gay men have formed totally monog- amous relationships on the model of marriage; while others, like a number of their heterosexual counterparts, have established an open relationship which attempts to balance commitment with some sexual freedom.

Sexual activity also cannot be separated out neatly from a whole web of needs, desires and fantasies with which it is customarily associated. All of us, whether gay, straight or bisexual, have somewhat idiosyncratic needs and expectations that we hope will be fulfilled within a sexual relationship or an individual sexual encounter.

Whatever diversity there may be between individual gay people in the ways in which they express their sexuality and the emotions associated with their sexual desires, they all share the problems that arise from the way in which homosexuality is represented and construed within our society. Homosex- uality has been a constant feature of human social life, but the meanings given to homosexuality have varied widely over cultures (Blackwood, 1985). Much recent writing on homosexuality has concentrated on trying to understand the cultural meanings of homosexuality, how a homosexual identity is defined and thought about within particular societies. Those writers who take what has been termed as a 'social constructivist' approach to the study of homosexuality have stressed the point that many of the features which we think of as charac- terizing homosexuality are in fact socially defined and specific to our own culture and historical period (see, for example, Weeks, 1986).

The social identity that has been thrust upon homosexual people is a heavily stigmatized one. The representation of the homosexual as different, objection- able or inadequate is built up from a number of different sources. For a start, in the Judeo-Christian tradition, as in a number of other religions, homosexual acts have been regarded as sinful and shameful. Closely linked to the view of homosexual acts as immoral is the deep-rooted belief that they are in some sense 'unnatural', that they go against the ordained order of nature. This belief can find no support whatsoever from the biological sciences which have revealed that homosexual behaviour can be found in very many animal spe- cies, as well as in almost all human groups. The scientific recognition that homosexuality can be seen as a normal variant of sexuality has had only a limited effect, however, in weakening the popular categorization of homosex- uality as an 'unnatural' way of behaving.

The view of homosexuality as unnatural and alien leads easily to an inability to empathize with gay people, and often an active revulsion against gay sexual practices (in particular against men having anal sex) and gay people as individuals.

Another source of stigma is the set of beliefs that associates homosexuality with effeminacy, with the failure to be a 'proper man'. Conventional views of homosexuality that we are all exposed to from childhood onwards deny the possibility that you can be very masculine in character and a homosexual. Homosexuality and the traditional definitions of masculinity are seen as being mutually exclusive.

Homosexuality has also been stigmatized as a result of the association that has been drawn between it and illness. From at least the mid-nineteenth century, homosexual acts and desires came to be viewed as a proper object for medical study. Doctors explained homosexual behaviour by attempting to define particular features which set homosexuals apart from heterosexuals, to explain homosexuality in terms of a personality or physical disorder. In other words, the emphasis shifted from regarding individual homosexual acts as immoral and shameful, to defining homosexuals as a group characterized by a specific illness. The view of homosexuality as a psychiatric disorder was maintained within the medical profession until comparatively recent times. It was only in 1974 that the US Psychiatric Association removed homosexual orientation from its list of mental disorders. Although nearly all mental health professionals nowadays would not see homosexuality in terms of an illness, the explanation of homosexuality in terms of a 'diseased or disordered state' has been widely disseminated during the twentieth century and has added to the stigmatization of a homosexual orientation.

A gay identity

The discussion of homosexual identity so far has focused on the socially stigmatized representation of gay people. Gay people, however, have forged for themselves a positive, self-affirming identity. The achievements of the Gay Liberation movement in North America and Western Europe in winning somewhat greater rights and respect for gay people are well known. Less attention is paid to the political and social achievement of gay liberation activists in disseminating a view of homosexuality to other gay people and the world at large, which presents it as a cause for pride and self-esteem, rather than humiliation and concealment.

Gay liberation was part of a wider movement for self-definition in the 1960s and very closely associated with feminist attempts to gain greater power for women to determine the shape of their sexual and personal relationships, and attacks on traditional stereotypes of what constituted acceptable masculine and feminine behaviour. As well as defining a homosexual orientation as a valuable and natural variant of human sexuality, the gay movement emphasized the importance of personal choice and self-definition in sexual matters, and celebrated the diversity of choice. It challenged the view of homosexuality as an inversion of gender, and to some extent sought to redefine the traditional terms in which masculinity and femininity have been viewed. At the same time, many gay men have claimed for themselves conventional definitions of masculinity and a strong gay identity.

Differing representations, different emotional reactions, to a homosexual orientation

This new gay identity has opened up the possibility for many people to see their sexuality in positive terms. For example, a very large proportion of the gay people surveyed in a large scale US study published in 1978 declared that they had no or very little regret about their sexual orientation (Bell and Weinberg, 1978). Of those subjects in this particular study who did report feeling a sense of regret about their sexual orientation, almost half of them cited rejection by society as the main cause of their lack of acceptance of homosexuality.

Acceptance of their homosexuality and consequent personal happiness is a possibility for many gay people, but there are some gay people who find it difficult to rid themselves of a feeling of guilt and to feel comfortable with their sexuality. They may find it difficult to escape the stigmatizing representations of homosexuality that have been described earlier in the chapter and to see themselves in more positive terms. Many of those who do feel positive about being gay may also have had to resolve an initial period of crisis in coming to terms with their sexuality. When one considers that for all of us in the later twentieth century Western world, our sexuality forms a very important part of our definition of self, problems in the acceptance of one's sexual orientation are likely to cause considerable unhappiness.

It is important not to think of the 'acceptance of homosexuality' from too individualistic a perspective, as something that an individual ought to be able to achieve for him- or herself. Problems in accepting sexuality may not necessarily have their source in a failure of self-knowledge or of the will to resolve personal feelings. Individual gay people may have received very real hurts and lack of acceptance from others which makes them unable to accept their own sexuality. They may also be living in social circumstances which make any public acknowledgement of their homosexuality impossible, and self-acceptance very difficult. Again they may have absorbed during childhood a set of beliefs about the nature and purposes of life which are now a deeply entrenched part of their way of responding to the world. These beliefs may make it very difficult for them to accept the homosexual desires which are part of their nature.

It also needs to be borne in mind that feeling comfortable about one's own sexuality need not be an all or nothing matter. We all show a lot of consistency in our attitudes and behaviour in situations that are highly similar, but often very little consistency across situations that are markedly different. Someone might find it very difficult to cope with being thought of as gay at work, but be quite happy about his sexuality in other contexts. By contrast, someone else might be very open and confident about being gay at work, but not be able to raise the issue with any members of his family. Helping responses will clearly vary depending on whether difficulties and anxieties concerning sexuality are confined to a particular social context or form a more general problem.

Anyone working in the area of HIV is likely to come across people who do need assistance in accepting their sexuality. Such assistance is likely to be of limited value, if the helper regards anxieties surrounding sexuality as a 'problem' that can be dealt with in isolation from the rest of the person's life. Any help that is given to someone to come to terms with his or her sexuality needs to be tailored to pay due regard to the person's general pattern of emotional needs, social situation and structure of beliefs.

'Understanding homosexuality'

It is customary at the moment for people who are being trained to work in the area of HIV to be exhorted that they must 'understand homosexuality'. One way of 'understanding homosexuality' is to try to gain some imaginative identification with the difficulties that gay people face as a result of prejudice and the crises that they may have to face in the process of coming to terms with their own sexuality and developing a positive view of themselves. The 'coming out' role-plays presented at the end of this chapter can be useful aids towards developing empathy with the way in which gay people have to negotiate their way through a problematic, and sometimes downright hostile, social world.

Looking at the understanding of homosexuality in a more intellectual sense, it would be unfortunate if people coming to work with gay men living with HIV felt that they needed to discover some essence of what homosexuality is about. The message of this chapter is that there is not some fixed template of knowledge that can be applied to every gay man and lesbian. There is a wide range of sexual desire, emotional needs, types of sexual expression and ways of construing identity that can be encompassed under the terms 'gay' and 'bisexual'. The diversity among gay people in the way in which they choose to express their sexuality, and the manner in which they think about their social identity, has been highlighted earlier in the chapter.

In terms of providing an appropriate helping response, this diversity among gay people in their emotional reaction to their sexuality and the meaning that they attribute to their sexuality needs to be emphasized. It is not sufficient for people in a helping position to be informed in general terms about the lifestyle and problems of gay people. They also need to think very closely about how the individual gay people that they are working with perceive their own sexuality, and to consider how thoughts concerning sexuality are influencing feelings and actions.

The impact of HIV on gay people

Problems arising from the way in which AIDS and homosexuality have been represented

Moving on from looking at homosexuality in general to focus in on the way in which HIV has affected the lives of all gay people, one immediate effect has been an increase in the stigmatization of homosexuality. This has come about as a result of the way in which AIDS has been represented. It is not only papers like *The Sun* which have talked about the 'Gay Plague'. However inaccurate this may be on a worldwide basis, the disease has been presented in the media as predominantly affecting gay men. The close associations that have been established between death, AIDS and homosexuality have made it possible to present gay people as a group as a potentially dangerous source of pollution.

Diseases and infections, such as HIV, can have many meanings, and social and personal anxieties associated with them. The disease can be seen not just as a threat to the physical body, but also as a punishment and as a source of personal, moral, social and spiritual danger. These meanings are also highly charged with emotion. People living with HIV, and by extension groups such as gay men who have been closely identified with the infection, have often been regarded with a peculiar dread and seen as alien and threatening. The stigmatization of the disease has reinforced the traditional stigmatization of homosexuals. It is only too easy for the pulpit, press and TV pundits to make a metaphorical leap from the threat that HIV infection poses to health to describe homosexuality in terms of moral and social danger, and to use revulsion against an ill-understood, threatening infection to reinforce revulsion against homosexuality.

Gay people who wish to promote a positive image of their sexuality have found it difficult to compete with this emotive rhetoric associating homosexuality with disease and danger. Simon Watney (1987, p.18) has written that: 'It is this new and fragile (if confident) gay identity which is now particularly at risk, not from Aids as such, but from the crisis of representation surrounding it.'

The negative representation of HIV and AIDS at a time when the government is expounding 'traditional values' and is doing its best to legislate the subject of homosexuality out of the classroom has created a difficult social climate for gay people. Although most gay people are not likely to feel any self-doubt as a result of the way in which HIV and homosexuality have often been represented in the past few years, it is possible that some gay people will be more likely to see themselves in negative terms.

Even people who do not ordinarily have problems concerning their sexual identity might well have temporary problems that result from the stress of receiving an HIV antibody positive diagnosis, or a diagnosis of HIV-related illness, which adds a new stigma to face and overcome. In seeking to give meaning to the situation they find themselves in, some people who discover that they are HIV antibody positive may wonder if something about their previous lifestyle has been 'wrong', and may feel some guilt about their sexuality. I have worked with individuals who have reacted initially to an HIV antibody positive diagnosis in this way.

If initial feelings of guilt and unhappiness about sexuality after receiving an HIV positive diagnosis are sustained over time, there may be a need to explore carefully with the individual concerned the ways in which he is thinking about both HIV and his sexuality. After this exploration, more positive ways of thinking about being gay can be introduced. However, as a previous section of the chapter indicated, helping people towards seeing their sexual orientation in more positive terms needs to be undertaken with a great deal of sensitivity. It must be guided by an appreciation of other difficulties in the person's life and an understanding of his general way of perceiving the world. Helpers require to be prepared to discuss anxieties concerning sexuality with a client, but this must not be seen as a 'task' that always needs to be undertaken. The client sets the agenda, not the helper.

Turning to look at a particular group of people who may have problems concerning how they feel about their sexuality as the result of an HIV positive diagnosis, some individuals have a style of thinking which leads them to feel that they must be at fault if some misfortune befalls them or people near to them. They tend to attribute all of their problems to internal causes, and don't give sufficient weight in their account of their problems to external events and to other people's actions. It is important with individuals who have this attributional style to point out that they may have sustained real hurts and are being presented with very bleak views of the nature and implications of homosexuality. It is only natural that such reactions and views should cause them distress, and lead them to view themselves negatively. Their difficulties are not their fault, or the result of some failure on their part.

Gay people with HIV-related illness also may be able to cope more effectively with their condition if they have a positive attitude to their sexuality and their energy is not dissipated in feelings of guilt and blame. Sheila Namir, writing about her work as director of a psychosocial AIDS study in Los Angeles, discusses how the social stigma attached to the disease makes coping with AIDS more difficult, and then goes on to describe how:

> If a person with AIDS internalizes the 'blame' for his illness, feelings of inferiority, inadequacy, and rejection are easily aroused and can seriously impair the ability to cope. Often, based on previous experience, the expectation of hostility arouses anger or a sense of guilt. In our study, we found that the more positive a person is about disclosing his

homosexuality to others, the less likely he is to use avoidance and isolation as a coping strategy, the less angry he feels and less anxious he is as
well. A positive attitude about one's homosexuality results in less mood
disturbance, depression, and fatigue. . . . Encouraging that positive attitude toward oneself helps to counter the stress on all coping strategies
(Namir, 1986, pp. 89–90).

A cautionary note needs to be added to Namir's comments, however. As was
discussed earlier, some gay men find themselves living in a social setting where
they cannot readily disclose their homosexuality to others.

The disclosure of their homosexuality is likely to be a particularly difficult
matter for a certain group of men infected with HIV – those who have had sex
with other men but who have no gay friends, and have avoided emotional
commitment and identification with gay men. Returning to the distinction
that was made earlier between sexual expression and identity, such men, often
married, who have been infected with HIV as a result of having unsafe sex
with other men, do not think of themselves as 'gay' and may find it very
difficult to come to terms with what they see as a very stigmatized identity
which has now been thrust upon them. Working with people in this situation
is challenging and requires a particularly high level of awareness and skill.

Assisting people infected with HIV, or who are very uncertain about their
HIV antibody status, to avoid a stigmatized view both of HIV and their own
sexual orientation may on occasion be a very necessary helping action.
However, even when gay people remain confident and assertive about their
sexual orientation, they may face real problems of discrimination and of being
treated in a stigmatized fashion. Often they may require help, advice and
support to deal with these problems. The next section of the chapter describes
the work that is being done by voluntary groups to provide counselling,
support and advice.

Positive responses to HIV

A number of gay men and women responded quickly to the arrival of HIV
infection in Britain in the early 1980s, setting up self-help organizations which
provide health education, and a wide range of services for people affected in
some way or other by HIV and AIDS. These groups also have an advocacy
role, and press for the rights and needs of people who are HIV antibody
positive or who are living with HIV-related illness. The best-known of these
organizations in the UK are the Terrence Higgins Trust based in London, and
Scottish AIDS Monitor. There are also groups which concentrate on the
needs of the individuals most directly affected by HIV. Body Positive groups
are run by and for people who are HIV antibody positive.

The organizations that have just been mentioned, and similar groups in
different parts of the country, now serve a much wider constituency than the

gay community. For the moment, though, it is appropriate to concentrate on the services that they offer to gay people. Within the gay community, they have been very successful in disseminating information and advice about HIV and safer sex. They can claim much of the credit for the fact that there has been a very marked change in the sexual habits of gay men towards sexual practices that carry no risk of transmitting HIV. They have set up organized support groups for gay men affected by the virus, and for their partners, as well as providing individual counselling and 'buddies', i.e. trained volunteers who can provide friendship, support and practical help.

Buddies can be of particular value to single gay men living with HIV who have no partner and may be socially somewhat isolated. Many gay people also live in parts of the country where there is no gay community to speak of, either in terms of organized gay groups or of informal networks of friendship among gay people. Contact with, and help from, voluntary organizations may be the only source of community support that such people have available to them.

Although the achievements which have been described in the last few paragraphs are impressive, the constraints which exist on positive responses by gay people to the challenges of HIV also need to be recognized. As the last paragraph indicated, the difficult social circumstances faced by gay people in the UK have meant that there are many areas where there may be no gay organizations and little of a sense of community among gay people. This lack of a strong community base in many areas on which to build an effective response to the challenges posed to gay people by HIV is a serious weakness.

Practical problems of discrimination and stigma

One area of services that voluntary HIV organizations provide which tends to receive less attention is advice on how to deal with problems of discrimination directly related to HIV, or indirectly as a result of being labelled as gay and therefore at risk of HIV infection. Such problems may arise in connection with employment, in housing, in obtaining mortgages, or in negotiations with insurance companies. The Terrence Higgins Trust, for example, has a legal centre and telephone helpline, and Scottish AIDS Monitor has a legal service ALBA (see Chapter 16). GLAD (Gay and Lesbian Legal Advice) run an advice helpline: 071-253-2043, Monday to Friday, 7 p.m. to 10 p.m.. LAGER (Lesbian and Gay Employment Rights) is a very valuable source of help for people with problems related to employment: 081-983-0696, Monday to Friday, 11 a.m. to 5 p.m.. Local gay switchboards, i.e. local helplines, can also often help to point people towards professionals and voluntary helpers in their area who can give good advice on practical matters.

As well as requiring advice on how to deal with discrimination that they have encountered, gay people may need to be given the opportunity to talk through such problems, and to vent their feelings of anger and frustration.

They may also find it useful to have someone with whom they can discuss plans and develop a set of tactics for dealing with a problem such as discrimination at work.

Moving on from dealing with discrimination to consider coping with prejudice in social life, it may be very helpful for someone who is gay and is HIV antibody positive, or is living with HIV-related illness, to have someone available who will not only provide emotional support but also help with the task of planning how best they are going to cope with social situations where they may encounter prejudice and rejection. The issues of who to tell and when about an HIV antibody positive test result and how to go about the matter have already been explored in Chapter 8.

A particularly challenging situation that many gay men living with HIV have to face is that of telling their family at the one time that they are HIV antibody positive and that they are gay. This may involve different scenarios; for example, telling a wife and children, telling an elderly parent, or telling a younger sibling. Although families have usually responded to such news in an accepting, caring fashion, some gay men living with HIV may have very reasonable fears that they will be shunned or will meet with a very mixed reaction from their family. It is appropriate that someone faced with having to make this double disclosure should receive very solid support from someone in a helping capacity. They also may sometimes require help with planning how the family should be told the news, and someone whom they trust present with them to assist in presenting the news to the family.

Problems of belonging to a group in which levels of uncertainty and stress are high

Having to tell your family that you are gay and are HIV antibody positive is likely to be a particularly stressful and challenging task. More everyday, routine examples of having to cope with a stigmatized social identity could be provided from the lives of very many gay men. There are also few gay men who have escaped experiencing some increase in stress which is directly related to HIV. The advent of HIV seems to have had a somewhat polarizing effect on the gay community, causing some people to retreat from any kind of public identification as gay, while others have found a new sense of commitment to, and concern for, other gay people.

However they choose to react to the existence of HIV, gay people cannot escape the problems of belonging to a group in which levels of uncertainty about the future and stress are high. Jeffrey Mandel reports the findings of a study in San Francisco where the disease bit early and hard into the gay community, in the following terms:

> The unexpected finding that healthy gay-identified men shared high
> levels of emotional distress with their sick gay and heterosexual counter-

parts reveals the powerful impact of the AIDS epidemic on those at high risk for the disease. Healthy individuals who experience profound psychosocial dilemmas as a result of the AIDS epidemic may need interventions to help them cope with their distress (Mandel, 1986, p.77).

The needs of gay men living with HIV-related illness, and the separate set of needs of gay men who know that they are HIV antibody positive, require an immediate response; and it is sometimes easy to overlook the difficulties faced by gay men who are healthy but suffer emotional distress from fears which centre on HIV. A large number of the gay men who have been sexually active in the years before safe sex became a routine response to avoid infection have at least occasional worries about their HIV antibody status. For some individuals, these fears can become a constant preoccupation, and they regard the future with the same uncertainty as people who have received an HIV antibody positive diagnosis. Chapter 7 has presented appropriate helping responses for working with the worried well. At the moment, I want to highlight the fact that for many gay men their antibody status is a source of stress, and for some a constant worry. It is important that the needs for counselling and for group support of gay men whose antibody status is unknown are not ignored.

Another source of distress for a considerable number of gay people at the moment is that of having to deal with the death of a number of friends or acquaintances within a relatively short space of time. This accumulating burden of grief and loss can be difficult to bear. The loss of friends, of people who could have been relied on for support in times of sickness and trouble, may also leave some individuals feeling socially isolated. The continuing deaths of people close to you also acts as a constant reminder of your own mortality, something which most young people in the post-war generations have not had to face. This continuing proximity of death can make life take on a very different aspect.

The needs of young gay people

Moving on to consider the way in which HIV has had an impact on young gay people, the advent of HIV and AIDS has increased the stigmatization of homosexuality and may make it more difficult for some young gay men to come to terms with their sexual orientation. They may also find it more difficult to 'come out' to family and friends than a previous generation of gay people did.

It would be unwise to assume that all young people who are nowadays coming to explore their sexual orientation are well-informed about HIV. Aside from requiring information about HIV and AIDS, young people may also have worries about HIV which need to be explored. The successful campaign that has been run within the gay community to inform people about

HIV and safe sex must be continued to reach new members of the gay community. The final report from project SIGMA, a large recent study of the sexual lifestyles of men who have sex with men, commented that 'if HIV infection is to be minimized, homosexually active under 21 year olds need to be targeted for health education initiatives which promote behavioural change' (Project SIGMA, 1990, p.135). However, targeting appropriate health education towards young gay men is a very difficult matter in the UK, given that homosexual activity is illegal under the age of 21.

It is worth noting that even within the efforts made by gay people themselves to provide health education about HIV and safer sex, there has been comparatively little attention given to the particular needs of black gay and bisexual men living in the UK. Any health education initiatives which are designed particularly to meet the needs of younger gay men, require also to consider how to provide appropriate information to younger black gay men.

The manner in which safe sex is presented to young gay people also requires considerable care. Young people, whether heterosexual or homosexual, who are just beginning to express their sexuality, can be a bit hesitant about defining the terms of a sexual relationship. Young gay men who are coming to terms with their sexual orientation may need to be encouraged to be assertive about safer sex. 'Safe sex' workshops where young people can explore ways of being assertive about having safe sex, and many feelings and issues around the expression of their sexuality, are likely to be a much more effective way of promoting behaviour change than simply providing information about safer sex in a didactic fashion. Safe sex is also not going to appeal to young people if safe has the connotation of dull. It needs to be presented as an attractive, erotic alternative.

Problems in changing sexual habits, and in the expression of sexuality

'Safe sex' workshops can also be useful to gay men who have been sexually active for quite a number of years and are having difficulties in adjusting to safe sex practices. Some men may experience considerable feelings of loss in making radical changes in their sexual habits. Changing sexual practices is often talked about in somewhat simplistic terms, as if it involved no more disturbance than changing a make of car. For all sexually active adults, pleasure and fulfilment become closely associated with some particular class of sexual acts, and it is not a trivial matter to divest that act of all of its pleasurable associations and to transfer these feelings to another sexual practice. Anyone in a helping capacity should be sensitive to the magnitude of the change that has been required of many gay men, and to consider how he or she would feel about undertaking similar changes in behaviour. Helpers also need to be alert to the difficulties that some gay men may face in *maintaining* a change to safer sex over a long period of time.

Turning from difficulties in changing behaviour, and in maintaining new behaviours, to actual problems in the expression of sexuality, fears about HIV have created a problem of loss of libido for quite a number of gay men. Others may have no loss of desire, but may have developed considerable anxiety about engaging in any sexual act, however safe. It is a difficult matter to acknowledge that you are having problems in your sexual life. Anyone in a helping role needs to ensure that they have built up a good relationship which provides sufficient security to allow someone to look at and then to begin to deal with anxieties concerning sex.

The impact of HIV on gay relationships

Problems with sexual expression, related to worries about HIV, clearly may bring tension into some gay relationships. At times, stated worries about HIV might also be used by one or both partners in a relationship to mask problems in sexual expression or emotional problems. A couple might use HIV-related fears as a way of avoiding change in an unsatisfactory relationship. Anyone in a helping role needs to proceed very carefully and sensitively in any case where worries about HIV are presented as the source of problems in sexual expression within the relationship.

Worries about HIV antibody status, or the knowledge that one or both partners in a relationship are HIV antibody positive, can place a lot of strain on any relationship, gay or heterosexual. Men in a partnership may wish to support each other but find that they are too preoccupied and stressed by their own individual worries to do so. It may be useful for them to have someone outside the relationship to whom they can ventilate fears and concerns.

It has been the author's own experience of gay men in relationships where both partners are HIV antibody positive that recriminations about who infected who do not tend to be a common problem. However, this may be a powerful source of rancour in some gay couples, at least for a time after receiving an HIV antibody positive diagnosis.

Worries which centre around HIV are added to the problems that arise from the fact that gay relationships are not valued by society at large. There is a lack of institutional supports or of any clear social guidelines, models, of how a relationship between two men should proceed. Consequently, a relationship between two men often demands more commitment, and more imagination in dealing with difficulties, than a heterosexual relationship.

Many gay men at the moment are showing a great deal of commitment and resourcefulness in looking after partners who are sick, or in coping with an uncertain future for their partner or themselves. This intrusion of sickness and mortality brings not only many hard everyday tasks of caring, but also a very distinct change to the terms and the character of the relationship. The following quote from a short story by Adam Mars-Jones captures the nature of this change very clearly: 'He thought with nostalgia of the time when people had got so exercised about who loved who, and how much. Now it was simply a question of what character of love would be demanded of him, and how soon' (Mars-Jones, 1987, p. 119).

The needs of partners who are caring for a person who has HIV-related illness are referred to in Chapter 14, where the need to respect the position of the partners of gay men with HIV-related illness, and to keep them informed of, and involved in, the treatment process are highlighted. It is also worth noting that quite a number of gay men may not have a regular sexual partner, but they do have a non-sexual, but close and emotionally sustaining friendship with another gay man or with a woman. The needs of the lover of a gay man with HIV-related illness might be considered by health professionals, but those of a very close friend might be overlooked.

The stresses faced by a gay helper/counsellor

As a final point, it may on occasion be necessary to remind some gay people who are very actively involved in a voluntary or professional capacity in caring for people that they also have needs of their own which deserve to be met. Gay people are likely to identify closely with the situation of gay men who have HIV-related illness and for that reason to be more empathic and effective as helpers. Sometimes, though, this closeness to the people that they are helping may be a source of considerable stress and grief. Gay helpers need to have a good support network themselves, and to establish a space in their lives which is free from the work of caring, and of personal anxieties concerning HIV. This issue of providing appropriate support for carers is dealt with in detail in Chapter 15.

Role-plays: Coming out

The following role-plays can be performed in small groups within the space of 3 hours, taking a short break at some point in the proceedings. They should only be attempted with a group of people who have already established trust and confidence in each other. They aim to give the participants at least some feeling of what it is like to come to terms with being gay, and of how their life could be changed by being gay. It is important that sufficient time is allowed after the role-play to take the participants carefully out of their role. Support might need to be provided for any individuals who have experienced a change in their understanding of their own sexuality as a result of undertaking the role-play.

The participants are asked first to put themselves into the position of someone who realizes that he or she is gay, but is daunted by the changes that a recognition of their sexuality may bring about in their life. They are asked to imagine for themselves a very concrete set of circumstances, or to use their own life, and to think very hard for 5–10 minutes about how they would feel if the people in their imaginary or real world saw them as being gay. What practical consequences also would there be? After this period of silent thought, the participants are asked to share with another member of the group what they had imagined and felt.

The participants are next asked to role-play in pairs trying to raise the subject in a tentative fashion with someone, for example with an older person who is a trusted friend. This is followed by 'phoning a gay switchboard to talk through feelings. Next, in groups of three or four, one member has to play the role of going into a gay bar for the first time and attempting to make conversation with people there. This is followed by a role-play in pairs where one of the pair have to make their first faltering attempts to tell someone of the same sex that they find them attractive. To finish off the set, the participants are asked in groups of two to play the part of telling a parent or a very close straight friend that they are gay. After each role-play, the participants are asked to share with their partner(s) how they experienced the role.

References

Bell, A.P. and Weinberg, S. (1978). *Homosexualities – A Study of Diversity among Men and Women.* New York, Simon and Schuster.

Bell, A.P. *et al.* (1981). *Sexual Preference: Its Development in Men and Women.* Bloomington, Ind., Indiana University Press.

Blackwood, E. (1985). *Anthropology and Homosexual Behaviour.* New York, Haworth Press.

Fisher, S. and Greenberg, R.P. (1977). *The Scientific Credibility of Freud's Theories and Therapy.* New York, Basic Books.

Kinsey, A.C. *et al.* (1948). *Sexual Behaviour in the Human Male.* London, W.B. Saunders.

Mandel, J.S. (1986). 'Psychological challenges of AIDS and ARC: Clinical and research observations'. In L. McKusick (ed.), *What to Do About AIDS: Physicians and Mental Health Professionals Discuss the Issues.* Berkeley, Calif., University of California Press, pp. 75–86.

Mars-Jones, A. (1987). 'A small spade'. In A. Mars-Jones and E. White, *The Darker Proof: Stories from a Crisis.* London, Faber and Faber, pp. 65–119.

Namir, S. (1986). 'Treatment issues concerning persons with AIDS'. In L. McKusick (ed.), *What to Do About AIDS: Physicians and Mental Health Professionals Discuss the Issues,* Berkeley, Calif., University of California Press, pp. 87–94.

Project SIGMA (1990). *Longitudinal Study of the Sexual Behaviour of Homosexual Males: A Final Report.* London, Project Sigma, Department of Social Science, South Bank Polytechnic.

Watney, S. (1987). *Policing Desire: Pornography, AIDS and The Media.* London, Methuen.

Weeks, J. (1986). *Sexuality.* Chichester/London, Ellis Horwood/Tavistock.

West, D.J. (1977). *Homosexuality Re-examined.* London, Duckworth.

TWELVE

Drug users and HIV

ALAN FERRY AND
CHARLES ANDERSON

Introduction

This chapter considers the problems faced by drug users since the arrival of HIV and issues raised in working with this client group. It looks at the influences which lead individuals to take drugs in a way which exposes them to the risk of HIV infection, and at the counselling repsonses that are required if any significant behavioural change is to be achieved. The chapter also draws attention to the needs of injecting drug users who are infected with HIV and of drug users with HIV-related illnesses.

The chapter draws on research evidence, on the experience that one of the authors has gained as a drugs worker, and on ideas suggested by colleagues. It presents a view based on everyday observation of the lifestyle of drug users.

Before examining drug use and HIV in greater detail, it is useful first to look at both the public response to drug-taking and at drug users' own self-perceptions.

Thinking about drugs and their effects

Drug use is hardly a new phenomenon, and it has not always been regarded as constituting a social problem. From the earliest human civilization onwards, a variety of psychoactive substances have been chewed, eaten or drunk to create a temporary alteration of perception or to improve communication with the gods. Michael Gossop (1982), in his book *Living with Drugs*, suggests that: 'The desire to experience some altered state of consciousness seems to be an intrinsic part of the human condition . . . drug taking still remains one of the easiest and most immediate ways of altering psychological states.'

Drug use may be a part of normal human behaviour, but drug-taking within most societies is governed by social rules which tolerate the taking of certain drugs but proscribe other drugs which are regarded as harmful to the individual and a social danger.

There are sound reasons for proscribing certain drugs, but it must be acknowledged that there is a lack of consistency in the way in which certain drugs are categorized as being a source of personal and social harm, while others, such as alcohol, are tolerated. The dividing line between legal and illegal drugs may on occasion appear to be a somewhat arbitrary one and difficult to justify in terms of differences in their toxicity or in their effects on behaviour. The illegal nature of much drug-taking has meant that people who are heavy or dependent users of a drug are as likely to receive a custodial sentence as they are to receive medical help or support and counselling within the community. Official responses have wavered between regarding drug use as a policing problem, a medical problem or a 'social' problem.

The association between the use of certain drugs, illegality and crime has powerfully determined the nature of the public perception of, and reaction to, drug users. They are seen as a threat and as a somewhat alien presence in society. The images of drug users as a source of dirt, danger and social disorder, who can corrupt and infect the 'normal' world have been given even more power with the advent of HIV and AIDS. Even in quite responsible reporting of HIV among drug users, one comes across phrases such as 'seed bed of infection'. Drug users are also often described as a group from which infection can 'leak' into the general community.

Much attention is also given in the press to the topic of how HIV-infected drug users who turn to prostitution to finance their habit may transmit the virus to their customers. This is a matter of serious concern, but the reporting of it almost always betrays a double standard. The woman is seen as the cause of disease, and the client's failure to act responsibly is ignored.

Exploring attitudes and beliefs

An essential part of any training course for helpers who wish to work in the field of drug use and HIV is the exploration of attitudes towards drug use, and of the everyday categories and metaphors that are used to explain the behaviour of drug users. Trainees require to look closely at how negative stereotypes of drug users may influence their feelings and actions. Individuals also need to be given sufficient time to examine and deal with any anxieties that they may have concerning working with drug users. It is important that they look at their own conceptions of what is harmful about drug-taking, at how they themselves explain dependent drug use, and at their goals and purposes in working in this area. Looking at their own pattern of use of legal everyday drugs, such as alcohol, tobacco, coffee and tea, and at the benefits they derive from these drugs is a good way in to prompting more reflective discussion of drug use. Similarly, it can be useful to get trainees to think about objects, people, situations in their life that they feel they are dependent on, then to consider why they are dependent on these things and what they gain from them.

The beliefs that trainees have about the ability and the personal responsibility of drug users to modify their behaviour, and about whether drug users should be 'directed' or gently assisted to gain more personal control, form another area that needs to be examined. Problems can ensue if beliefs about personal responsibility, control and ability to change in relation to drug users are not examined in some depth. For example, there might be a serious mismatch between an agency which has the goal of self-empowerment and a worker who has an implicit model of addictive behaviour which views drug users as being incapable of change without the assistance of an authoritative professional.

As well as exploring how stereotypes of drug users affect their own thoughts, feelings and behaviour, trainee helpers need to consider how these powerful, negative images affect drug users themselves. Some drug users can see themselves as 'just junkies' – a label which has significant connotations of a lack of control. They may not see themselves as being capable of changing dangerous aspects of their behaviour, such as sharing needles which might be contaminated with HIV.

Despite legal constraints, public disapproval and possible exposure to a variety of economic, health and social problems, many people do become involved in the use of illicit drugs. The illegal nature of drug-taking makes it difficult for professional or voluntary helpers to gain access and then to maintain a relationship with this client group. Drug users prefer to keep a low profile about that part of their lives and it is therefore difficult to quantify the number of users of illicit drugs with any degree of accuracy. As an example of the likely numbers of drug users in a major British city, Sally Haw conducted a field survey of heroin use in Glasgow in 1983 and estimated that there were 5000 people using that drug then (Haw, 1985). Unofficial estimates made by drug workers in Glasgow since then point to an increase in the number of drug users rather than a reduction. The existence of a fairly large community of drug users is not unique to Glasgow. Throughout the UK as a whole, therefore, we are talking about quite a large population which needs to be reached to prevent the further spread of HIV in its midst.

What drugs can offer

Attempts to identify a personality type or specific personal attributes which are associated with addiction to drugs have not been particularly successful. The reasons that people have for taking drugs are many and varied. Drug users state boredom, curiosity, emotional and physical pain, peer group pressure and the immediate effect of well-being provided by the drug as some of the reasons for becoming involved in drug-taking. If we stop to consider the reasons that most of us have for the more modest consumption of legal drugs, we are likely to come up with a similar set of reasons.

The negative aspects of the use of illegal drugs are obvious. However, the existence of a fairly large population of drug users strongly suggests that individuals do find positive benefits from drug-taking. The next section of the chapter will describe how it does not make sense to think of drug use simply in terms of hopeless dependence. The connections between drug use, pleasure, comfort and social belonging need to be recognized. Counselling of drug users whose habit is endangering their health requires to focus on the attractive parts of drug-using as well as the negative aspects. Individual drug users can be helped to look carefully at the benefits which they gain from drug-taking and then to explore how they might retain these benefits while using drugs in a safe fashion, and possibly also reducing their dependence on drugs.

Aside from appearing to offer pleasure, comfort and excitement, drugs often give users a sense of social purpose and allow them to identify with a peer group. Someone who is using drugs heavily needs to make a lot of money every day and is as busily and as purposively employed as a worker in a regular occupation. Very often the pursuit of money for drugs involves users in illegal activities such as shoplifting, prostitution and dealing in drugs themselves. Many drug users will have spent at least one period in prison. Organizations working with HIV positive drug users therefore need to ensure that they have good relations with local prisons to allow access to their clients while they are serving a sentence.

Variations in drug use

The common picture held of drug users is that occasional initial use leads on to a continuous downward descent towards hopeless dependence. In fact there is variability in the pattern of drug consumption of many drug users if they are observed for a number of years (Robertson, 1987, p.14). Periods of heavy use may alternate with periods of much lighter and more controlled use of drugs, or even with periods of abstinence. Helpers and the family of drug users need to be alert to this variability in the pattern of drug-taking and to the fact that a relapse into heavy drug use does not necessarily mean that the person is irretrievably dependent on drugs.

As well as these variations in the pattern of drug-taking of individual drug users, there is considerable variability in the types of drug used in different areas and in the methods of drug-taking. The particular drugs used will depend on the local supply of illegal drugs, police policy and activity, the prescribing practice of doctors, and the traditions of the drug subculture in the area.

Heroin is the drug that is most associated with illegal use. It is a powerful painkiller and gives a very immediate effect of euphoria. There are a wide number of street names for the drug, the most commonly used being 'smack'. Heroin is often in short supply, and other drugs with, opiate-like, painkilling properties are frequently used. These drugs are obtained from legal sources but then traded illegally. Examples of such drugs are *buprenorphine,* which has the trade name *Temgesic,* and *dextropropoxyphene,* which has a number of proprietary names including *Distalgesic. Dipipanone,* which has the trade name *Diconal,* is another drug that is used to provide some of the effects that heroin gives. The *benzodiazapine* family of tranquillizers, such as *Activan, Librium* and *Valium,* are another category of drugs that are commonly abused.

Cannabis, in addition to being a drug that is used frequently within the drug-using community, is also in demand by young people and particular ethnic groups who do not perceive themselves as being drug users and who would not be prepared to take any other illegal drugs.

The drugs described so far work by depressing the activity of the central nervous system. There are also stimulant drugs which give the user a sense of excitement, a feeling of energy and self-assurance. The most widely used stimulant drugs are *amphetamines,* known in street language as 'speed' or 'uppers'. *Cocaine* is a stimulant drug. It has not been used widely in the UK; but the supply of cocaine, and in particular of a type of cocaine known as 'crack', has increased considerably in recent years. A stimulant drug which is not frequently used, but which can produce dangerous alteration of mood is *phencylidine hydrochloride* (PCP), also known as 'angel dust'. Like *LSD,* it is also a hallucinogen.

A frequent concern among people who are just beginning to work with drug users is that they will not be familiar with the terms used for drugs and drug-taking within the local drug-using community. Using a term for a drug that is outdated, is not used in that locality or is the wrong name for the drug, may lead the client to regard you as a fraud. It is appropriate to use the correct name such as heroin or amphetamines if you are unsure of the slang term. Ask what is meant if an unfamiliar name is used to describe a drug or a related subject.

Most of the drugs that have been listed above can be injected, including stimulants such as amphetamines. The sharing of injecting equipment, known colloquially as a 'set of works' or simply 'works', has been the principal means of transmission of HIV among drug users. HIV is a blood-borne infection and the sharing of needles, known colloquially as 'spikes', allows blood from an HIV-infected individual to be directly introduced into the bloodstream of another drug user.

The likelihood of the transmission of HIV by sharing needles and syringes is increased in areas where the practice of 'flushing out' has been common. The aim of this exercise is to make sure that all of the drug is injected into the bloodstream. 'Flushing' involves the drug user drawing blood into the syringe and then reinjecting it into the body. A small quantity of blood is left in the syringe which will then be injected into the bloodstream of the next user of the syringe.

*Regional variations, and the need for helping strategies tailored
to local circumstances*

It has already been noted that there are distinct regional differences in the preferred methods of drug-taking. Within a very large city such as London there are also distinct differences between different social and ethnic groups in the types of drug taken and the means of drug-taking. Even injecting drug users do not form a homogeneous group in terms of drug-taking practice. In some areas the sharing of needles has been normal practice, whereas in other cities the sharing of drug-using equipment has been confined to a minority of IV drug users.

These variations in the method of drug-taking are reflected in differences in the incidence of HIV infection among drug users in differing parts of the country. The highest incidence of HIV infection among drug users is in Edinburgh, which has been described in the press as the 'AIDS capital of Europe', with very high levels of infection also being common in Glasgow and Dundee. In Edinburgh, injection was the preferred means of drug-taking, there was a great scarcity of syringes and a local tradition of sharing 'works'. A study conducted in the mid-1980s which tested blood samples from 164 IV drug users in an Edinburgh general practice for HIV antibodies, found that 51% of the subjects were seropositive (Robertson *et al.*, 1986). It was suggested that by the date of publication of the study, 85% of this population might have been infected with HIV (ibid.).

Outside of the Scottish cities, estimates of the level of HIV infection among IV drug users are less reliable, but tend to show a much slower but still considerable increase in infection. A study by Coleman and Curtis (1988), which looked at the equipment-sharing practices and sexual behaviour of 162 IV drug users, found that 39 individuals accounted for 90% of all equipment-sharing contacts and that 4 individuals accounted for 90% of all sexual contacts. Coleman and Curtis suggest that the concentration of high-risk behaviour in a minority of IV drug users has contributed to the comparatively low overall incidence of HIV infection among drug users in London.

Regional differences in the level of HIV infection and in the methods of drug-taking among drug users means that different areas will have different priorities in the health education and care of drug users. For example, in areas where the intravenous injection of drugs is already common, a great deal of effort needs to be put into educating drug users about safe injecting practices and into helping them to obtain sterile syringes. In areas where intravenous drug use is less common, it is possible to put more effort into emphasizing the dangers of injecting and the benefits of safer methods of administration of drugs.

Services available to assist drug users

The services that are available for drug users also vary considerably from region to region. Anyone commencing work in this area needs to become acquainted with the range of services available within their locality. A role that drug workers are often forced to adopt is that of acting as advocates not just for individual drug users, but for the needs of the whole community of drug users within their area, pushing for a better and more co-ordinated range of services.

Drug treatment clinics

In some areas, drug treatment clinics exist. These are often part of a hospital and can prescribe drugs to their patients if this is considered to be appropriate. The prescribing policies of individual drug treatment clinics also serve to define to a certain extent the local response to meeting the challenge of HIV among drug users. Particular clinics may offer drug users detoxification programmes in which the supply of prescribed drugs is reduced sharply within a short period of time, longer-term programmes of dose reduction and drug maintenance programmes.

Maintenance prescribing and HIV

There has been a debate for many years prior to the advent of HIV on the merits and dangers of 'maintenance prescribing'. Some experts acknowledge the usefulness of drug maintenance in individual cases but are highly critical of the use of the practice as a general strategy for dealing with drug use (see Robertson, 1987). The term maintenance prescribing refers to the practice of attempting to keep the drug use of a client in a reasonably controlled state over a long period of time by prescribing an opiate, normally methadone, which is meant to free the drug user from the need to take illegal drugs. The methadone that is prescribed in maintenance programmes is customarily taken orally.

Current interest in methadone maintenance programmes has centred around the potential that they seem to provide for substituting safe oral administration of opiates for unsafe injecting of illegal drugs. Some research work has suggested that methadone maintenance programmes can bring about a significant reduction in the intravenous use of drugs (Ball *et al.*, 1988; Des Jarlais and Friedman, 1988). However, it would be very unwise to see methadone maintenance as a universal solution to the problem of preventing the transmission of HIV through the intravenous use of drugs. A proportion of drug users in oral methadone maintenance programmes continue to inject drugs, sometimes in an unsafe way. Where methadone maintenance is provided, it tends to be only one component of a wider programme of providing counselling, support and some structure to the drug user's life. In their report on a 3-year study of methadone maintenance programmes in three US cities, Ball *et al.* (1988) note that:

> Although both the short-term pharmacological and the long-term re-habilitative aspects of methadone maintenance are significant in success-ful treatment, the latter seem more important with respect to reducing IV use. Thus pharmacologic intervention is seen as a necessary but not a sufficient condition for successful methadone treatment. The sufficient aspect is long-term rehabilitation.

Needle-exchange schemes

Aside from local drug treatment clinics, which will adopt differing policies on prescribing, a number of needle-exchange schemes have been set up in the past few years in areas where there is a high level of intravenous drug use. Needle-exchange schemes often provide counselling and an entry point to medical care as well as sterile injecting equipment and advice on safe injecting practice. An evaluation of these needle-exchange schemes is being conducted and early results suggest that they have in general achieved contact with a sizeable number of clients (Stimson *et al.*, 1988, 1989). The schemes will have to be greatly expanded, however, if they are to reach the bulk of drug injectors.

GPs and drug users

For the majority of drug users, health care and the legal supply of drugs is obtained from GPs. Some GPs in areas where there is a high proportion of drug users are very knowledgeable concerning the lifestyle of drug users and provide them with a sympathetic and highly skilled service. However, the attitudes of GPs towards drug users, and their level of knowledge concerning problems relating to drug use, are very variable. An important action that a helper may sometimes need to perform for a drug user is to direct him or her to a practice where their needs will be responded to appropriately.

Voluntary drug agencies

Many of the agencies that exist to help drug users are run by voluntary groups. These voluntary groups customarily take the form of community-based 'street agencies', which aim to provide specialist advice, assistance with legal, finan-cial and housing problems, counselling, and support to drug users and their families (Ettore, 1988). Most of the projects which offer residential rehabilita-tion in a drug-free environment are also run by the voluntary sector. One important gap in the provision of services which has been identified by drug workers in various parts of the country, is the lack of accommodation for short-term care and support to drug users who are experiencing a crisis, as opposed to therapeutic communities which have the aim of achieving abstinence from drugs. Short-term 'crisis' care and housing would be a particularly valuable resource for drug users who have just received an HIV antibody positive diagnosis.

Outreach workers

Many drug users do not make contact with drug agencies, not even with a street agency based in their local community. Accordingly, drug agencies, particularly those in the voluntary sector, often employ outreach workers. These outreach workers set out to make contact with, and to provide advice and support to, drug users who have no contact with any of the helping services. Sometimes ex-drug users themselves are employed very successfully in this role. The advent of HIV has led to demands for more effort to be directed towards outreach work and to a modest expansion in the numbers of outreach workers. There is also scope for making more use of properly trained part-time volunteers within local communities in an outreach role.

Support groups and organization by drug users themselves

It has been a common assumption among drug workers in the UK that self-help groups for drug users are difficult to establish and require a considerable input from professionals to ensure their success. This assumption has been challenged in the last few years with the emergence of a number of small self-help groups for HIV antibody positive drug users throughout the UK. Some of the groups are specifically for women who are HIV antibody positive drug users. There is also a national support and advocacy organization, MAIN-LINERS, run by people who have contracted HIV infection as a result of intravenous drug use. MAINLINERS offers a variety of services to drug users who are HIV positive. A contact address and number for MAINLINERS is provided in Chapter 16. Drug workers can play an important role in encouraging HIV antibody positive users to set up such groups, in providing them with guidelines on how to run successful groups, and on occasion acting initially as facilitators of such groups. Acting as a facilitator to such a group is a very difficult balancing act – providing enough support and direction to get the group flowing well, but avoiding being too directive and intrusive and thereby defeating the purpose of the group.

Self-help groups require to be sensitive to the somewhat different sets of needs of people who have recently been diagnosed as HIV antibody positive, those who have known of their antibody status for a longer period of time, those who are beginning to become quite unwell, and those who have serious HIV-related illnesses. A group will be likely to experience more success if the participants agree on a set of aims at the outset and try to stay focused on these positive aims. It is also useful if a group has some definite structure. This will help the group to weather crises and difficult periods. At the same time, it is important that this structure is sufficiently flexible. Group members need to be able to reconsider objectives and to accommodate new members.

As an example of a successful support group, Greif and Price (1988) describe the HERO Program, a community-based support group for HIV antibody positive intravenous drug users in Baltimore, Maryland. This group has the aims of providing support, education and outreach to others.

Two points that emerge from the account given of the HERO Program are worth emphasizing. First, the group doesn't confine itself narrowly to allowing the sharing of information and the expression of anxieties and problems. It is also very much centred on action. Greif and Price describe how 'Throughout the group, the emphasis is on action, that is, what is the member going to do about his or her situation and how will he or she help others.' The second point is that although the group as a whole has positive goals for changing behaviour, the members do not behave in a judgemental fashion towards those individuals who find it very difficult to meet these goals. 'Even though there is a clear message to change drug-abusing and HIV-spreading behaviour, members are supported by the others regardless of their behaviour.'

Responding to the presence of HIV among intravenous drug users

Harm-reduction aims and strategies

There has been a longstanding, vigorous debate among professionals and policy makers in the area of drug abuse over what are the most appropriate goals for working with drug users. Some workers have set themselves the aim of getting drug users completely off drugs and helping them to remain abstinent. Others have set themselves the more limited, and they would argue also more realistic, aims of helping drug users to gain greater control over their use of drugs and to use drugs in ways which are less likely to cause them physical harm. This second set of aims for drugs work which centres around harm and risk reduction has gained wider acceptance since the arrival of HIV, with risk reduction being defined largely in terms of discouraging the sharing of needles.

Changes in needle sharing

A number of recent studies conducted both in the UK and the USA (Des Jarlais and Friedman, 1988; Power et al., 1988; Robertson et al., 1988; Stimson et al., 1988) provide evidence that there has already been a substantial change away from the sharing of needles, the principal means by which HIV has been transmitted among intravenous drug users. This does not mean, however, that efforts to change behaviours that may transmit HIV can be relaxed. Although many current intravenous drug users may have moved away from sharing needles, the sharing of needles does still occur.

Newcomers to IV drug use also need to be alerted to the danger of sharing needles. Given that the introduction to the IV use of drugs is likely to take place within a group, young people starting off using drugs intravenously may be at particular risk of HIV transmitted by the sharing of needles. Many young people use drugs, and needles, on a very experimental basis and do not go on to a more sustained use of drugs. Young people in this category are not likely to see themselves as drug users and may avoid recognizing the risks involved in injecting drugs.

A group who are at particularly high risk are IV drug users who are in prison. IV drug use within prisons is relatively common and the sharing of a very few sets of injecting equipment among a large number of prisoners means that the risk of transmission of HIV is very high. It can be very distressing for drug workers to see their clients who had moved to safe injecting practice, revert to sharing equipment when they go to prison.

Assisting change towards safer injecting practices

It was stated earlier in the chapter that different areas will have different priorities in the education and care of drug users. In areas where the IV use of drugs is an established practice, the emphasis needs to be on encouraging the safer injecting of drugs. Although needle sharing may be a well-established social practice among some populations of drug users, the reason for sharing needles is usually the pragmatic one of needing to inject drugs and a lack of availability of clean needles. Reporting the work of their own and other studies, Selwyn *et al.* (1987) conclude that: 'our finding that a substantial percentage of needle-sharers report doing so more out of expediency and the need to inject than out of ignorance or social enjoyment is perhaps relevant to the current debate on the merits of increasing the availability of sterile needles to IV drug users as a means of reducing the transmission of HIV infection'.

The useful role that needle-exchange schemes have played in providing sterile injecting equipment and more general help has already been mentioned. However, they do not exist in all areas, and it may be necessary in some areas for drug workers to assist drug users to make contact with sympathetic GPs or pharmacists who are willing to supply sterile drug-using equipment in exchange for used syringes and needles.

Cleaning injecting equipment

The urgent message to IV drug users is not to share syringes and needles. However, it is important that drug users who may find themselves sharing needles as a result of a lack of a personal supply of sterile equipment know how to clean the equipment that they are using. There was controversy for a time over the most appropriate method of sterilizing injecting equipment. The method that was once recommended, of washing out and then taking the syringe apart and leaving it in boiling water for 5 minutes, is no longer given prominence in current government guidelines. Although this was an ideal method of sterilization, it has proved impractical as it damages many syringes, and is also a somewhat complicated procedure to put into practice.

Current advice suggests methods that may be less foolproof in terms of sterilization, but are simpler and more practicable. First, users are advised to clean injecting equipment as soon as possible after it has been used, as this makes it much easier to remove the blood. Two methods of cleaning are now suggested:

1. Put a generous squirt of washing-up liquid into a cup and add cold water. Draw the liquid right up the needle and into the syringe. Flush it all away (not back into the cup) then draw some more liquid in and flush that away. Then flush the works through with cold water two or three times (Department of Health, 1989).
2. Draw concentrated bleach (like Domestos) from a cup or other container up the needle and into the syringe, and then flush it away (not back into the bleach container). Do this again, and then flush the works through with cold water two or three times (ibid.).

Assisting users to say no to the sharing of needles

Aside from the practical advice detailed above that drug workers can give to help drug users to avoid the risk of becoming HIV infected, they can also provide counselling which assists a move towards safer drug use. Some drug users who are well aware of the dangers of sharing needles may still find it difficult to say no to peers who pressure them to share equipment with them or to borrow their personal 'set of works'. It can be difficult to say no to a friend, a relation, and in particular to a partner in a sexual relationship. Drug workers can work with a client to help him or her to acquire the necessary skills and responses to be assertive about safer drug use and to be able to negotiate successfully on the subject with peers. This process of helping someone be more assertive about not sharing equipment might take the form of previewing social situations where it would be difficult to say no, and acting these situations out to a successful conclusion.

It is important, however, that drug workers do not see the process of helping someone to change their risky drug-taking behaviours simply in terms of acquiring a new, more competent set of social skills. They also may need to work with the client to explore the everyday beliefs that they have about the risk of becoming infected with HIV which may be acting as powerful barriers against change (Aggleton *et al.*, 1989). The challenge posed to health education by general 'lay beliefs' about disease and particular lay beliefs about HIV and AIDS is examined in more detail in Chapter 6. As an example here, some drug users may see infection as a matter of luck or chance: 'If it's going to happen to you, it'll just happen.' It may require very careful work to challenge and to attempt to change such fatalistic beliefs.

Difficulties in changing behaviour towards safer drug use may also be associated in some people with a very low sense of self-efficacy, with a lack of belief in their own ability to influence events. Self-initiated change may be regarded by such people as a very difficult business and its success only a remote possibility. Clients who belong to this category of people will require to have reflected back to them strongly a genuine interest in them as individuals and a belief in their capacity to change and to influence events. In addition to emotional support, help with practical matters such as housing which may give them some real control over their environment, and assistance with problem solving, may lead some clients with low self-efficacy to believe that they can exercise more control over the shape of their lives.

Assisting change towards safer sex

Because the sharing of needles has been the principal means of transmission of HIV among drug users, the encouragement of safer injecting practice has necessarily been the principal focus of attention of drug workers. It is important, however, that this emphasis on the need to change unsafe drug-using behaviour is matched by an equal effort to bring health education about the sexual transmission of HIV and assistance in moving towards safer sex to the drug-using community. More outreach work which concentrates on bringing education about safe sex, giving family planning advice and distributing condoms to drug users in their own community is required. As in working with other groups, it is important that safe sex is presented in attractive and erotic terms.

Drug workers also need to be very clear about their own aims in presenting information about safer sex to drug users. Some recent writing on HIV has stressed the fact that there can be a double standard in the provision of health education in this area, with the general population being encouraged to take steps to protect themselves while 'at risk' groups are seen as having a duty to change and are actively *directed* to change their behaviour (Patton, 1989; Watney, 1989). Drug users deserve to be accorded the same rights and responsibilities in the health education that they receive as other sections of the population.

Workers can explore with individual drug users their current feelings about sex, including anxieties that they may have, and sometimes may assist them to resolve any difficulties they have about practising safer sex. Well-organized self-help groups for drug users can also provide the opportunity for the discussion of sexual behaviour and a mutual sharing of problems.

It needs to be emphasized, however, that change in this area may be a difficult matter for some clients and that considerable sensitivity and skill is required on the part of the counsellor or the facilitator of a group. Many male drug users have been brought up in a 'macho' culture which inhibits the open discussion of sexual feelings and anxieties. They also may perceive any change towards safer sexual practices as an imposition on their sexual freedom. Some women drug users, or non-drug-taking partners of male users, may fear that if they insist on safer sex their relationship may end, or at least deteriorate in quality. Such fears are *not* always irrational or unjustified.

Women, drugs and HIV

The above illustration indicates just one of the painful dilemmas which the arrival of HIV has brought for women drug users. It has been estimated that about 30% of heroin users are female (Robertson, 1987). Such women have to live with a great deal of prejudice, as the stereotypes held of women who take drugs tend to be more negative than those of male users. It is worth noting that some male drug users are themselves not altogether immune to the influence of these general negative views of women who take drugs.

Drug-using women may wish to have safer sex, but those who turn to prostitution to finance their drug habit may not always have sufficient power over the running of their own lives to be able to insist that their clients use condoms. Some men offer to pay a very much higher rate for sex without a condom. Drug-using women can find it difficult to resist such financial inducements or can be forced by partners who rely on their earnings to engage in riskier sexual practices.

Women who use drugs and who have children often find themselves isolated, with few sources of social and practical support. They may on occasion be concerned about the effect that their drug use may have on their children, but also be reluctant to seek help and thereby draw attention to themselves and risk the possibility of their children being taken into care. From their perspective, it may seem like a 'Catch 22' situation. For HIV positive women, there are also all the anxieties that arise from considering what will happen to their children if they themselves become sick or die, or how they will cope if the child becomes seriously ill.

Strong emotions and a large amount of prejudice are often aroused by the subject of women who have children and who continue to use drugs. It can be difficult even for professionals not to make snap judgements based on a superficial assessment. Workers may not gather sufficient data on which to reach a well-principled decision about the future of the offspring and the mother. A calm, clear-sighted view which considers a wide range of factors, and looks at matters from the perspective of the mother as well as of that of the child, is required in any assessment of the child-rearing practices of a drug-using mother.

A very careful, yet succinct discussion of the issues involved in working with drug users who have children together with a clear set of guidelines for assessing the effects of parental drug use on child care is provided in Griffiths and Pearson (1988, ch. 10).

Turning to the matter of working with HIV positive women who become pregnant, there is a concern on the part of some drug workers that such women have on occasion been pressurized to have an abortion without being given sufficient opportunity to explore their own feelings or express their desires. HIV positive drug users deserve to be accorded the same rights and respect as other women who, for quite different sets of reasons, have to make difficult decisions which centre around the future health of their unborn child and their own safety. There is a need to apply the well-established principles of *genetic counselling* which have been developed over the years to advise women, and to enable them to explore and become clear about their own feelings and wishes, where there is a risk of a baby being born with a serious defect or disease. Counselling in this area, and in more general family planning work, requires the development of a particular set of skills and a great deal of sensitivity. Drug workers need to keep themselves informed of counsellors in their locality who possess the necessary skills and personal qualities to assist HIV positive women or drug users who are uncertain of their antibody status, to come to a decision about pregnancy which feels comfortable and is practicable for them personally.

Drug users and HIV testing

The issue of according drug users the same rights and consideration as other groups in the community, applies as much to testing for HIV antibodies as it does to providing counselling on pregnancy and termination.

Some health-care professionals have advocated the use of HIV antibody testing as a means of getting IV drug users to change their behaviour away from practices which involve a risk of transmitting HIV. Knowing that one is HIV antibody positive may lead an individual towards adopting sexual and drug-taking practices which reduce the risk of the transmission of HIV. However, this is only one of the potential outcomes of testing. The shock of receiving a positive test result, or the reassurance of 'safety' that can be gained by some individuals from a negative result, might lead to more 'risky' behaviour rather than less.

Behavioural change is also only one of the issues which is addressed in the general discussion of the benefits and disadvantages of HIV antibody testing. Other considerations predominate in this debate. It is difficult therefore to justify a narrowing of the concerns of the debate on testing to a focus on bringing about behavioural change in the case of drug users.

Aside from questions concerning the justice of having different agendas for testing for different groups, there is little evidence available at the moment to support the utility of using testing as a general policy for bringing about behavioural change. The studies which have reported a strong linkage between learning about one's antibody status and changing to safer injecting practices were conducted within treatment settings and provided considerable testing counselling (Casadonte *et al.*, 1986; Cox *et al.*, 1986). One cannot, therefore, easily separate out the effects of the specific counselling and general support provided from the knowledge of test results *per se*.

Reviewing these and other studies, Des Jarlais and Friedman (1987) conclude that:

> When HIV antibody testing is done without these extensive [counselling and treatment] supports, there appears to be no net positive effect on AIDS risk behavior, and a potential for harm to the individuals participating. Even with the intensive supports, antibody test feedback is likely to produce increases in anxiety and depression. In terms of reducing AIDS risk behavior, it is probably a mistake to think of antibody testing as a prevention technique.

It is important that the pre-test counselling which drug users receive takes into account the considerations which are discussed in Chapter 7, and that it is carefully tailored to the individual needs and situation of the client.

Working with drug users who are HIV positive or who have AIDS

Drug users who do receive an HIV antibody positive test result very often require a great deal of support to enable them to cope. In common with all other individuals who receive an HIV antibody positive result, they are likely to require solid emotional support and someone who will listen and respond sensitively to their feelings of shock, grief, anger, isolation and uncertainty. It will also be useful for them to learn techniques which will assist them in coping with episodes of panic and feelings of anxiety. A considerable amount of time may need to be spent by drug workers helping in a more structured way by focusing on *problem solving* with the drug user. This will involve encouraging clear thinking and moving towards possible solutions of some of the practical and emotional difficulties which HIV has brought into the drug user's life (see pp. 15–16). For drug users who develop serious HIV-related illnesses, the types of support and the counselling actions which are described in Chapter 9 will be required.

Counselling work with a drug user who is HIV antibody positive or who has an HIV-related illness is likely to be more successful if it takes a broad focus, and considers how the user's own responses are determined in part by the reactions of family and friends. It may also be necessary to help an individual drug user to harness informal sources of support more effectively, and to work towards repairing family relationships which are the source of considerable tension or grief.

Help with housing and other pressing practical problems

For many drug users, the uncertainty and emotional turmoil which commonly follow an HIV antibody positive test result or the diagnosis of AIDS, are exacerbated by the fact that there is a lack of stability in the external circumstances of their lives and many pressing practical problems. Counselling and emotional support are likely to have a very limited impact, if practical problems are not addressed at the same time.

As a consequence of the illegal nature of drug-taking, it is common for drug users to have often quite severe *legal* problems. Drug workers need to maintain good contacts with community law centres, or sympathetic, effective individual solicitors, to assist their clients to deal with this particular set of problems.

Dealing with *financial* problems and with difficulties concerning *welfare rights* is an area where drug workers need to have considerable competence. The regulations governing welfare provision, and the interpretation of these regulations, are quite complex, so it is useful if one member of a drugs agency can specialize in this type of work.

One of the most urgent problems that is quite commonly faced by drug users, is that of *homelessness*. Given the reluctance of private landlords and of some housing bodies to rent accommodation to drug users, it can also be a very difficult problem to solve. Some local authorities in areas where there is a high incidence of HIV infection among drug users have taken steps in the past few years to ensure that there is a stock of housing reserved for HIV antibody positive drug users and that users are well supported within this accommodation. However, such provision of public housing does not exist in many areas, and drug agencies frequently face the tasks both of maintaining good relations with local housing departments and of acting as advocates for the housing needs of drug users.

Drug users can be somewhat neglectful of matters such as obtaining an adequate diet, and do not always place a high priority on looking after their health. This lack of attention to *health care* is of particular concern in the case of individuals who are infected with HIV, given that it is generally accepted that it is desirable to follow sensible guidelines to maximize the body's immunity.

Change towards a healther lifestyle can be very difficult for some drug users. Drug workers, however, can do much useful, patient work in this area. They can help individual HIV antibody positive drug users to build up the motivation to make some changes in their lifestyle. Those individuals who have the motivation to change can be given advice about healthier living and assisted with problem solving about how to put this advice into practice.

Drug users also may need to be encouraged to seek *medical care* promptly when a problem develops, rather than waiting until it becomes acute. Some drug users find it difficult to maintain a consistent pattern of contact with a GP or hospital; and, as a result of mutual mistrust, difficulties in communication and relationships between drug users and medical staff can arise. Professional and voluntary drug workers can help here by accompanying a drug user on a clinic visit which he or she finds stressful. On occasion a drugs worker may need to act as an intermediary between the drug-using patient and a doctor, to help communication to flow well and to ensure that no misunderstandings develop. There also may be times when a drugs worker may have to act as an advocate for drug users to ensure that they receive appropriate medical care and that tey are kept well informed about their treatment and health status.

Issues concerning drug treatment programmes and HIV positive drug users

The preceding sections of this chapter have emphasized that drug workers need to be able to provide a wide range of practical help and of types of counselling if they are to respond appropriately to HIV antibody positive drug users. However, a considerable amount of a drug worker's efforts will need to remain focused on helping the drug user to manage his or her drug use.

The topic of helping drug users to move towards safer injecting practice has already been discussed. At the moment, we want to look at harm reduction not in the sense of reducing the transmission of HIV infection, but of helping HIV antibody positive drug users to use drugs in a way which will be less injurious to their physical health and will allow them to cope more successfully with the stresses of living with HIV infection.

It seems reasonable to suggest that a move away from the intravenous use of drugs is likely to be of some benefit to the health of an IV drug user. However, there is not yet clear evidence to suggest that the continued injection of drugs has a particularly strong damaging effect on the immune system of HIV-infected individuals. Some studies, such as that by Des Jarlais *et al.* (1987), have suggested that continuing to inject drugs after HIV infection could be a co-factor in leading to a faster decline in the efficiency of the immune system. However, in their review of studies in this area, Des Jarlais and Friedman (1988) conclude that: 'current epidemiologic data . . . indicate that continued injection at most operates as a modest co-factor for HIV immunosuppression, and perhaps only at high frequencies of injection'.

The extent to which work with an HIV antibody positive drug user needs to centre on the matter of drug use itself requires careful assessment. In cases where someone has reacted to the news of an HIV antibody positive test result by using drugs very heavily and in an uncontrolled manner, it may be a priority to bring about some changes in drug use. More effective coping will only be possible when drug use becomes less chaotic. On the other hand, some HIV antibody positive individuals who are managing to use drugs in a way which is fairly controlled, may find attempts to reduce or eliminate their drug use extremely stressful. The stress of changing their pattern of drug use might hinder their attempts to cope with being HIV positive.

Drug treatment plans will also be affected by constraints such as prescribing practices in the locality and the availability of places in rehabilitation centres which offer an appropriate treatment regime. Any assessment which aims to identify the most suitable response to the drug use of an HIV antibody positive user, needs to look carefully not just at the individual's own resources and motivation, but also at possible sources of social support and of practical help.

The type of counselling offered to those HIV positive drug users who do wish to reduce or even eliminate their use of drugs, needs to be carefully tailored to the particular stage of change in drug use that has been achieved. There is fairly general agreement among researchers that changes in addictive behaviour are best thought of as occurring in distinct stages. A particularly influential model of the sequence of changes which may be observed in addictive behaviour is that produced by Prochaska and DiClemente (1986). They identify four stages of change:

precontemplation → contemplation → action → maintenance

Individuals may proceed through these stages in a linear sequence, or more likely revolve through them several times before they achieve relative freedom from a particular addiction. In the *precontemplation* stage, an individual is involved in drug use and is not actively considering any form of change. In *contemplation*, the individual is actively considering change and acquiring motivation. This stage forms a preliminary to that of *action*, where change in drug-taking is initiated. *Maintenance* is concerned with sustaining successful change and with avoiding relapse.

For clients who are at the *precontemplation* stage identified by Prochaska and DiClemente, the most helpful action is likely to be concentrating on establishing a warm, caring therapeutic relationship. Such a relationship can be used to communicate respect for and some identification with aspects of the client's life. It can also provide a secure environment in which feelings, including those which are acting as barriers to change, can be explored; and in which change can begin to seem less threatening.

For clients who have reached the stage of *contemplation*, the addition of a more structured and active intervention may be required, to assist with the process of re-evaluating their lifestyle, their aims and their sense of self. As well as assisting in this process of re-evaluation of goals and gaining motivation for change, it may be important to work to encourage clients to develop a better sense of self-efficacy, a belief in their ability to act successfully and to influence events.

Encouraging the development of a greater sense of self-efficacy remains crucial at the *action* stage, as does strong emotional support to enable the person to feel secure enough to risk putting major changes into practice. Much help is needed also in solving how best to tackle situations which will bring temptation, how to reward and reinforce successes, and how to evaluate progress and stay on course. In the *maintenance* stage, clients can be helped to preview situations which might lead them to relapse and to develop responses to cope with these situations. The knowledge that someone will be around to give solid support at times of temptation or crisis is also valuable.

Working together to help drug users with HIV-related illnesses

A considerable number of different professional, and possibly also voluntary, workers may be involved in the care of drug users who have HIV-related illnesses: infectious diseases consultants and other hospital staff, GPs, home helps, district nurses, social workers and workers from drugs agencies. Problems can arise if there are inconsistencies in treatment among these different groups of workers, or a lack of clear communication.

It can be difficult to set up interdisciplinary teams, and general liaison work and case conferences can take up quite a lot of time. However, in terms of improving the efficiency of the services and the quality of care, the investment of effort and time is well worthwhile. The manner and the spirit in which such interdisciplinary teams are organized does require careful thought. Even when a team has the very explicit aim of responding sensitively to the expressed needs of drug users with HIV-related illness, there can be a tendency to discuss the patient in terms of a problem to be successfully 'managed'. It is important that interdisciplinary teams are structured in a way which allows the ill drug user to voice his or her feelings and wishes and to take part in the formulation of a plan for treatment and the provision of services.

Training and support needs of drugs workers

The existence of a multidisciplinary team and an established network of people who can contribute their own particular set of skills to the care and assistance of drug users, can provide much needed resources and support to individual drugs workers. However, with the advent of HIV, drugs workers themselves need to develop new skills, to have the opportunity to reassess their priorities, and to plan carefully to meet anticipated needs within their local community. Workers, who commonly have a heavy workload, will not be able to meet these new demands if training, together with support and counselling for their own emotional needs, is squeezed into marginal time. Adequate time for staff development and an effective support scheme for staff need to be provided by agencies, if workers are to cope with the challenges posed by the presence of HIV infection among drug users.

References

Aggelton, P. *et al.* (1989). *AIDS: Scientific and Social Issues. A Resource for Health Educators*. Edinburgh, Churchill Livingstone.

Ball, J.C. *et al.* (1988). 'Reducing the risk of AIDS through methadone maintenance treatment'. *Journal of Health and Social Behavior,* **29**, 214–26.

Casadonte, P. *et al.* (1986). Psychological and behavioral impact of learning HTLV-III/LAV antibody test results'. Paper presented to the *International Conference on AIDS,* Paris, June.

Coleman, R.M. and Curtis, D. (1988). 'Distribution of risk behaviour for HIV infection amongst injecting drug users'. *British Journal of Addiction,* **83**, 1331–4.

Cox, C.P. *et al.* (1986). 'Psychological and behavioral consequences of HTLV-III/LAV antibody testing and notification among intravenous drug abusers in a methadone program in New York City'. Paper presented to the *International Conference on AIDS,* Paris, June.

Department of Health (1989). *Cleaning Injecting Equipment.* Internal Report.

Des Jarlais, D.C. and Friedman, S.R. (1987). 'HIV infection among intravenous drug users: Epidemiology and risk reduction'. *AIDS,* **1**, 67–76.

Des Jarlais, D.C. and Friedman, S.R. (1988). 'HIV and intravenous drug use'. *AIDS,* **2**, S65–S69.

Des Jarlais, D.C. *et al.* (1987). 'Development of AIDS, HIV seroconversion, and potential factors for T4 cell loss in a cohort of intravenous drug users'. *AIDS,* **1**, 105–11.

Ettore, B. (1988). 'London's voluntary drug agencies. 1. Funding and organizational management'. *The International Journal of the Addictions,* **23**, 1041–56.

Gossop, M. (1982). *Living with Drugs.* London, Temple Smith.

Greif, G.L. and Price, C. (1988). 'A community-based support group for HIV positive I.V. drug abusers: The HERO Program'. *Journal of Substance Abuse Treatment,* **5**, 263–6.

Griffiths, R. and Pearson, B. (1988). *Working with Drug Users.* Aldershot, Wildwood House.

Haw, S. (1985). *Drug Problems in Greater Glasgow.* Report of the SCODA Fieldwork Survey in Greater Glasgow Health Board. Glasgow, SCODA.

Patton, C. (1989). Keynote address presented to the *Third Conference on the Social Aspects of AIDS,* London, February.

Power, R. *et al.* (1988). 'Drug injecting, AIDS, and risk behaviour: Potential for change and intervention strategies'. *British Journal of Addiction,* **83**, 649–54.

Prochaska, J.O. and DiClemente, C.C. (1986). 'Towards a comprehensive model of change'. In W.R. Miller and N. Heather (eds), *Treating Addictive Behaviors: Processes of Change,* pp. 3–27. New York, Plenum Press.

Robertson, J.R. *et al.* (1986). 'Epidemic of AIDS related viruses (HTLV III/LAV) infection among intravenous drug users'. *British Medical Journal,* **292**, 527–9.

Robertson, J.R. *et al.* (1988). 'HIV infection in intravenous drug users: A follow-up study indicating changes in risk-taking behaviour'. *British Journal of Addiction,* **83**, 387–91.

Robertson, R. (1987). *Heroin, AIDS and Society.* London, Hodder and Stoughton.

Selwyn, P.A. *et al.* (1987). 'Knowledge about AIDS and high-risk behavior among intravenous drug users in New York City'. *AIDS,* **1**, 247–54.

Stimson, G.V. *et al.* (1988). 'HIV transmission risk behaviour of clients attending syringe-exchange schemes in England and Scotland'. *British Journal of Addiction,* **83**, 1449–55.

Stimson, G.V. *et al.* (1989). 'Syringe-exchange schemes in England and Scotland: Evaluating a new service for drug users'. In P. Aggleton *et al.* (eds), *AIDS: Social Representations, Social Practices*. London, Falmer Press, pp. 186–98.

Watney, S. (1989). 'Mosquitoes, door-knobs, oral sex and polls: Theorising rumor in relation to perceptions of risk concerning HIV transmission'. Paper presented to the *Third Conference on the Social Aspects of AIDS*, London, February.

THIRTEEN

People with haemophilia and HIV

PATRICIA WILKIE

Introduction

Haemophilia is a life-long inherited or genetic disorder affecting males from birth and transmitted to them by their mothers. People with haemophilia have a partial or complete lack of one of the clotting factors normally present in the blood (Factor VIII or Factor IX). The result of this deficit is that the blood clotting time is delayed. Haemophilia is often classified as *severe, moderate* or *mild* according to the amount of clotting factor present in the blood. The proportion of haemophiliacs in these groups is: severe and moderate both 40% and mild 20%. Those with severe haemophilia, which usually manifests itself in early childhood, suffer from internal haemorrhages into the muscles and the joints, in particular the elbows, knees and ankles. These bleeds frequently occur spontaneously without the person having been injured, are very painful and, if left untreated, can lead to the development of a painful and crippling arthritis. More mildly affected people need special care only for major operations or after a serious accident. Those moderately affected may bleed excessively after dental extraction or accident.

Treatment of haemophilia

The key to modern treatment in haemophilia is the use of blood transfusion and blood products. Prior to this treatment, the choices of treatment were immobilization of the affected limb or injured part of the body, bed rest and possibly the local application of snake venom. The current treatment is the replacement of the missing clotting factor by intravenous injection. Since 1973, it has become possible for people with haemophilia to treat themselves promptly at home with an intravenous injection of Factor VIII or Factor IX.

Consequently, less time is spent travelling to hospital for out-patient treatment as well as time spent as an in-patient, thus reducing long absences from school and work that had been such a problem for those with haemophilia. Furthermore, prompt treatment reduces pain caused by a bleed into a joint and helps prevent the development of arthritis.

Blood products

The clotting factor used in the treatment of haemophilia bleeds is taken from the blood donated to the Blood Transfusion Service. Hundreds of donations are pooled for each batch of Factor VIII, and therefore any infective agent which is present in a single donation, e.g. hepatitis or HIV, will contaminate the whole batch. The number of donations required to produce an infusion of Factor IX is less than that required for Factor VIII.

In the UK, the Blood Transfusion Service has been unable to supply sufficient blood products for the treatment of the UK haemophiliac population despite the promises of successive governments and pressure for self-sufficiency in volunteer donor blood products. In May 1987, only 20% of the existing need for Factor VIII and Factor IX was supplied by the UK Blood Transfusion Service. Although Scotland was in a better situation, the net result was the extensive importation of blood products from abroad, in particular the USA, where blood donors are paid for their donations. In these circumstances, it is believed that donors are more likely to carry infections than donors from the voluntary donor system. It is hoped that the introduction in 1985 both of the system of screening blood donors for HIV and the heat-treatment of blood products to destroy HIV will ensure the future safety of the treatment of haemophilia with blood products. In a process not dissimilar to the pasteurization of milk, blood products are heat-treated at 60°C for 10 hours in an aqueous solution.

In the UK, there are approximately 5000 people with haemophilia. Up to January 1991, there have been official reports of 228 people with haemophilia who have AIDS, of whom 156 have died of AIDS. There are 1253 people with haemophilia who are HIV antibody positive.[1] However, it is estimated that the actual number of known HIV-infected haemophiliacs is greater as a number of persons known to be HIV antibody positive but for whom the exposure category is unknown are thought to have haemophilia.

The majority of haemophiliacs infected with HIV are the more severely affected who have received greater amounts of blood products. Since the introduction of HIV antibody testing of blood donors and the heat-treatment of blood products, the risk of transmission of HIV by blood products used in the treatment of haemophilia or by blood transfusion has been virtually eliminated.

Living with haemophilia

Living with haemophilia can be very frustrating for the affected person and his family. Bleeds are invariably unpredictable and this means that there is often uncertainty about making and keeping plans. Until recently, people with haemophilia had difficulty in attending school regularly and this in turn led to problems in finding suitable employment (Markova and Forbes, 1984). As a result, people with haemophilia have been concerned about whether or not to inform employers or future employers about haemophilia. They fear discrimination. Some haemophiliacs have lost their jobs after having told their employer that they had haemophilia. On the other hand, lack of disclosure about their condition can lead to inappropriate work and working conditions, e.g. heavy lifting, which contributes to more bleeds and further absences from work. Many people with haemophilia have been unemployed at some stage in their lives. The Haemophilia Society has recently estimated that 30% of HIV positive haemophiliacs are unemployed. Also, few of the more severely affected people with haemophilia have been able to continue working to the normal retirement age with the resulting full pension. Thus many people with haemophilia have faced shortages of money at some stage in their life.

People with haemophilia and their partners have had to consider whether or not to have children. While the sons of a man with haemophilia will not have haemophilia themselves, all his daughters will be carriers of the gene causing haemophilia and can therefore pass on the gene to their sons. Whether or not to take the risk of having a carrier daughter is a difficult decision for these families, and there is no easy solution. For those who decide to have a family, there is often anxiety about the health of the father with haemophilia. There is also the possibility of guilt regarding passing on the disorder to the next generation should this couple have an affected son.

Many of the more severely affected people with haemophilia have experienced life-threatening situations. Some have suffered from and survived major bleeds, such as cerebral haemorrhage, which remains one of the major causes of death for those with haemophilia. Some have had hepatitis contracted from infected blood products. Others have developed inhibitors to the blood products with the result that the treatment becomes ineffective. Thus many of those with severe haemophilia have faced their own mortality and have also known of the premature death of a contemporary.

Haemophilia and HIV

In recent years, the improvements in the treatment for haemophilia have resulted in considerable optimism in the haemophilia world. The expectation of life has been approaching that of normal. Many of those with haemophilia have found it possible to obtain life assurance and a new generation of haemophiliacs have been able to anticipate living a 'normal life', attending school on a regular basis and obtaining employment appropriate to their ability. Then, in 1982 in the USA, when Acquired Immune Deficiency Syndrome was being recognized as a major clinical problem, a person with haemophilia was first diagnosed with a similar immune deficiency syndrome. It took some time before the hypothesized viral transmission of this new disease was accepted by the scientific and medical communities and transfusion-related AIDS was recognized. The very therapy that had so dramatically affected the medical management of haemophilia had become an instrument for a potentially fatal disease. And so, from the outset of the AIDS epidemic, people with haemophilia were recognized as forming one of the major risk groups, along with members of the gay and intravenous drug-using communities.

Haemophilia by itself has implications not only for the affected person but also his family. HIV and HIV-related illnesses are likely to have a profound effect on all members of the family of a person with haemophilia who is HIV antibody positive. In the next section, particular problems facing different members of the family of a person with haemophilia and HIV-related illnesses are addressed.

For the person with haemophilia who has become HIV antibody positive, the infection was iatrogenically acquired, i.e. the infection would not have been transmitted to the patient had he not been receiving sound and professionally recommended treatment (Moser, 1969). It is therefore not surprising that haemophiliacs should feel extremely angry and disillusioned because the main cause of the problem has been attributed to imported blood products. Furthermore, for many years successive governments have failed to fulfil their promise that the UK should be self-sufficient in blood products. The reaction of those with haemophilia to the diagnosis of HIV includes the emotions and feelings expressed by others in the same situation and is described in Chapter 8. In addition, because of the way in which the infection was contracted, the following reactions are also common.

Anger, disillusionment and fear

These emotions are frequently expressed and may partially be explained because the source of the problem has been imported blood products. When the link between these blood products and HIV was first made public, some patients with haemophilia cut back on their treatment. Some also refused to take imported blood products.

Disbelief at the seriousness, or potential seriousness, of HIV

This reaction is possibly different from the denial frequently expressed by other HIV positive people on learning of the diagnosis. Many people with haemophilia have survived serious bleeds and other life-threatening illnesses.

Initially, HIV was perceived by many as being no different from these bleeds and other serious haemophilia-related illnesses from which they had survived.

Reappearance of stigma

Recent improvements in treatment and in the expectation of what someone with haemophilia could hope to be able to do has resulted in less stigma being associated with haemophilia. The association of HIV, AIDS and haemophilia has quickly reversed this trend. In recent years, people with haemophilia and their families have been more willing to explain what it means to have haemophilia. It has been observed that since the appearance of HIV, there is a tendency to deny or to hide the existence of haemophilia. Common explanations for joint pain are 'arthritis', an 'old football injury' or 'got it in the army', rather than haemophilia.

Feeling powerless

Many people with haemophilia feel that they cannot complain about what they see as the injustice of having acquired HIV through blood products. They say that medical and nursing staff do not always seem to understand. In some cases hospital staff appear to think that the person with haemophilia is blaming them personally. This is not usually the case. The person with haemophilia just wishes some explanation for what has happened to him. In addition, people with haemophilia also fear that their situation is not generally understood and that if they complain or criticize staff for having acquired HIV, they may be accused of being ungrateful for the care and resources that they have already had. Furthermore, it is well known that patients do not wish to criticize staff who look after them and those with haemophilia are no exception.

Intolerance of gay people and intravenous drug users

This sentiment has been expressed by some patients who do not like the association between those with haemophilia, members of the gay community and intravenous drug users. Often this intolerance is expressed even more strongly by supporting family members and partners of those with haemophilia. Sometimes there is a reference to the HIV positive haemophiliac as the 'innocent', a phrase that has been much used in the media. The presence of these often strongly expressed anti-gay sentiments can make life difficult for those who have haemophilia and are gay.

Desire for compensation

The Haemophilia Society lobbied very hard on behalf of HIV positive haemophiliacs for 'recompense' and in 1987 £10 million was awarded by the government. A new organization, the Macfarlane Trust, was established to distribute this sum of money to HIV positive haemophiliacs. In 1989, the government paid a further £24 million to the Macfarlane Trust. Many haemophiliacs or parents on behalf of younger HIV positive haemophiliacs had filed writs seeking compensation for having acquired HIV iatrogenically. The writs were taken out against the health authorities, the Blood Transfusion Service and in some cases individual doctors. The mere taking of such action, although usually not directed against individual doctors, caused tension and at times upset the relationship between the patient and the medical staff caring for him. The government has always insisted that compensation was a matter for the courts.

In 1989, the Haemophilia Society launched a campaign to persuade the government to settle out of court the many claims for compensation which had already been started. The government believed its case, based on the level of medical knowledge at the time the contaminated blood products were supplied, was strong. Furthermore, there was concern about the precedent in other medical negligence cases if they conceded to the haemophilia case. This stance came under very considerable political and public pressure, and in December 1990 a £42 million settlement was awarded to the HIV positive haemophiliacs.

Blood products

All people with haemophilia should be given an opportunity to discuss their views about the safety of blood products. A 'one off' discussion is often inadequate as anxieties may arise when new AIDS figures appear in the national press. While some patients need to be able to cut down on their treatment, it is essential that bleeds are treated. It has been emphasized that to the best of our knowledge, the combination of the heat-treatment of blood products and the screening for HIV in blood donors appears to have been successful in ensuring the safety of blood products.

The young HIV positive haemophiliac

Young HIV positive haemophiliacs will be known to the unit or department where they have been receiving their treatment before they contracted HIV. This is helpful, as in most units the same staff will continue to be involved in their care should they develop HIV-related illnesses. It is, however, extremely important that parents are given sufficient information about their child's health and illness and whatever support they may need, so that they as parents can help their child live as normal a life as possible.

Informing children that they have HIV

There has been considerable discussion about the most appropriate way in which to tell children that they are HIV positive. While it is hoped that there will be no more HIV positive haemophiliac children, the experience of the haemophilia population may have relevance for those involved in the care of non-haemophiliac HIV positive children. Most parents wish to tell the child themselves. The difficulty is to know when to tell the child. It is also necessary to consider what the child might already know. Young children do understand the implications of serious illness (Burton, 1975) and children with haemophilia are usually well informed about the condition and its medical management. However, it is quite common for information about the child's progress and his illness not to be given directly to the child. When there is information that has not yet been discussed with the child, conversations may stop when the child is within earshot. Furthermore, the routine when they attend the clinic may have changed. For example, the nature of the examination may be slightly different or the clinic visits may be more frequent. Children do pick up odd pieces of information in hospital. They hear discussions between other parents in the waiting room and some of this may not be accurate nor relevant to that particular child. Furthermore, some children may think that they are not making progress.

The great majority of HIV positive children will have been exposed, to a greater or lesser extent, to media coverage of HIV and AIDS linking haemophilia and AIDS. Primary school haemophiliac children report that they have been subjected to jokes about AIDS. Some children have complained that they have missed out on certain activities at school because the other children say that they have AIDS whether they are HIV antibody positive or not. Furthermore, discussions about HIV and AIDS have been introduced into the syllabus of many schools. It is necessary to consider the effect of such information being discussed in class on an affected child. If parents are informed about this discussion in advance, they can work out what is the best course of action for their child. For some children, it may be better that they do not attend that class, although by not attending they can be seen to be different, while others can join their classmates.

It is also not known what sort of information about HIV the child has picked up at home from parents and from sibs. Children glean information not only from what has been said explicitly but also from making inferences. Children will make deductions from the behaviour of family members in certain circumstances. For example, how does the family deal with programmes about HIV on television or the radio in the presence of the affected child? Is the family able to continue to watch or listen 'normally' or do they in some way give a clue to the child that something is amiss?

While there is no published evidence, it is very likely that the majority of school age haemophiliac children do know of their HIV positive status even if they have not been told 'formally'. The evidence for this is based on information from parents who have not said anything to the child but suspect that the child does know. What is known is that it can be detrimental to the child for the parents not to inform him about a serious problem concerning his health when he suspects that there may be something wrong (Burton, 1975).

It is understandable that parents may be reluctant to tell their child about HIV. Some parents have said that they see little point in giving this potentially distressing information and in discussing complex issues with a child who may not live long enough for the issues to become relevant. In her study of the inherited disorder cystic fibrosis, Burton (1975) suggests that not telling the child tends to isolate him depriving him of knowledge and making the whole subject of his illness taboo. Children mature at different rates, but it may be kinder for children to know of their HIV status before they leave primary school. After primary school, it is more difficult to influence the child's environment. When children go to secondary school they are exposed to a wider social environment. They will have more teachers and will meet more children. It will therefore be more difficult to know what information about HIV they are acquiring.

Confidentiality and the young HIV positive haemophiliac

Some parents feel that it is better for the maintenance of confidentiality if education authorities are not told about their child's antibody status. Other parents believe that a well-informed teaching staff can be extremely supportive. It is hoped that teachers and other school staff are now able to deal with cuts involving blood calmly and sensibly without singling out the HIV positive child for special treatment.

Parents need also to decide which members of their family to tell of their child's HIV status, which friends and which neighbours. While the child remains asymptomatic for HIV, it may be easier not to disclose the information. However, because the child has haemophilia and this is likely to be generally known and because of the publicity that has been given to the association between HIV and haemophilia, many people may suspect and parents have been put under considerable pressure to tell. Some families who have been open about the situation have met with very considerable consideration and support. Others have been stigmatized. HIV positive children need to be able to play with other children and parents may be anxious to know what to say. It is important that those working with the family can help parents decide what is the best strategy for them.

Parents of an HIV positive haemophiliac child

It is known that bringing up a child with a chronic illness can put a considerable strain on family life and on marital relationships (Hewitt and Newson, 1970), and bringing up a child with haemophilia is no exception. Parents have had to adjust to the problems that haemophilia may cause their child and to the expectations of what 'might have been' if their son had not had haemophilia. Some fathers find it very difficult to accept that they have a son with haemophilia whom they believe may not be able to participate in traditional male activities. HIV can cause these feelings to resurface. Fathers also say that they are left out, or not sufficiently involved, in the care of their son. The mother takes the child to the hospital and it is invariably the mother who is trained to give the child his treatment until he is able to do it himself.

Mothers of a son with haemophilia often feel guilty and responsible for their son's condition because the gene carrying haemophilia is transmitted through the female. In many instances, HIV in their son has reawakened this feeling of guilt. It is not uncommon in families where there is a child or children with an inherited disease for the parents to blame each other or each other's family as being the cause of the problem. The appearance of HIV can rekindle these feelings and be the cause of dissension between the parents. Mothers of young sons with haemophilia on home treatment are taught to give the treatment to their son until he is able to inject himself. Many of these mothers have expressed the fear that they may have been the person 'responsible' for giving the infusion of contaminated blood products and they are tormented by this thought.

Helpers need to consider these issues when working with parents of a haemophiliac son who is HIV positive as well as looking at the following points.

The parents' relationship

Are the parents able to communicate with each other? Have the parents been able to talk together about the fact that their son has contracted HIV – a stigmatizing condition for the affected person and his family. Have the parents been able to talk about how they will deal with HIV-related illnesses and the possible premature death of their son from AIDS? Have parents been able to discuss their feelings about this situation with each other? In some cases, parents will be the natural parents of the child, in other cases there may be a step-parent and in other cases a single parent will be looking after the child. These different domestic circumstances can create different problems for the parents and for the child.

Needs of the parents for information

Parents need information about their son's illness and the stage of illness. It is unlikely that parents of young children will experience difficulty in obtaining information as doctors would normally discuss the child's progress with them. Difficulties can arise with teenagers who may now be attending an adult hospital and seeing the doctor on their own. While it is important not to undermine the developing independence of the young person, it is equally important that parents receive appropriate information. It cannot be assumed that the young person will be able or wish to tell his parents about what is happening to him.

Parents need support

Parents need to be encouraged and helped to take some leisure time. The combination of haemophilia and HIV infection in one of their children can become overwhelming. The formation of a parents' group where parents of affected sons can meet each other to discuss their difficulties can be extremely supportive. The groups can take different forms and while they may initially be led by a counsellor, parents may continue to meet on their own.

Anger

Parents feel very angry about the fact that their son has contracted HIV. It has already been mentioned that some parents are taking legal action on behalf of their son(s). Some parents have also sought some media exposure. The combination of these actions can sometimes make it difficult for parents to have a dialogue with medical staff and helpers may need to assist parents to channel their anger. In situations where there are one or more HIV-infected sons, and there are no other children, it is not surprising that parents feel angry about the very real possibility of losing all of their children.

Infection control

The chances of transmission of HIV among non-sexual household contacts of an infected person are negligible. Nevertheless, some parents do express concern about the possible transmission of infection. This was particularly obvious at the beginning of the epidemic. One mother reported that when she first learned that her son was HIV positive, she spent much time wiping surfaces with disinfectant even though she understood how the infection was transmitted. Another mother who also understood the method of transmission reported that when she first learned that her teenage son was HIV positive, she poured bleach into the toilet on each occasion after her son had been to the toilet. Gradually these mothers were able to put infection control into perspective. However, in turn, these parents need to be able to explain to friends, relatives and visitors how HIV is transmitted and reassure them.

Protectiveness

Previous studies have reported the tendency for mothers of haemophiliac sons to be over-protective, discouraging their sons from being involved in activities that may be harmful to haemophilia (Markova *et al.*, 1980). It was the author's experience from working with HIV positive haemophiliacs and their families that parents, and in particular mothers, became very protective towards their HIV positive sons. One mother said that the only time that she was really happy was when she knew that her son was safely at home. She worried about what would happen if he had an accident and was concerned that other people could be put at risk. One father was similarly concerned and began to attend football matches with his son. In both these cases, the parents were aware that their behaviour could be restricting their sons. Parents may need help to work out an appropriate balance between giving freedom to their son and maintaining some peace of mind for themselves.

Informing other children in the family

Parents may need help in deciding when is the most appropriate time to inform other children in the family that their brother has HIV. Initially, parents have to come to terms with the information themselves and there is a tendency to ignore the needs of other children who may be well aware that there is something wrong. It is also important that parents continue to inform the other children about what is happening to their brother. Parents may need to be reminded to spend time with their other children who may feel 'left out', as so much attention is focused on the person with HIV. This is particularly true during acute episodes of illness. In some families, there is more than one haemophiliac son, but only one has HIV. In this situation, parents may need help in dealing with the relationship between the brothers.

Informing others

Parents often ask who outside the immediate family should know that their son is HIV positive. As most relatives, friends and neighbours will know about haemophilia, they often ask leading questions. Some parents feel that it is in the best interests of the child to maintain confidentiality. Other parents believe that it may be necessary to share the information with friends or neighbours who look after their son from time to time. Many parents have expressed relief when they have told others about the situation. These parents have found it easier when their child is ill as these friends are understanding and offer very considerable support. Parents who have lived in an area for a long time and who have decided to tell their neighbours have also found much support. Helpers may need to work with parents to assess the advantages and disadvantages of telling people and which people should or should not be informed.

HIV positive adolescents

Adolescence is a period of finding independence and becoming sexually aware. HIV can impose very great restrictions on a person's sexual activities and on their independence.

Part of HIV counselling involves giving information to the person in order to prevent the spread of HIV. It is important when working with this age group first to establish at what stage they are at in their own sexual maturity. It is unwise to assume that all 16-year-olds are sexually experienced. It is possible that in the presence of a chronic illness such as haemophilia, young children are less sexually experienced than their peers who do not have haemophilia simply because haemophilia is time-consuming. Adolescents frequently resent questions about any sexual activity they may or may not have had. This is particularly apparent when information about the sexual prevention of HIV is being given to the young person by several people – his parents, a counsellor and perhaps even other members of the clinical team. Studies prior to the advent of HIV have shown that adolescent haemophiliacs have low self-esteem and are hesitant about making relationships (Molleman and van Knippenberg, 1987).

In counselling these young people, it is important to have a very positive approach about what they can do. For example, they can have friendships with girls and they can have a sexual relationship if that is what they and their partner wish. Factual information about safer sex should also be given once a good rapport and feeling of trust has developed between the young person and the helper. It is important that young people who are not yet ready for a sexual relationship do not feel pressurized by the assumptions of parents and caring staff that they should be having a relationship.

When a young haemophiliac is old enough he will transfer from a children's hospital or unit to an adult hospital where he will attend as an adult patient in his own right and not necessarily accompanied by his mother. It has to be assumed that any information about his condition will be given to the young person himself. His parents are anxious to learn about his condition and ask how he got on at the clinic. Frequently, the young person is off-hand in his response and this can lead to a tension between parents and son who is not intentionally being difficult. He may just wish to forget about the clinic visit and questions remind him of the underlying problem. On the other hand, he may not have any information.

Adolescent haemophiliacs with HIV are concerned about what they will do in the future. Their peers will be talking about plans for jobs, careers, earning money and holidays. For some of these adolescents, haemophilia will have already altered their expectations of what they can do. It is possible that HIV will put additional restrictions on them, preventing them from gaining greater independence. These young people may need help in selecting a career and finding a job as well as encouragement to believe that they have a future.

Adolescence can be a very lonely time, particularly for those who think that they are in any way different from others. Having HIV exacerbates the feeling of isolation and complicates the life of the young person. A feature of adolescence is a desire to be the same as one's peers. Having HIV makes the young person different. One young man admitted that he had spent much time examining his face, neck and back and had come to believe that the acne that he had developed was the early signs of AIDS. He did not wish to discuss his fear with his parents. Nor did he wish to raise it with the medical staff in case his worst fears were realized. The problem only surfaced when a member of staff made a chance remark about how common acne was among people of his age. It is likely that adolescent girls exchange confidences with their friends, but this may be less common with adolescent males and particularly those who may already feel different or not part of the gang because of haemophilia. HIV will isolate them even further from their peers. It is important that helpers are perceptive and enable the young person to express his feelings and gain confidence. Invariably, the responses of these young people are normal re-actions to an exceptionally difficult situation.

HIV positive adult haemophiliacs

The reactions of a person with haemophilia to the news that he is HIV positive are very similar to the reactions of a non-haemophiliac when found to be HIV positive. There are, however, problems which are particularly perti-nent to the haemophiliac population and which helpers should consider over and above the issues discussed elsewhere in this book.

Some of these particular problems have been briefly described at the begin-ning of the chapter. We have already referred to the fact that for the HIV positive haemophiliac the infection was iatrogenically acquired. It is therefore not surprising that haemophiliacs should feel extremely angry and disillu-sioned. The initial reaction of many haemophiliac patients when the link between blood products and HIV first became known was to cut back on their treatment (Madhok *et al.*, 1986), with some patients refusing to take imported blood products. However, this situation gradually stabilized as those with haemophilia accepted that the greatest danger to them was untreated bleeds. Blood products usage among those with haemophilia has returned to pre-HIV usage (Madhok, personal communication).

When HIV was first diagnosed in the UK haemophilia population, many HIV positive haemophiliacs expressed disbelief at the seriousness, or the po-tential seriousness, of HIV. This could be interpreted as a form of denial which is a common response when people first learn that they are HIV positive. Many people with haemophilia have survived serious bleeds and other life-threatening illnesses. It is therefore possible that HIV is perceived by some HIV positive haemophiliacs as being no different from other life-threatening illnesses that they have already experienced. If the person has survived episodes of these other life-threatening illnesses, why should he not survive HIV-related illnesses? Another explanation suggested by Markova *et al.* (1990) is that if someone has little control over their situation, one expedient is to degrade the importance of such a condition and thus regain some control over it.

The counselling needs of HIV adult haemophiliacs are varied and will depend upon their circumstances. These may include whether they have a stable relationship and where they live, their state of health, whether they have a job and are able to continue with it.

The person in a stable relationship does not have to worry about making relationships and telling a new partner about haemophilia and HIV. On the other hand, he may be deeply concerned about the possibility of having already transmitted the virus to his partner. When the partner is discovered to be HIV positive, the guilt of the haeomophiliac is very intense. In these circumstances, both partners may require help to work through their feelings and then to make practical arrangements for the future.

When the partner is HIV negative, there is a great sense of relief. But then couples have to face the reality of how to continue with a sexual relationship in the presence of HIV. In some cases, the woman has been sterilized on completion of the family. Frequently, these women say that they are for the first time really enjoying their sex life free from the fear of becoming pregnant. (It is not uncommon to find among couples where the male has severe haemophilia that the female is sterilized, the operation being considered less risky and problematic for the female than for the male partner who has severe haemophilia.) It may take some time for these couples to resume a sexual relationship practising safer sex. Some HIV positive haemophiliacs have explained that they feel very guilty about the restrictions that haemophilia has imposed upon their marriage and on family life. They talk about periods of illness and periods of severe pain from bleeds and the resulting disruption of family arrangements and the additional responsibility placed on their partner. Concern about the sexual transmission of HIV to their partner adds another very great restriction upon their lives.

Men express concern about what should happen to their children. There is concern about when or at what age the child should learn that his or her father has HIV. Some parents have said that the need to discuss the matter with the children has coincided with a period of high media publicity about HIV, AIDS and haemophilia. In some cases, children have asked their mother whether their father has HIV. Parents have found this an extremely difficult subject to raise with their children. They have often been surprised at how relatively easy it was to talk about it and subsequently parents have thought that their children had some inkling that their father had HIV. However, it is not simply a matter of telling children that their parent has HIV. Parents need also to have some sort of plan of how to help children cope with this knowledge and of how they themselves will deal with subsequent questions that may arise. It is important that the child's future security is clarified, particularly when both parents are affected.

HIV positive haemophiliac men with a family express great concern about money and how the family will manage financially in the future. Some of these men are still in employment. But unemployment is high in the haemophilia population and in particular among older men who have not had in their youth the advantage of the modern methods of treatment. Married men who have been working and who have a mortgage are particularly concerned about the repayment of the mortgage in the event of them having to give up work. It should be remembered that it is unlikely that these men will have been able, because of haemophilia, to obtain mortgage protection in the form of life assurance (Wilkie, 1987). In some families, the wife or female partner has already become the main breadwinner as her partner has been unable to work regularly or has had to give up work prematurely because of haemophilia. In addition, the reversal of the traditional male/female roles with the female partner being the major breadwinner can cause problems for some men who may already have low self-esteem.

Some HIV positive haemophiliacs were in a relationship when they learned that they had HIV but were not necessarily living with their partner nor had necessarily envisaged a long-term commitment to that partner. It has been this author's experience that men in this situation acted with great responsibility, informing current partners and in some cases previous partners of their risk and telling them where they could have counselling and testing for HIV if they wish. These men said that they feared rejection by their girlfriend and that it took considerable courage to tell them about HIV. Some of these young men develop longstanding relationships with the intention of getting married after they had learned that they had HIV.

The HIV positive adult haemophiliac who was not in a sexual relationship when he learned that he had HIV, like those who do not have haemophilia and who have HIV, may experience difficulties when getting involved with a new sexual partner. It is not always possible to hide the disability that haemophilia can cause. For example, bleeds into a joint can cause stiffness or a limp. It has been observed that since the appearance of HIV, there has been a tendency for people to deny the existence of haemophilia. Men with haemophilia have often said that they are likely to have more success with women if they hide the fact that they have haemophilia. It is not surprising that they feel that the combination of haemophilia and HIV will not help them in making a relationship. As one man said: 'What bird would want to get involved with an HIV positive haemophiliac?' A direct consequence of this problem is that some men have found it possible to have a relationship for one night only. Safer sex can be practised and there is no need for the man to offer any information about himself. However, if this pattern continues it becomes very difficult for men to develop more meaningful relationships.

Loneliness can be a problem for unemployed haemophiliacs with HIV and particularly when the partner goes out to work. Some men have said that they do not feel so lonely providing that they can continue to drive and afford to keep their car (often adjusted for disability) on the road. Having haemophilia can be time-consuming and not everyone has been able to develop interests and hobbies. Some men who live in smaller communities have found support from neighbours and other local people. On the other hand, some have declined the offers of help from local people for fear that once it is known that they have HIV or AIDS they will be stigmatized. The Haemophilia Society provides a most articulate lobby for those with haemophilia. But it does not necessarily provide a local network of support for those with HIV as the gay community has in some areas. The centre where the person attends for the treatment of his haemophilia may provide, or be prepared to provide, support outside the hospital. However, not all haemophiliacs wish this, seeing it as an over-medicalization of their lives.

In any case, not everyone lives near the treatment centre. While there are over 1200 HIV positive haemophiliacs, they are geographically dispersed and, therefore, cannot form a homogeneous group. In some cases, support has very successfully been found through other organizations such as Scottish AIDS Monitor or the Terrence Higgins Trust.

Note

1 Statistics prepared from voluntary confidential reports by clinicians and sent to the PHLS Communicable Diseases Surveillance Centre and to Communicable Diseases Scotland, and published by the Department of Health, 21 January 1991.

References

Burton, L. (1975). *The Family Life of Sick Children*. London, Routledge and Kegan Paul.

Hewitt, S. and Newson, J.E. (1970). *The Family and the Handicapped Child*. London, Allen and Unwin.

Madhok, R. *et al.* (1986). Changes in factor use subsequent to publicity of AIDS in haemophilia. Poster presentation to the *International Conference on AIDS*, Paris, June.

Markova, I. and Forbes, C. (1984). 'Coping with haemophilia'. *International Journal of Applied Psychology*, **33**, 457–77.

Markova, I. *et al.* (1980). 'Impact of haemophilia on child-rearing practices and parental cooperation'. *Journal of Child Psychology and Psychiatry*, **21**, 153–62.

Markova, I. *et al.* (1990). 'Self and other – awareness of the risk of HIV/AIDS in people with haemophilia and implications for behavioural change'. *Social Science and Medicine*, **31**, 73–9.

Molleman, E. and van Knippenberg, A.D. (1987). 'Social and psychological aspects of haemophilia'. *Patient Education and Counseling*, **10**, 175–89.

Moser, R.H. (1969). *Diseases of Medical Progress: A Study of Iatrogenic Disease*. Charles C. Thomas, Springfield, Ill.

Wilkie, P.A. (1987). 'Life assurance, HIV sero-positivity and haemophilia'. *Scottish Medical Journal*, **32**, 119–21.

FOURTEEN

Particular issues in working with partners

PATRICIA WILKIE

Social and legal context

HIV has very great implications not only for someone living with HIV but also for his or her partner, and this has been referred to in most of the preceding chapters. Many of the helping actions identified in earlier chapters will be required in working with the partner of a person who is living with HIV. There are also a number of special considerations that need to be taken into account in helping work with a partner, and these considerations are explored in this chapter.

The needs of the partner and the effect of the knowledge of his or her HIV status will vary depending upon a number of factors including who is the partner; whether the partner is male or female; whether they are gay, lesbian or heterosexual; the antibody status of the partner; the strength of the relationship, the commitments of the relationship and how long the couple have been together; whether the couple have dependent children; and the legal status of the relationship.

The lack of formal legal recognition of a relationship and the way in which society devalues particular types of sexual relationships, may set very distinct limitations on the resources and strategies for coping of some partners of people living with HIV. For example, a woman who is living with, but not married to, an HIV positive man may have to face more practical worries about the future financial security of herself and her children than a married woman. She may also receive less support from friends and family. In Chapter 11, Charles Anderson has highlighted the problems that arise for gay people from the fact that gay relationships are not valued by society at large. He comments that, as a result: 'a relationship between two men often demands more commitment, and more imagination in dealing with difficulties, than a heterosexual relationship'. Aside from the problems that arise from the general lack of social valuing of gay relationships, gay partners may find themselves excluded at times of acute illness. The needs and wishes of a gay partner of someone living with HIV may not always be recognized by medical staff, or by the family of the HIV positive person. Helpers need to be alert to the way in which the resources for coping with HIV are affected by the legal and social status of a relationship.

Learning that a partner is HIV antibody positive

Many individuals will learn about the HIV positive status of a partner directly from the partner. However, others will learn from a third party including medical and counselling staff. There are many reasons why an affected person may find it difficult to tell a loved one that he or she is HIV antibody positive, including fear of what HIV may do to their relationship. Some individuals have said that with the knowledge of hindsight their HIV antibody positive partner was trying to tell them and that hints were being dropped. Good HIV testing counselling procedures recommend that there should be a discussion between counsellor and client about informing partners. In an ideal world, relationships are built on mutual trust between the partners. Unfortunately, it will remain difficult for some individuals to learn of the HIV antibody positive status of their partners.

Some individuals, on learning that their partners are HIV antibody positive, may not immediately appreciate that they also are at risk of having already contracted HIV. In view of the very great publicity about the sexual transmission of HIV, this may seem surprising. One woman said that when she first learned that her partner was HIV antibody positive, she felt very angry that it had happened to him, frightened and fearful of the future. It was some days later before the further implications that she too might have been infected began to sink in. This pattern is not uncommon. A possible explanation for this reaction is denial; but an equally possible explanation is the amount of information held by, or given to, the partner and the way in which the partner learned about the HIV diagnosis.

Partners themselves need independent counselling, information and advice. Some partners may not wish to consult the same doctor or unit as their already diagnosed partner. In counselling people who have been given an HIV antibody positive test result, information should be given about choices that are available to their partners for counselling. Partners need to decide whether or not they wish to be tested for HIV and to work through the implications for them and their relationship if they are HIV antibody positive and have been infected by the person in their current relationship.

Emotional aspects

Many of the emotions felt by partners and the problems they face when their partner is HIV antibody positive or has HIV-related illness will be similar, regardless of their sexual orientation or special circumstances. These emotions will include fear of illness in a loved one, fear of being unable to cope with illness, fear of stigma, fear of becoming infected with HIV, uncertainty about the future, fear of the death of the person living with HIV and fear of being on one's own.

Difficulties may arise in the way that the partner learns about HIV. The HIV antibody status of the person living with HIV may have been known to both partners at the beginning of the relationship. There are also situations where at the beginning of the relationship neither partner is aware of any problem, the original infection having been contracted by the HIV antibody positive partner some time, even years, previously. The diagnosis of HIV infection is very often traumatic, but in these circumstances the source of the infection can be attributed to an event that happened before the couple met, thus reducing the possibility of recrimination between the partners.

The situation where the couple has been together for some time and the infected partner contracted HIV as a result of an affair which was unknown to the other partner can be very difficult emotionally. Sometimes, the partner who has been diagnosed as HIV antibody positive is able to tell his or her partner about HIV. In other cases, some considerable time may elapse before the partner is told about HIV. In these circumstances, partners may feel a variety of emotions including anger that their trust has been broken, sadness, fear and even contempt for their partner. It is often necessary for the partner to work through these emotions before he or she is able to absorb the implications of HIV.

Sometimes, the news of the HIV antibody positive diagnosis involves a female learning for the first time that her male partner is bisexual. Bill Kirkpatrick describes situations where the sexual orientation of a son was unknown to the family before the onset of HIV-related illness. He suggests that, 'three facts are forced into parents' awareness at the same time: your son is gay, your son has a partner and your son is dying' (Kirkpatrick, 1988, p. 54). The situation of the female partner described above is not dissimilar. Her partner is bisexual, her partner may have a male partner, and her partner is HIV antibody positive. The female partner may or may not have contracted HIV from her partner and may or may not have already transmitted the infection to a child.

In the scenario described in the last paragraph, the female partner, the male partner and the person living with HIV may all separately experience the need to gain support and counselling from a helper. Some confusion and possible damage in relationships may result, however, if one helper tries to meet the needs of all of these three people who are trying to cope with HIV. Helpers may need to define their role very clearly and indicate whether their helping efforts are focused primarily on the needs of a person living with HIV, or on the needs of his or her partner. Where helpers are working with both partners in a relationship to assist them to deal with difficulties in their relationship, they need to be vigilant that they maintain an impartial stance. The danger of being 'drawn into' a disagreement between partners must be avoided.

The emotional needs of a partner who is HIV antibody negative are considerable and will change according to the state of the HIV antibody positive partner's health. It will take some time for partners to come to terms with the diagnosis. Some may never do so and some relationships may end. When this happens, unaffected partners can feel very guilty.

The problems for an HIV negative partner of sustaining a sexual relationship with their HIV antibody positive partner should not be underestimated. Some couples succeed in maintaining very happy long-term relationships where safer sex is always practised. Others find emotional, and possibly also sexual, adjustment difficult and the relationship breaks up. Some couples find it difficult to maintain practising safer sex and decide to take risks 'just this once'. Some female partners would like to have a child by their HIV antibody positive partner, and are prepared to take the risk of unprotected intercourse to conceive.

The longer the HIV positive individual remains asymptomatic, the easier it may be for the relationship. Concerned partners will always have a niggling doubt at the back of their mind. However, the partner should not get lulled into a false sense of security and stop practising safer sex.

Partners may need support when they are looking after a partner who is ill, particularly in the terminal stages of illness. Partners need strength to give support, love and comfort when they are caring for someone who is ill. Some partners will also have the responsibility of dependent children. Just as the person living with HIV or HIV-related illness can be helped to take control of his or her life and make plans, so too can the partner. It can be very helpful to a person with HIV-related illness, in the terminal stage of illness, to know that his or her partner has made plans for the future.

Information and confidentiality

One of the difficulties that some individuals face is how to get information about the health and the prognosis of their partner. This happens when the couple are unable to talk about it together. This is not uncommon in any serious, or potentially serious, situation. There are many possible reasons for this behaviour. The person with HIV-related illness may simply be denying the situation. Alternatively, the person with HIV-related illness may not know what to say to his or her partner and some may assume that the partner may know. Some people regard their own illness as a very personal matter, the details of which they do not discuss even with a partner. Others may fear the dependency and changing relationship within the partnership which could result from the illness. Sadly, there is sometimes evidence of HIV-related brain damage which can affect the ability to reason and communicate.

The doctor caring for the person with HIV-related illness is not necessarily the doctor to the partner. Sometimes staff involved in the care of an individual with HIV-related illness are not aware that his or her partner does not know what is happening. They may not even know of the existence of a certain partner. The personal and family life of patients attending departments of genitourinary medicine in large cities is not necessarily known to staff. This is in contrast to someone attending a GP who may also be the doctor to other members of the patient's family.

It can be difficult for the partner to get information when the partner has no legal or 'official' status and when the wishes of the person with HIV-related illness have not been made clear. For example, the estranged husband of a woman dying of AIDS is contacted as the next of kin by the hospital. The longstanding lover is ignored. As an earlier section of this chapter indicated, this problem can be particularly acute for gay couples where partners have found themselves excluded by the family of an individual with HIV-related illness from access to their lover at times of crisis in the illness and at death. When the family neither recognizes the validity of their gay son's lifestyle nor the rights of his partner to be involved in the care of his lover and in making decisions about the estate, then acrimony is likely to occur.

Doctors are bound by confidentiality to the patient and counsellors are in a similar position. HIV has highlighted issues about confidentiality that have been unquestioned for a long time or have been taken for granted. For example, how confidential is medical information. Relatives of terminally ill patients certainly know that doctors break confidence in preferring to discuss the patient's prognosis with the relative rather than the patient (Gillon, 1985). In the circumstances where an HIV antibody positive partner refuses to inform his or her partner about HIV, how does the partner learn? This situation may face some doctors and helpers with an ethical dilemma.

In situations where helpers are providing support to both partners in a relationship, they need to state very clearly how they will protect confidentiality while assisting communication between the partners. At the same time, they need to recognize that problems may arise if other voluntary or professional helpers working with this pair of partners are guided by a less strict definition of confidentiality.

Practical problems

There are certain practical issues facing couples where a partner has serious HIV-related illness. These issues are similar to those facing people when a partner is suffering from other serious, life-threatening illnesses. Often the couple have been able to discuss some of these problems together. However, it is often therapeutic for the partner to discuss these issues with a helper. Such discussion can help to give the partner a feeling of control over the situation and may also facilitate further discussion between the partners. The following matters may need to be considered.

Housing

If the couple live in local authority housing, in whose name is the house registered and is it worthwhile looking at ways in which this can be changed? If the couple are living in rented accommodation, in whose name is the rent agreement? If the couple are in privately owned accommodation, do they have a mortgage and, if so, is it a joint mortgage or is it in the name of one partner only?

Financial arrangements

Clearly questions about housing are related to the financial arrangements that the couple may have and there will be wide variations in these. For example, who pays which bills? Where the partner does not have financial independence from the partner living with HIV, he or she may wish to consider what sort of financial arrangements should be made should the partner living with HIV become ill. This is particularly relevant when there are dependent children. Female partners who have not had employment outside the home can be helped to find some sort of work compatible with the needs of the family.

It may not be appropriate to discuss these housing and financial issues with all partners. Helpers may also need to consider the timing of such a discussion in the counselling process. For example, when people living with HIV are apparently well and asymptomatic, their partners may not wish to acknowledge that their future health is uncertain. Such discussions of practical matters may be both pressing and difficult if the individual with HIV infection becomes very ill, or develops HIV-related psychiatric and neurological problems.

References

Gillon, R. (1985). *Philosophical Medical Ethics*. Chichester, John Wiley.
Kirkpatrick, B. (1988). *AIDS: Sharing the Pain. Pastoral Guidelines*. London, Darton, Longman and Todd.

The needs of the helper

FIFTEEN

Organizing support for helpers

NORAH SMITH

The helping environment should be one in which support exists at several levels. The careful selection of trainees is crucial, followed by training long enough for intending helpers not only to acquire the necessary knowledge and counselling skills, but to explore their own motivations, attitudes and feelings. This allows people time to decide whether HIV work is really for them. Beyond initial training, there should be ongoing training events and group and possibly individual supervision, as well as a support group and ideally the opportunity for individual consultation with experienced counsellors.

The supportive organization creates a sense of security by being clear on issues of accountability, making supervision compulsory and possibly also setting standards for record-keeping. It will also be part of a network capable of offering alternative provision (e.g. to clients' relatives) when pressures on helpers become too great, or where their involvement is not appropriate.

Supportive and supervision groups

All counsellors need to receive both supervision of their activities and personal support. Groups that are established for helpers working in the area of HIV may focus either on providing support for helpers or on supervision.

The supervision group is primarily task-oriented, offering technical information and practical advice, extending the teaching aspects of the training. Groups established during training may form the basis of supervision groups once helping is begun, but there are also advantages in combining new with more experienced counsellors whose range and depth of contribution may be rewarded by the renewed enthusiasm gained from beginners. Supervisors would be experienced counsellors/trainers with expertise in the HIV field. The emphasis in supervision tends to be on the cognitive and problem-solving aspects of the task and the main focus is largely on the *client's* needs.

The needs of the *helper* are the main concern of the support group, where feelings can be ventilated, the irrational can be tolerated and explored, and insecurities can be voiced in a safe and non-judgemental setting. The off-loading of issues and feelings reduces emotional tension and workers discover that their problems and frustrations are not unique.

This chapter deals primarily with support groups, first making a case for establishing them in addition to providing supervision, then exploring their function and the task of setting them up. Finally, it looks briefly at group processes and at some of the issues that can arise within groups. Some of this discussion is, of course, relevant to groups whose primary focus is supervision.

Why support?

Positive diagnosis

Helping individuals to cope with the shock of an HIV antibody diagnosis, and to live with uncertainty, anxiety and the implications for work and social life demands considerable resources. The helper needs to be able to develop and sustain a relationship at a time when the client may be least able to respond. Working with individuals who may be experiencing very considerable emotional distress and fears of loss of personal control requires training and support to enable helpers to withstand these distressing feelings, and to respond appropriately to their clients.

Clients who are living with HIV or who have HIV-related illnesses are more likely to encounter public fear and rejection than compassion, and as a group they face tremendous scapegoating. Helpers themselves may on occasion have to deal with negative or ambivalent reactions to their work from family and friends and might feel themselves isolated and without sufficient support at home. Helpers who are very conscious of, and empathic with, the difficulties that their clients may be experiencing in their social lives, may themselves feel somewhat out of sympathy with the wider society.

The anger of the recently diagnosed HIV antibody positive client may sometimes be focused in the first instance on the helper. This anger may be expressed in terms of rejection of certain aspects of the helper, e.g. sex, sexual orientation and race.

Hospital care and terminal illness

The needs of a person developing health problems requiring in-patient hospital care are likely to be somewhat different from those of a person who is asymptomatic. Helpers need to be flexible to adapt to this new situation. A group can provide the supervision that ensures that helpers respond to this transition appropriately, while at the same time providing personal support.

Working with the terminally ill raises a number of issues, both in the helping and for the helpers themselves. Often those who take up caring roles (especially those attracted to work with the dying) are strongly idealistic. Over-idealism, too, can be a source of stress and may impair the helper's work. The possiblity of models of adjustment being imposed on clients in a way which is not responsive to their own expressed needs has been discussed in Chapter 1. Group support can encourage the helper to relinquish perfectionist goals and focus on the possible. Support is needed to enable helpers, carers, to sustain the capacity to tolerate despair and to avoid unhelpful defensive strategies in cases where illness progresses.

Macks and Turner (1986, p. 121) point out that:

> The key to successful clinical work with AIDS patients lies in our willingness to look at our own attitudes and fears about death and dying The feelings of helplessness, loss of control, dependency, uncertainty, and guilt that *we* experience in working with a person with AIDS require particular attention. Clinicians at risk for AIDS themselves face the added difficulty and responsibility of sorting out their own feelings in their work with clients.

The role of the support group in this sphere is obvious, for the benefit of both helper and client.

In hospital settings, hierarchical issues can make it difficult for medical and non-medical carers to join in creating and sustaining support groups. Medical staff in particular may be reluctant to acknowledge the need of support. The airing of emotive issues may risk interdepartmental conflict. Organizational factors, e.g. finding a suitable time for members of the group all of whom will have busy schedules and who may work in different places, may also discourage the formation of a support group. Only if support is seen as a priority will problems of allocating time in institutional and agency settings be seriously worked on. The findings by Antony Grey (Convenor of the British Association of Counselling AIDS panel) that the presence of support and supervision groups in the hospital setting leads to a reduction of absenteeism is of note in this context (NACAB, 1988: video).

A high level of personal commitment to clients with serious HIV-related illnesses may easily lead to emotional depletion, particularly if several deaths occur within a short period. Often those in caring roles find it hard to seek help for themselves because there is a stigma of disapproval, as in the case of doctors (Bailey, 1985, p. 24) and of social workers who are 'not allowed' not to cope.

Statutory services

Carers in statutory agencies commonly find that supervision is their only legitimate source of support. An exploration of feelings is secondary to goal and task-oriented work and indeed the expression of feelings may be interpreted as an inability to cope. Feelings may thus go unvalidated and unacknowledged in professions such as social work where there is an expectation that workers should be equal to any task. Anxiety and self-blame in this group may be higher than among voluntary carers and the need for support may be concealed for fear of adversely affecting career prospects. In some agencies, there may be token acknowledgement that support groups are valuable, but the implicit message – often conveyed by relegating meetings to lunchtimes – is that support comes only after work for others is done. The tacit message that care for the carers smacks of self-indulgence encourages inappropriate defensive reactions to stress and inhibits individuals from taking personal responsibilty for maintaining their health and inner resources.

The voluntary sector

In the voluntary sector, ongoing training, supervision and support is essential to prevent helpers from falling back on an unreflective, possibly inappropriate response at the expense of a more thoughtful, skilled intervention.

Helpers who are exhausted or disillusioned are likely to create distress and disturbance within the organization, if they do not leave helping work altogether. Their feelings, if they do leave, are liable to be of failure and guilt, while for the organization there will be waste in terms of training and human resources. To ignore the need for support is costly to the individual, to the agency and to society. Part of an effective system of support may involve scheduling 'time out' from helping work for volunteers who are finding that they are very tired or are having considerable difficulties in coping. Such a system is preferable to allowing them to continue to 'burn themselves out' and then have to cope with feelings of inadequacy.

The function of the support group

It is helpful to have a variety of sources of support so that the counsellor can choose what best suits his or her individual needs, but ongoing support and supervision should not be regarded as optional. Lopez and Getzel (1987, p. 51) describe support strategies in the Gay Men's Health Crisis in New York, the largest US volunteer agency serving gay and non-gay people living with HIV. They emphasize the sustaining value of intensive training and regular group support and supervision meetings: training and supportive work done in groups brings home the fact that no-one can work closely with people who have serious HIV-related illnesses alone or in isolation from members of the team, which includes care-giving buddies, crisis workers and section leaders.

Dealing with unexpected reactions

While attitudes and motivations will have been examined during training, reactions cannot always be anticipated. Sexual orientation, drug use, social class, gender or race may evoke responses that catch the helper off-guard and the support group is a place where feelings can be identified and analysed. Only when we recognize and cope with our own anxieties are we able to achieve the emotional stability needed to care for others.

Unconscious mirroring of client/counsellor dynamics

A phenomenon of which support groups should be aware is that of the 'reflection process' identified by Searles (1955) and elaborated by Mattinson (1975, p. 11): 'The process at work currently in the *relationship between* client and worker are often reflected in the *relationship between* worker and supervisor.' In her role as supervisor, Mattinson discovered that the behaviour of the student in supervision sessions revealed not only the student's difficulties, but enacted the difficulties of the client, presenting a model of what the client was trying to do in the interaction with the worker.

Knowledge of the possibility of re-enactment of a client's difficulties in the supervision session offers a useful tool to the supervisor. It allows the supervisor to gain insight into the difficulties of both helper and client. Members of a support group need to be alert to behaviour that is uncharacteristic and which may be an example of the re-enactment by the helper of the difficulties of the client.

Maintaining boundaries and sustaining morale

There is often strong identification with clients and the support group can help prevent boundary issues from becoming blurred. Experienced helpers are able to assist new workers to accept how little they may feel they can achieve at times, particularly in areas of deprivation. Strong support is needed for all individuals working in situations where the clients' external resources are inadequate and there are few possibilities for clients to gain greater control over their lives.

Providing feedback

Feedback plays an invaluable role in creating accurate and adequate self-evaluation and in enabling helpers to come to terms with their limitations and to perceive the impact and quality of their work. Saretsky (1977) and Inskipp (1986) have useful sections on feedback, which Saretsky (1977, p. 48) describes as a communication giving information as to how a person affects others and which helps him consider changing his behaviour. Inskipp (1986, p. 43) emphasizes the need, if it is to be helpful, for feedback to be given in a concerned and supportive way and to include positive as well as negative observations.

Setting realistic goals

One of the most important functions of the support group is to provide mutual help in setting realistic goals. Cherniss (1980, p. 160) points out that common sources of stress are excessive, self-imposed demands arising from unrealistically high goals. The support group can help a worker to clarify and to become more aware of his or her personal goals and can encourage alternative sources of satisfaction where counselling work appears to be the primary or sole source of need fulfilment.

Avoiding burnout

Another important function of the support group is to help to combat burnout. In the words of Antony Grey, burnout 'is characterised by disturbing feelings of helplessness and despair' and is the likely outcome 'of not being sufficiently in touch with your own feelings, not having clear boundaries to your relationships with clients, and not having an effective support system' (HMSO, 1987, p. 119). Maslach's (1979, p. 117) research shows that burnout rates were lower for carers who had access to a support group 'especially if it was well developed and supported by the parent institution'.

Claus and Bailey (1980) emphasize the importance of perception in coping with difficult situations. What one person perceives as negatively stressful, another will see as a challenge. The individual suffering from burnout '*perceives* environmental stimuli as taxing the physiological, psychological, or social systems' (Claus and Bailey, 1980, p. 10).

The support group is a place where perceptions can be explored and where signs of stress can be detected before burnout is reached. Cherniss (1980) warns that burnout is highly contagious and difficult to reverse, and advocates prevention as being more effective and less costly than cure. Consciousness-raising 'must be the first step in any effort to deal with the problem of burnout in a community agency' (Cherniss, 1980, p. 159). A group that encourages 'both emotional support and positive problem-solving' will foster 'an attitude of enquiry' towards negative reactions (to clients or colleagues, for example) and towards sources of stress, frustration and satisfaction (Cherniss, 1980, p. 164).

Cherniss (1980, pp. 17–18) distinguishes between three stages in burnout: stress ('imbalance between resource and demand'); strain, the short-term emotional response to stress, in the form of anxiety, tension, fatigue and exhaustion; and defensive coping, evidenced in changes in attitude and behaviour.

Identifying defensive coping

Defence mechanisms, as described by Freud, are psychological processes whereby a person unconsciously deceives him- or herself about the presence external threats or frustrations. This can be seen as a form of coping, but the threat is only *perceived* to have been changed and is not changed in actuality.

Defensive coping is frequently demonstrated through detachment, leading to loss of concern for the client (defending against awareness of responsibility and therefore of inadequacy or failure). Intellectualization is another way of achieving detachment from threatening feelings or events, so that we can remain emotionally untouched. Cynicism and pessimism may be employed to reduce guilt and frustration.

Defence mechanisms can be inferred from the discrepancy between what a person says about him- or herself and the circumstances of his or her actual behaviour. The support group can both note these as warning signs of stress and help each other to avoid maladaptive ways of reducing it. Bailey (1985, p. 59) argues that long-term defensive coping (for example, when dealing with death and dying) can lead to stored-up stress and consequent increased risk of burnout.

Not all attempts to combat stress are unconscious, of course. Carers may try to avoid personal pain by denying their clients the opportunity to fully express feelings of grief, sadness and anger. Support groups can attempt to identify if a counsellor is in fact acting in this self-protective way and denying clients the opportunity to express and thereby begin to resolve difficult feelings.

Combating negative thinking

Under stress the focus may become 'What's wrong with me?' and support groups can help to change the question to 'What can I do about the situation?' Zastrow (1984, pp. 145–46) refers to the kind of thought that characterizes burnout, such as 'What's the use, whatever I try won't work' and 'I'm going to give up – am no longer going to make an effort'. He argues that burnout is 'caused by two types of factor: distressing events and by a certain kind of self-defeating thought about distressing events' (Zastrow, 1984, p. 147). He groups stress reduction strategies into three categories: (1) organizational strategies to reduce stress and burnout; (2) individuals' strategies for changing distressing events; and (3) individual's strategies for altering negative thoughts about distressing events.

Looking first at organizational strategies, support groups can become pressure groups if necessary, to achieve organizational cooperation in the form of reducing the size of case-loads, improving work conditions (such as private rooms set aside for counselling), diluting the hours of stressful work by providing variety in the case-load, introducing and implementing 'time-outs', and expanding the training programme.

Individuals' strategies can be fostered within the supportive and non-judgemental atmosphere of the group, which can assist members to think positively about themselves and their work. They can be helped to identify and explore difficulties and to take responsibility for doing something about them. The group can encourage the making of contracts, the negotiating of tasks and adherence to limits and boundaries. The ability to say 'no' is often essential for self-preservation. Exercises such as those described by Dickson (1982) or Phelps and Austin (1975) can usefully be tried out in groups.

The altering of negative thoughts can be achieved with the help of the group, who can encourage relaxation, meditation, exercise, autogenic training and the positive use of leisure time. Pelletier (1978) and Chaitow (1984) elaborate on these methods and are useful guides to stress reduction. Particularly helpful on burnout in general are Cherniss (1980), Pines *et al.* (1981), Zastrow (1984) and Bailey (1985).

Setting up support

Negotiating the purpose of the group and defining boundaries

Groups may be part of the organizational structure or pioneered by helpers themselves. In either case, it is important for members to formulate a very clear remit. The expectations of members need to be explored and the purpose of the group negotiated and defined. The frequency and duration of meetings should be established and time boundaries adhered to. This differentiates group time from ordinary social contact and reinforces the role of the group as not simply a place to let off steam, but as a setting in which the focus is on making sense of the experiences shared. Maintaining time boundaries in the support setting will contribute an aspect of order and security. Boundaries relating to the function of the group also need to be observed: a support group, for example, is not a psychotherapy group and individuals should be encouraged to seek help elsewhere if necessary.

Confidentiality

Overt rules for the group have to be established. These rules will include not only the boundary issues discussed in the last section, but also the need for confidentiality both in relation to clients and to the individuals in the group. The rights of clients must be protected and strict confidentiality maintained (see Chapter 1).

Information about group members must also be treated as confidential. Anxiety about confidentiality may be particularly acute for members who are, say, part of a small gay community, who have used drugs, or who are themselves HIV antibody positive. Only when the group is felt to be truly safe can it function effectively.

Size and composition of the group

Too large a group can be intimidating and a membership of five or six is probably ideal. Lopez and Getzel (1987, p.52) emphasizes the advantages of

heterogeneity of membership in helping to clarify values: 'The more opportunities the team provides volunteers to face and handle differences among
themselves (including race, age, class, and gender differences), the more effective are volunteers when engaging and working with persons with AIDS.'

Deciding on leadership

The group must decide whether or not to have a leader. If it decides to have a
leader, the leader's role must be defined. The existence of a leader relieves
individual members of the full responsibility of attending to group processes
and with the agreement of the group the leader may draw attention to under-
currents (arising from, say, envy or competitiveness) if these are interfering
with the task. It seems important that he or she should not impose ways of
working and should not function as the 'expert' (though the group may seek
this at times). A valuable role is that of finding ways of developing and
sustaining a strong sense of purpose, and of making the most of members'
strengths and abilities. The leader can play a useful part in fostering a trusting
environment in which members take personal responsibility for what they
want to happen.

Functions of leadership

The 'maintenance' and 'task' functions of leadership have been distinguished
(see, e.g. Claus and Bailey, 1980, pp. 169–70; Balgopal and Vassil, 1983, p.
213 ff). Maintenance functions are concerned with the relationships and com-
forts of group members and are demonstrated, for example, when the leader
encourages spontaneity, cooperation and the expression of feelings, or tackles
disharmony. Task functions are those of energizing and co-ordinating and are
seen when the leader questions or confronts members, interprets their behaviour, clarifies, explains or summarizes.

Selecting a leader

A strong argument can be made for choosing a leader from outside the agency.
Such a person need not be an expert in the area of HIV counselling, since
supervision will also be available; he or she is there to help understanding of
what is going on within the group and to enable individual members to gain
support for their personal needs. The leader's detachment from the agency can
free members to be more open. In addition, boundary issues are likely to be
more clear to an outside leader, who is in a better position to help boundaries
to be maintained.

Adapting to available resources

Poor finances or a scarcity of suitable outside group leaders may restrict options; and arrangements appropriate to the circumstances of individual organizations need to be evolved. For example, in an agency with several support groups, each group might nominate a member who would meet on a regular basis with representatives from the other groups and an outside consultant. The consultant would have contact with the groups when necessary and would offer crisis intervention. Financially well-off organizations (if such organizations exist!) might employ a counsellor for the sole purpose of being available to the helping team, as an addition to the support system.

Self-review

Self-review is an important aspect of group functioning and it is helpful to establish this explicitly in the planning stage. This involves setting aside time on a regular basis to check out whether or not the group is functioning according to its remit and whether the expectations of members are being met. It may be that the remit changes as the group develops and it is important that it continues to be clearly formulated.

Group processes

Growing together as a group evolves in stages, from tentative beginnings through gradual shedding of façades to more open communication as trust develops.

At first, there are anxieties over acceptance and members are concerned to defend their public image and to avoid conflict. As trust grows, people can more freely voice true feelings, attitudes, perceptions and motivations. There may be a stormy period, but such a period is often necessary for growth and the group will be enabled by it to move on creatively and spontaneously. Growth is often painful, frequently involving issues of vulnerability and control, and good leadership can help the group to weather these difficulties. It is also useful to be able to refer back to the original remit and to review progress in the light of members' expectations.

Exercises can be helpful in increasing group cohesion. Saretsky (1977) suggests ways of promoting empathy, trust and acceptance, and exercises relating to various aspects of group development are described by Remocker and Storch (1982) and Ernst and Goodison (1981). Exercises on specifically HIV- and AIDS-related issues are included in Dixon and Gordon (1987).

Problems and issues

It is useful to be alert to aspects of relating in groups that can cause difficulties if they are not acknowledged and dealt with. Some of these are outlined in the next few sections.

Differing approaches

Conflicts between members may arise from differences in views of counselling (psychodynamic *vs* behavioural, for example) or from differences in personal values. Friction may also arise where group members come from different backgrounds. Conflict between members is not necessarily a bad thing and can lead to change and growth. It therefore needs to be confronted and worked with rather than defended against. Disagreement over theoretical issues on occasion can be a cover for personal dislikes, and leaders need to be sensitive to this. An advantage of having several small support groups within an organization is that where personal antagonism seems insuperable there is the option to change groups.

Prejudices

Groups can create an atmosphere of artificial cosiness and a tendency to believe that 'we all think the same way'. This may slide imperceptibly into the delusion that 'we have no prejudices' and the effective support group is one in which people are sufficiently aware and feel safe enough to say 'I don't think like that'. Prejudices are often revealed through choice of words and there are particular problems of communication in HIV helping (see Chapter 6) which groups can tackle. Consider the use of 'junkie', 'victim', 'sufferer', and 'promiscuous' for example, and the difference between 'living with' and 'dying from'.

Scapegoating

Scapegoating is an (often unconscious) strategy to deal with difficulties or conflicts arising in groups. Designating one person as the cause allows emotion to be released and the rest of the group may work harmoniously together at that individual's expense. Constructive tackling of the difficulty itself, however, will have been hindered. Here again, good leadership can stimulate awareness and encourage positive action.

Covert rules

There are also rules of the group that are covert, such as 'this is a group where you only talk about problems' or 'being a good member means producing the most distressing or horrific story'. It is easier in a group with a leader for these 'rules' to be spotted, since the leader is more free to attend to process as well as content.

Conclusion

This kind of group, then, is a very necessary safe environment in which the helper's needs for support are understood, accepted and met. The expression of feelings is seen as a healthy outlet and not as a failure to cope. Organizations that make support groups an integral part of their structure help to promote high morale and effective caring, benefiting clients, helpers and the organization itself.

References

Balgopal, P.R. and Vassil, T.V. (1983). *Groups in Social Work: An Ecological Perspective*. London, Macmillan.

Bailey, R.D. (1985). *Coping with Stress in Caring*. Oxford, Basil Blackwell.

Chaitow, L. (1984). *Your Complete Stress-proofing Programme: How to Protect Yourself Against the Ill-effects of Stress*. Wellingborough, Thorsons.

Cherniss, L. (1980). *Staff Burnout: Job Stress in the Human Services*. Sage Studies in Community Mental Health 2. Beverley Hills, Sage.

Claus, K.E. and Bailey, J.T. (eds) (1980). *Living with Stress and Promoting Well-Being*. St Louis, C.V. Mosby.

Dickson, A. (1982). *A Woman in Your Own Right*. London, Quartet Books.

Dixon, H. and Gordon, P. (1987). *Working with Uncertainty: A Handbook for Those Involved in Training on HIV and AIDS*. Cambridge, FPA Education and AIDS Education Unit, Cambridge Health Authority.

Ernst, S. and Goodison, L. (1981). *In Our Own Hands: A Book of Self-Help Therapy*. London, Women's Press.

HMSO (1987). *House of Commons Third Report from the Social Services Committee Session 1986–87: Problems Associated with AIDS*, Vol. 2. London, HMSO.

Inskipp, F. (1986). *Counselling: The Trainer's Handbook*. Cambridge, National Extension College.

Lopez, D. and Getzel, G.S. (1987). 'Strategies for volunteers caring for persons with AIDS'. *Social Casework: The Journal of Contemporary Social Work,* **68**, 47–53.

Macks, J. and Turner, D. (1986). 'Mental health issues of persons with AIDS'. In L. McKusick (ed.), *What to do about AIDS: Physicians and Mental Health Professionals Discuss the Issues,* pp. 111–24. Berkeley, Calif., University of California Press.

Maslach, C. (1979). 'The burn-out syndrome and patient care'. In C.A. Garfield (ed.), *Stress and Survival: The Emotional Realities of Life-threatening Illnesses*. St Louis, C.V. Mosby, pp. 111–20.

Mattinson, J. (1975). *The Reflection Process in Casework Supervision*. London, Institute of Marital Studies/Tavistock.

NACAB (1988). *A Positive Approach: A Video Training Package for Carers and Counsellors of Those who are HIV Positive or Who have AIDS*. London, NACAB Vision.

Pelletier, K.R. (1978). *Mind as Healer, Mind as Slayer: A Holistic Approach to Preventing Stress Disorders*. London, Allen and Unwin.

Phelps, S. and Austin, N. (1975). *The Assertive Woman*. California, Impact Publishers.

Pines, A.M. and Aronson, E., with Kafry, D. (1981). *Burnout: From Tedium to Personal Growth*. New York, Free Press.

Remocker, A.J. and Storch, E.T. (1982). *Action Speaks Louder: A Handbook of Nonverbal Group Techniques*, 3rd edn. Edinburgh, Churchill Livingstone.

Saretsky, T. (1977). *Active Techniques and Group Psychotherapy*. New York, Aronson.
Searles, H.F. (1955). 'The informational value of the supervisor's emotional experiences'. In H.F. Searles (ed.), *Collected Papers on Schizophrenia and Related Subjects*. London, Hogarth Press/Institute of Psychoanalysis, pp. 157–76.
Zastrow, C. (1984). 'Understanding and preventing burn-out'. *British Journal of Social Work*, **14**, 141–55.

Sources of information
and services

SIXTEEN

Resources

Keeping up to date

Chapter 6 emphasized the importance of helpers keeping up to date with recent developments (social as well as medical) in the area of HIV. A good general guide to recent developments is provided in the regular (17 issues a year) *AIDS Newsletter*, which is published by The Bureau of Hygiene and Tropical Diseases, Keppel Street, London WC1E 7HT. Tel.: 071-636-8636.

Although its price is beyond the budget of an individual helper, the *National AIDS Manual*, which is published in two volumes, is an essential reference book for any voluntary or statutory agency which is providing a service to people living with HIV infection. The two volumes contain up-to-date information on all aspects of HIV infection, and a comprehensive listing of national and local organizations which can provide services to people living with HIV. Regular updates to the manual are produced. The *National AIDS Manual* is published by NAM Publications Ltd, PO Box 99, London SW2 1EL.

For helpers who wish to keep up to date with new developments and issues in the treatment of HIV and HIV-related illnesses, there is a useful US publication which appears regularly: *AIDS Treatment News*. It can be obtained from John S. James, PO Box 411256, San Francisco, Calif. 94141, USA.

Another source of information on recent work on the trialling of treatments for HIV and HIV-related diseases is the *AIDS/HIV Experimental Treatment Directory* which is compiled and published by the American Foundation for AIDS Research (AmFAR). It can be obtained from AmFAR, 1515 Broadway, Suite 3601, 36th Floor, New York, NY 10036, USA.

Organizations

There are now many organizations throughout the UK which are exclusively concerned with meeting the needs of people who are living with HIV and HIV-related illness. There are also very many organizations, which although not exclusively concerned with HIV, can provide useful services to people who are living with HIV. The following short list only identifies some of the most important agencies in the area of HIV. National organizations such as the *Terrence Higgins Trust, Scottish AIDS Monitor* and the *National AIDS Helpline* are likely to be able to direct enquirers towards local sources of help and services. There are also now many local helplines. These helplines are listed in the *National AIDS Manual*.

A national 24-hour helpline offering information about HIV and related matters, on a free 0800 number, is provided by the *National AIDS Helpline* on 0800-567-123. Minicom facilities for people who have hearing difficulties are provided on 0800-521-361 (daily, 10 a.m. to 10 p.m.).

The National Aids Helpline is answered at specific times by people who speak the following languages.

- *Cantonese* and English, on 0800-282-446, on Tuesdays, 6 p.m. to 10 p.m.
- *Arabic* and English, on 0800-282-447, on Wednesdays, 6 p.m. to 10 p.m.
- *Bengali, Gujarati, Hindi, Punjabi, Urdu* and English, on 0800-282-445, on Wednesdays, 6 p.m. to 10 p.m.

The Terrence Higgins Trust (THT), 52–54 Gray's Inn Road, London WC1X 8LT. Tel.: Office, 071-831-0330; helpline, 071-242-1010. Provides a wide range of services to people living with HIV, their partners, friends and families, including buddying, practical help, face-to-face counselling, support groups, welfare rights advice. THT is also a leader in the dissemination of information about HIV. It has a safer sex roadshow, and is involved in outreach work. It runs a Legal Centre. It also has a legal advice helpline: 071-405-2381, Wednesdays, 7 p.m. to 10 p.m.

Scottish AIDS Monitor (SAM), Scottish AIDS Monitor National Office, PO Box 48, Edinburgh EH1 3SA. Tel.: 031-557-3885. Scottish AIDS Monitor is a national Scottish charity which provides a wide range of services including buddying, individual counselling, buddying in prisons and other prison work, welfare rights advice, and a support group for family, friends and partners of people living with HIV. SAM is also very actively involved in health education and in the production of health education materials. It runs a Safer Sex Roadshow. There is an associated legal service *ALBA* (Advisory Legal Bureau on AIDS) which provides legal advice from solicitors.

Body Positive groups which are self-help organizations for people who are HIV antibody positive now exist throughout the UK. As well as running support groups, many of them offer a number of services to HIV antibody positive people. There is a *National Network of Body Positive Groups* to promote effective networking between the different HIV self-help groups throughout the UK: National Network of Body Positive Groups, c/o Positive Birmingham, PO Box 2015, Birmingham B3 1QD. Tel.: 021-212-1814.

The central London *Body Positive* organization has a helpline run by people who themselves are HIV antibody positive: 071-373-9124, daily 7 p.m. to 10 p.m. They also run a drop-in centre: 071-835-1045.

Positively Women, 5 Sebastian Street, London EC1V 0HE. Tel.: 071-490-5515. Positively Women provides a range of counselling and support services to women living with HIV.

Positive Partners, 8 Manor Gardens, London N7 6LA. Tel.: 071-272-4231; helpline, 071-249-6068. This is a self-help group for people living with HIV and their partners, relatives and friends. Associated with Positive Partners is *Positive Children*, which is concerned with responding to the needs of children living with HIV or who have a parent or guardian who is living with HIV, and to the needs of parents with children who are HIV antibody positive.

The Haemophilia Society, 123 Westminster Bridge Road, London SE1 7HR. Tel.: 071-928-2020. Gives advice and information about HIV to people with haemophilia, their families and friends as well as information about haemophilia. As well as the reference centres where those with haemophilia receive their medical treatment, the Haemophilia Society will give information about regional branches and small groups. The Haemophilia Society has spearheaded the campaign for recompense for haemophiliacs infected with HIV.

AVERT (the AIDS Education and Research Trust), PO Box 91, Horsham, West Sussex RH13 7YR. Tel.: 0403-864010. Funds research, including educational projects, and has produced a number of very useful publications such as a teaching pack: *AIDS: Working with Young People*.

Family Planning Association Education and Training Department, FPA Education Unit, 27–35 Mortimer Street, London W1N 8RJ. Tel.: 071-636-7866. The FPA education and training department has been actively involved in creating HIV awareness courses and in other HIV training projects. They can give advice and assistance with sex education programmes.

Crusaid, 83 Clerkenwell Road, London EC1R 5AR. Tel.: 071-831-2595. Crusaid is a national HIV funding charity with an individual hardship fund for people living with HIV, which it administers in consultation with other agencies. It funds projects concerned with services for people living with HIV.

National AIDS Trust (NAT), 14th Floor, Euston Tower, 286 Euston Road, London NW1 3DN. Tel.: 071-383-4246. A major national fund-raising agency which gives grants to voluntary agencies.

Immunity, 260a Kilburn Lane, London W10 4BA. Tel.: 081-968-8909. A health education and HIV research charity which publishes educational materials. It also runs a full-time legal centre which provides advice for people with legal problems related to HIV.

Brook Advisory Centres: Central office and enquiries, 153a East Street, London SE17 2SD. Tel.: 071-708-1234. There are Brook clinics in several cities. They provide confidential advice on contraception, pregnancy, termination of pregnancy and sexual problems for young people. The clinics are run by women.

Women's Health and Reproductive Rights Information Centre (WHRRIC), 52 Featherstone Street, London EC1Y 8RT. Tel: 071-251-6580/6332. Deals with women's health issues, all aspects of women's reproductive rights, and advice to women on HIV. Gives detailed information on artificial insemination.

Family Planning Clinics can be found throughout the UK, and are listed in local telephone directories under 'Family Planning'.

SCODA (Standing Conference On Drug Abuse), 1–4 Hatton Place, London EC1N 8ND. Tel.: 071-430-2341/3. Plays a co-ordinating role for non-statutory drug agencies in England, produces a guide to drug ervices (including syringe exchanges) in England, and can advise on referrals.

Scottish Drugs Forum, 266 Clyde Street, Glasgow G1 4JH. Tel.: 041-221-1175. Can supply information on drug services and drugs education within Scotland.

Mainliners, Mainliners Ltd, PO Box 125, London SW9 8EF. Tel.: 071-274-4000. A self-help agency which provides counselling, support groups for users and ex-users, a telephone helpline and other services to anyone affected by HIV and drugs.

DAWN (Drugs, Alcohol, Women, Nationally). Omnibus Workspace, 39 North Road, London N7 9DP. Tel.: 071-700-4653. Provides information and assistance to women experiencing problems related to alcohol or other drugs.

AIDS and Housing Project, 16–18 Strutton Ground, London SW1P 2HP. Tel.: 071-222-6932/6933. Provides a number of services to further the aim of providing people living with HIV with appropriate, good-quality accommodation.

Benefits Research Unit, Department of Social Administration, University of Nottingham, Nottingham NG7 2RD. Tel.: 0602-484848, ext. 3645. Provides training courses on welfare rights and benefits issues for people living with HIV.

Gay Bereavement Project. Tel.: 081-455-8894. Gives telephone counselling and support to bereaved lesbians and gay men.

CRUSE, Cruse House, 126 Sheen Road, Richmond, Surrey TW9 1UR. Tel.: 081-940-4818. CRUSE is a national organization, with a large number of branches, which offers bereavement counselling and support.

Panos Institute, 9 White Lion Street, London N1 9PD. Tel.: 071-278-1111. A unit of the Panos Institute is concerned with gathering and disseminating information concerning HIV in developing countries. It is also concerned with investigating and highlighting HIV-related discrimination worldwide.

ACT-UP (AIDS Coalition to Unleash Power), BM Box 2995, London WC1N 3XX. Tel.: 071-490-5749. ACT-UP Scotland, PO Box 135, Edinburgh EH8 9XJ. ACT-UP is an activist organization which aims to protest and take direct action against discrimination and a lack of government response to HIV-related issues. It also seeks to promote the rights of people living with HIV.

Landmark, 47a Tulse Hill, London SW2 2TN. Tel.: 081-678-6825. An important drop-in and day centre for people living with HIV which provides a very wide range of services.

BHAN (Black HIV/AIDS Network), BM BHAN, London WC1N 3XX. A national organization which provides a wide range of services to Black and Asian people living with HIV, including HIV support groups, and support for carers, relatives and friends. It is also involved in health education work.

Blackliners Helpline. PO Box 1274, London SW9 8EZ. Tel.: 071-738-5274, Monday to Friday, 9.30 a.m. to 4.00 p.m. Provides a telephone helpline, individual counselling and practical help for people living with HIV in the Black and Asian communities.

ACET (AIDS Care Education and Training), PO Box 1323, London W5 5TF. Tel.: 081-840-2616. ACET is a Christian charity with a number of branches which provides practical home care and nursing, and financial assistance to people with HIV-related illness.

London Lighthouse, 111–117 Lancaster Road, London W11 1QT. Tel.: 071-792-1200. Lighthouse provides residential care for people with HIV-related illness, including terminal care, a home support service, a drop-in centre, support groups, training and a number of other services.

Name index

Subject index